Aids to Acute Medicine

Volume 1

(A highly informative and mostly note-type discussion of selected common topics of acute medicine for easier learning)

Dr Bimalendu Pramanik

MBBS MRCP (Ireland)

ISBN-13:
978-1545093542

Notice

Medicine is an ever-changing branch of science. Although the information believed to be reliable has been included in this book, practitioners are encouraged to evaluate the information contained herein with their own knowledge and experience along with other current sources; it is particularly important before prescribing any drug. Readers must check the current guidelines from the manufacturer of the drug, and other reliable sources for information on its safe use such as indication, contraindication, dose, method of administration, adverse effects etc. Moreover, this book is an individual creation and there is a possibility of human error.

Although possible best efforts have been made to provide accurate information, the author and publisher of this work do not warrant that the information contained in this work is complete and accurate in all respects. The author, publisher, distributor or any other parties involved in the preparation or distribution of this book will not be liable for any form of loss, damage, or problems arising from the use of information contained herein.

The Author and Publisher

Printed by CreateSpace, An Amazon.com Company.

Available from Amazon.com and other retail outlets.

Preface

The most important goal of doctors who are placed for their general medicine training is to learn high-quality care of acute medical conditions. To provide the high-quality care, a more comprehensive knowledge of the management of commonly encountered acute medical problems is very important. A single study material where adequate information needed for that level of care is available in a highly integrated and easily understandable format is very desirable; it can make these busy trainee doctors' learning easier and faster. But in many areas of acute medicine, available study materials have some obvious limitations in this regard; either they do not have sufficient information required for these doctors or it is time consuming to find the necessary information in them because of their presentation styles. 'Aids to Acute Medicine' is intended to minimize these problems.

This volume of the book contains infectious disease, and electrolyte and acid-base disorder related chapters. The topics in this book have been selected considering the potential need of trainee doctors of internal medicine. **Pediatric age group has not been included in any discussions in this book.**

Target audience:

- The main target audience is the trainee doctors (eg, Interns, Residents and Registrars) enrolled in Internal Medicine department. This book would also be very useful to non-consultant doctors of other medical disciplines who regularly manage acute medical problems.
- Other intended audiences include junior doctors of all disciplines; general practitioners/ family physicians; nurses; senior medical students; clinical pharmacists; and physicians' assistants. They will find a lot of useful information on the topics discussed in this book. Also, senior doctors, especially of medical disciplines, will appreciate this book as a very useful material for quick refreshing of their knowledge and teaching juniors.

Key features:

- **The content of the book is designed for high-quality care** that is going on in hospitals or health systems with adequate facilities. However, in some cases, separate suggestions have been included for health system with limited resources.

- **A vast amount of clinically useful information on the discussed topics is available in an easily understandable format;** so users do not need to go through too many sources spending a lot of time for the required information on those topics.

- **Reliable information:** The most common sources of information are Medline indexed journal articles and publications of well-known professional bodies (of developed countries) relevant to the topic. During preparation of the manuscript, when any information appeared doubtful, alternative sources were checked for accuracy before including that in this book. The whole content has been revised carefully several times up to this final version.

- **Required information can be found easily.** There are enough headings and sub-headings; the presentation is mostly note-type, avoiding long paragraphs; question and answer style has been used in some cases; abundant tables and flow charts have been used; treatment portion of all chapters has an additional 'treatment summary'.

- **Specified references:** Each chapter has a reference section at the end. The referencing style that is commonly seen in medical journal articles (numbered citations) has been used in all chapters to specify the information sources.

- **Junior doctors will be less dependent on their seniors for their learning** if they go through this book carefully.

Acknowledgement:
I am grateful to my teachers, friends, colleagues and others who have helped me to learn.

I would greatly appreciate your comments and suggestions to improve this work.

Dr Bimalendu Pramanik, MBBS, MRCP (Ireland)

Contents

Abbreviations (page 6-8)

Section 1: Infectious diseases

Section 2: Electrolyte and Acid-base disorders

Abbreviations

ABG	Arterial blood gas
ACS	Acute coronary syndrome
AFB	Acid fast bacilli
AIDS	Acquired immunodeficiency syndrome
ALT	Alanine aminotransferase
APTT	Activated partial thromboplastin time
AST	Aspartate aminotransferase
ATS	American Thoracic Society
BID/BD	Twice daily
BP	Blood pressure
BTS	British Thoracic Society
CAP	Community acquired pneumonia
CBC	Complete blood count
CDC	Center for Disease Control and Prevention (USA)
CKD	Chronic Kidney Disease
CMV	Cytomegalovirus
COPD	Chronic obstructive pulmonary disease
CRP	C-reactive protein
CT	Computed Tomography
CXR	Chest X-ray
DM	Diabetes Mellitus
DVT	Deep vein thrombosis
EBV	Epstein-Barr-virus

ECG	Electrocardiogram
ESR	Erythrocyte sedimentation rate
FBC	Full blood count
FNA	Fine needle aspiration
GFR	Glomerular filtration rate
GIT	Gastrointestinal tract
GI	Gastrointestinal
GGT	Gamma Glutamyl Transpeptidase
HAP	Hospital acquired pneumonia
Hb	Hemoglobin
HIV	Human immunodeficiency virus
ICU	Intensive care unit
IDSA	Infectious Diseases Society of America
IM	Intramuscular
IV	Intravenous
LDH	Lactate dehydrogenase
LFT	Liver function test
MRI	Magnetic Resonance Imaging
MRSA	Methicillin-resistant Staphylococcus aureus
MSSA	Methicillin-sensitive Staphylococcus aureus
NG	Nasogastric
NHS	National Health Service (UK)
NICE	The National Institute for Health and Care Excellence (UK)
NSAID	Non-seteroidal anti-inflammatory drug

OD	Once daily
PO	By mouth
PPI	Proton pump inhibitor
prn	As needed (Latin: pro re nata)
PT	Prothrombin time
QID	Four times daily
RBC	Red blood cell
SLE	Systemic lupus erythematosus
SO2	Oxygen saturation (with Pulse Oximetry)
T_3	Tri-iodothyronine
T_4	Thyroxine
TB	Tuberculosis
TID	Thrice daily
TSH	Thyroid stimulating hormone
USG	Ultrasonography
UTI	Urinary tract infection
VAP	Ventilator associated pneumonia
VDRL	Venereal disease research laboratory
WBC	White blood cell

Section 1: Infectious diseases

Chapter 1

Fever

Fever

Normal Body Temperature

Normal body temperature is variable. However, generally an oral temperature between 97 °F (36.1 °C) and 99 °F (37.2 °C) is considered as normal.[1]

Factors associated with variation in normal body temperature

(All temperature given below is oral. *Rectal temp is usually 0.4°C (0.7°F) higher than oral temperature*[2])

Normal body temperature varies with time of the day, age, sex, ethnicity, phase of menstrual cycle, activity, meal, Body Mass Index (BMI), WBC count etc. It also varies from person to person.[1-4]

- **Time of the day:** Diurnal variation in body temperature is typically 0.5°C (0.9°F). Body temperature is low at 6 am and high at 4-6 pm. Generally considered maximum normal oral temperature at 6 am is 37.2°C (98.9°F) and at 4 pm is 37.7 °C (99.9°F).[2]
- **Sex:** Overall, women have higher body temperatures (roughly 0.3°F – 0.5°F) than men; the difference is relatively high in 20 –50 age groups (about 0.5°F) compared to above-50 age groups (about 0.3 °F).[3]
- **Phase of menstrual cycle:** In women during childbearing age, early morning temperature is usually lower in the two weeks before ovulation; then the temperature rises with ovulation by approximately 0.6° C (1° F) and remains at that level until menstruation.[2]
- **Age:** In both sexes, body temperature decreases significantly with age; the difference between the oldest (80+) and the youngest groups (20-40 years) is approximately 0.3°F in the respective sex.[3]
- **BMI:** In both sexes, obesity is associated with a higher mean body temperature. Generally, obese individuals have approximately 0.3–0.5°F higher mean temperature than normal individuals of the same sex and age.[3]
- **Activity:** Core body temperature increases with exercise; however, it comes back to normal quickly after stopping the exercise.
- **Meal:** Body temperature increases after eating or drinking anything with calories.
- **Ethnicity:** Generally, black people have a slightly higher temperature than their white counterpart.[4]
- **WBC count:** Body temperature increases slightly with increasing WBC counts (even within the normal range of WBC); the highest variation within the normal range of WBC is approximately 0.4°F.[3]

***In both sexes, a small percentage of normal people have body temperature <96°F,** and the proportion is greater in males than females. In both sexes, the proportion slightly increases with age. (Prevalence: 20-59 age groups, 11% male and 6% female; 60 + age groups, 13% male and 10% female).[3]

Definition of fever

- Generally, for young adults (<40 years), an early morning oral temperature higher than 37.2°C (98.9°F) or an overall oral temperature higher than 37.7°C (99.9°F) can be considered as fever.[4] Also, the following thermometer readings at any time of the day irrespective of age and sex are usually regarded as fever:[5]
    - Oral temperature ≥ 100°F (37.8°C)
    - Rectal, ear or temporal artery temperature ≥ 100.4°F (38° C)
    - Armpit temperature ≥ 99° F (37.2° C)
- Ideally, before recognizing a temperature as fever possible normal variation for that individual should be considered as much as possible.

Low-grade fever: Range of temperature from 99.5°F (37.5°C)/ 100°F to 101°F (38.3 °C) can be defined as low-grade fever.[6,7]

Hyperpyrexia: Hyperpyrexia is defined as a fever with body **temperature > 41.5°C (106.7°F).** It can be due to severe infection but more commonly occurs in CNS hemorrhage.[2]

Notes:

1. The elderly has reduced ability to develop fever, and severe infection may cause only modest fever.
2. Although hypothalamic disorders can cause fever, in most cases, hypothalamic damage causes subnormal, not supranormal, body temperatures, which is contrary to the common belief.[2]

Pyrexia/ fever of unknown origin (PUO/ FUO)

Definition

Various definitions have been proposed for PUO/ FUO. Simply PUO/ FUO can be defined as a fever [of 38.3°C (101°F) or more on several occasions] for at least three weeks without a specific diagnosis despite reasonable diagnostic evaluations.[8-11]

The requirement of a temperature ≥38.3 °C (101°F) eliminates the possibility of 'habitual hyperthermia', which is an exaggerated circadian variation in normal body temperature (described later after investigations).[11]

The requirement of the first three weeks time has been left for the resolution of most acute, self-limiting conditions and completion of the initial diagnostic workup.[11]

Epidemiology

The exact incidence and prevalence of FUO are unknown; however, the prevalence may be about 3% among hospitalized adult patients.[9]

Classification of PUO/ FUO (Information from references 9,12,13)

FUO can be divided into four categories.

Classic FUO

- Fever $\geq$ 38.3°C (101°F) on several occasions
- Duration $\geq$ 3 weeks
- Diagnosis uncertain after appropriate diagnostic evaluation for three days in hospital or three out-patient visits

Nosocomial FUO

- Hospitalized for >48 hours
- Fever $\geq$ 38.3°C (101°F) on several occasions
- No infection (fever) present or incubating at the time of admission
- Diagnosis uncertain after 3 days despite appropriate diagnostic evaluation, including microbiological cultures incubating for $\geq$ 2 days

Neutropenic (Immunodeficient) FUO

- Fever $\geq$ 38.3°C (101°F) on several occasions
- Neutropenia (with Absolute Neutrophil Count < 500/ mm^3)
- Diagnosis uncertain after 3 days despite appropriate diagnostic evaluation, including microbiological cultures incubating for $\geq$ 2 days

HIV-associated FUO

- Confirmed HIV infection
- Fever $\geq$ 38.3°C (101°F) on several occasions
- Duration of fever as outpatient $\geq$ 4 weeks, or as inpatient $\geq$ 3 days
- Diagnosis uncertain after 3 days despite appropriate diagnostic evaluation, including microbiological cultures incubating for $\geq$ 2 days

Notes

1. For all categories of FUO, a fever of $\geq$ 38.3°C (101°F) on several occasions is required.
2. To fulfill the criteria for nosocomial FUO and neutropenic FUO, no specified duration of fever is needed.
3. For all categories of FUO, at least three days' appropriate diagnostic evaluation is required.

Why the four categories of FUO have been introduced

Actually, when the FUO was first defined in 1961, there was only one type of FUO, which was mostly like currently defined 'Classic FUO'. The last three categories of FUO (mentioned above) have been defined later. The reasons why they should be considered separately are:[12]

- The etiologies of the last three groups of FUO differ from those of classic FUO;
- The diagnostic approaches to them are also different.
- The patients with the last three categories of FUO are at increased risk for rapid deterioration because of their weak immune system. Therefore, empiric antimicrobial treatment is usually considered promptly for the last three categories of patients whereas in classic FUO empiric therapy is considered cautiously.

Here only 'Classic FUO' has been described.

Causes FUO

- A wide range of disorders cause FUO and the causes are influenced by regional diseases.

- **FUO is more commonly due to an atypical presentation of a common disease rather than a rare disease.**[11]
- Recent studies show that in developed countries, the percentage of FUO cases due to infection and malignancies has decreased because of widespread use of modern diagnostic technologies, while the noninfectious inflammatory diseases and undiagnosed category have increased.[8,9,11] However, this trend is not true for developing countries, where infections (particularly tuberculosis) and neoplasms still comprise a higher proportion of FUO cases.[11]

Infections (20 – 30%)(Information from references 9,10,11,14)

- ***Site specific***
  - Abscesses : particularly abdominal*; dental; CNS etc
  - Heart valves: Infective endocarditis*
  - Bone and joint infections
  - Head and neck: eg, chronic sinusitis
  - Prostatitis
- ***Organism specific***
  - Tuberculosis* (especially extrapulmonary, or disseminated)
  - Viral infections: Epstein-Barr virus, cytomegalo virus, HIV etc.
  - Deep fungal infections: Histoplasma, aspergillus, candida etc.
  - Toxoplasmosis
  - Q fever
- ***Infections of specific geographic areas*** *(involving* residents or travelers returning from the endemic areas)
  - Malaria, rickettsial infections, enteric fever, brucellosis, amoebic liver abscess, Leishmaniasis etc.

Connective tissue diseases (15- 30%) (Information from references 9,10,11,14,15)

- Temporal arteritis/ polymyalgia rheumatica* (almost exclusively affects above-50 age group)
- Systemic lupus erythematosus (SLE)*
- Adult Still's disease*
- Vasculitic conditions: Polyarteritis Nodosa (PAN)*, Wegener's granulomatosis, microscopic polyangitis
- Rheumatoid arthritis
- Mixed connective tissue disease (MCTD)
- Cryoglobulinemia*
- Polymyosistis
- Bechet's disease

Malignancy: (10-30%)(Information from references 9,10,15)

- Hematological: Lymphoma*, leukemia and myeloma
- Solid tumors: Renal cell carcinoma, hepatocellular carcinoma, colon cancer, pancreatic cancer etc.

Miscellaneous (10-25%)[9,11,14,15]

- Gastrointestinal: Chronic liver disease- eg, granulomatous hepatitis and alcoholic liver disease; inflammatory bowel disease;
- Respiratory: Sarcoidosis; extrinsic allergic alveolitis
- Cardiovascular- Deep vein thrombosis/ pulmonary embolism; atrial myxoma; aortitis
- Endocrine: Thyrotoxicosis; thyroiditis
- Hematological: Thrombotic thrombocytopenic purpura; Graft-versus-host disease;
- Hereditary: Familial Mediterranean fever; periodic fever syndromes;
- Drug fever*
- Factitious fever*

Undiagnosed (10-50%)[8,11]

*Relatively common causes in the specific group.

Notes:

(1) Drug fever

- It is a fairly common condition.[16]
- Almost any drug, especially antimalarials, sulfonamides, amphotericin B, Gold and penicillamine, can cause drug fever.
- Probably the most common mechanism of drug fever is drug-induced antibody mediated immunologic reaction. However, the drug's pharmacologic action, its thermoregulatory effects, local complications after parenteral administration, or an idiosyncratic response may also cause drug fever.[17]
- The latency period in drug fever (from starting a new drug in a nonsensitized individual to the development of fever) is highly variable; however, in most cases, it is 7-10 days.[16,17]
- Drug fever has no classic presentation. It is a diagnosis of exclusion, so delayed diagnosis or misdiagnosis is common.
- In the presence of leukocytosis, elevated CRP or ESR, careful evaluation to rule out infection is very important before considering the fever as drug fever.
- Rechallenge with the offending drug usually causes recurrence of the fever within a few hours which confirms the diagnosis. However, rechallenge is controversial, as it can induce more severe drug reaction.[16]
- Drug fever usually resolves within 48 hours of discontinuing the offending drug.[17]

(2) Familial Mediterranean Fever (FMF) (Information from 2, 10 18)

- FMF is also called recurrent polyserositis.
- FMF is characterized by recurrent episodes of fever with abdominal pain and tenderness due to acute peritonitis; other forms of serositis such as pleurisy and arthritis may also be present.
- If not treated, episode of symptoms usually lasts 24-72 hours.
- Although FMF occurs almost exclusively in people of Mediterranean ancestry, people without a known Mediterranean ancestry are affected occasionally.

Clinical evaluation of a patient with FUO

A good concept of a wide range of possible causative diseases of FUO and the diagnostic yields of the tests used is very important to manage FUO cases.[12] Thorough history taking and physical examination can give some clues to the diagnosis in many cases.

Information on the following history points should be collected:

- About the fever itself:
  - Onset: Sudden/ gradual with reaching a peak over several days;
  - Duration
  - Recorded maximum temperature
  - Pattern: continued/ intermittent
  - Associated chills and rigors
- Associated other symptoms: cough, headache, vomiting, dysuria, rash etc
- Review of systems: ask about main symptoms related to all systems
- Food related information: Eating undercooked meat or fish, unpasteurized milk etc
- Contact history: any febrile patient especially patients with TB; contact with birds and animals
- Recent travel including recreational activities at the travel spot- swimming, sexual exposure etc.
- Past medical history: Malaria, TB, connective tissue diseases, liver diseases, neoplasia, diabetes mellitus, HIV status etc.
- Past surgical history: History of any recent surgery; any prosthetic devices in place such as heart valves or joints
- Obstetric and gynecological history: (History of multiple pregnancy loss may be related to connective tissue disorders)
- History of recent hospitalization; living in a nursing home;
- Drug history: All drugs with dose, duration, therapeutic response especially antibiotics, antimalarials and immunosupressives; drug allergy
- History of immunization and use of prophylactic drugs
- Family history: eg, Familial Mediterranean Fever
- Social history: Alcohol and illicit drug use; sexual exposure; sexual practices (eg, anal sex may lead to rectal abscess)
- Occupational history including exposure to birds or animals

Physical examination:

- Thorough physical examination of all systems is very important.
- **The aspects of physical examination that can be missed easily include**:
  - Temporal artery examination (particularly important when age > 50) for tenderness, nodularity, and pulse volume (normal/ reduced / absent; asymmetry);
  - Digital Rectal Examination (DRE) particularly for any clues to prostate diseases (eg, prostatitis, prostatic abscess); also it is very important to detect rectal pathology including rectal abscess which may be the cause of fever in individuals involved in anal sex.
- Thorough physical examination should be repeated on regular basis (preferably daily) to detect possible emerging features.

Notes

1. Objective evidence of fever is important for defining FUO, particularly when the patient does not look really sick; hospital admission may be needed for this purpose.
   - Some patients have habitual hyperthermia (described later below the investigations) and some have factitious fever; in both the conditions, patients do not really have fever.
   - When factious fever is suspected temperature measurement should be supervised.

2. The pattern of fever is not a reliable indicator of the nature and severity of the disease and it has little or no diagnostic value. However, in malaria endemic area, a fever with rigors is often due to malaria; a patient with abscess may have a high swinging temperature with rigors.

3. The temperature may be found normal in a possible febrile patient if the patient is on NSAIDs or steroid.

4. Sometimes, a temperature chart can provide some clues to the cause of fever; for example **relative bradycardia** may be related to an infection with intracellular organisms[9] such as:
   - Typhoid fever
   - Brucellosis
   - Legionellosis
   - Psittacosis
   - Q fever

Investigations (Information from references 2, 8-14, 19)

- There is no widely accepted specific set of investigations for FUO.
- If clinical evaluation gives clues to a possible diagnosis or a possible organ system involvement, that should be investigated with priority. But **when there is no clue, the investigations can be performed in the three steps described below.**
- If any diagnostic clues are found at any stage of the evaluation, appropriate tests should be performed.
- The diagnostic approach are also depends on general condition and comorbidities of the patient. In an unstable patient or a patient with other serious comorbidities, all possibly useful investigations should be performed quickly.

Step1 **(Minimum investigations)**

- CBC with Peripheral blood smears
- C reactive Protein (CRP); Erythrocyte sedimentation Rate (ESR)
- Urine analysis; Urine culture
- Urea, Creatinine and electrolyte (U&E); Blood glucose
- X-ray chest (CXR)
- Tuberculin skin test/ Interferon-Gamma Release Assay (IGRA)

- Liver function test (LFT)
- Muscle enzymes- Creatine kinase (CK), Lactate dehydrogenase (LDH)
- Rheumatologic markers: ANA, RF and ANCA
- Ultrasonography (or CT) of the abdomen and pelvis
- Blood culture- three sets from different sites, both aerobic and anaerobic; to allow the growth of slow-growing organisms, blood culture should be held by the laboratory for two weeks.
- Serologic tests for Epstein-Barr virus, cytomegalovirus and human immunodeficiency virus
- Malarial screen: Thick and thin blood film, usually for patients in malaria endemic areas or travelers returning from those areas; ICT for malaria is also highly sensitive and specific.
- Sputum for Gram stain, AFB, fungus, cytology and culture (If Cough and sputum is present)
- Screening tests (mainly serology) for possible regional infections;

***When the above investigations fail to reveal any clues to the diagnosis, the fever then actually meet the criteria for FUO; in such cases,* consider step 2 investigations below.**

Step 2

- Echocardiography (preferably transesophageal; may be useful even in negative blood culture and in the absence of audible murmur)
- Serum ferritin
- Thyroid function tests
- CT abdomen and pelvis; and chest with contrast
- Serum protein electrophoresis
- Cryoglobulin (useful to rule out some forms of vasculitis)
- Serologic tests for toxoplasmosis, brucellosis and coxiellosis;
- Bone marrow biopsy
- Temporal artery biopsy (if age >55 years)
- FDG-PET scan or other nuclear scintigraphy (helps to detect the site of infection, inflammation and malignancy; order only if ESR/ CRP is raised)

If still the diagnosis remains uncertain, consider step 3 investigations below.

Step 3 (These investigations are not performed in all cases; instead, they are usually considered when information obtained from clinical evaluation and already performed test results justifies)

- **Lumber puncture** (to exclude meningitis in the presence of headache)
- **Lymph node biopsy** (if lymphadenopathy present; palpable inguinal lymph nodes usually not diagnostically useful)
- **Liver biopsy** (in the presence of abnormalities in LFT or imaging);
- **Laparoscopy or exploratory laparotomy** (considered rarely as the last means to establish a diagnosis when abdominal pathology is suspected; direct visualization and biopsy from the suspicious tissues may be helpful)

Notes:

1. Abnormal LFT in FUO:
   - Nonspecific abnormalities in liver enzymes are common in FUO (in one study, among 27% of all patients with FUO) and usually do not contribute to the final diagnosis directly.[8]
   - In FUO patients with abnormal liver enzymes, liver biopsy can be considered only: (a) when there is other finding(s) that justifies liver biopsy, or (b) when noninvasive and relatively less invasive investigations (of step 1&2) have failed to establish a diagnosis.

2. Biopsy of skin rash may be helpful in the diagnosis of some collagen vascular diseases or infections.[10]

3. Temporal artery biopsy may be helpful even in the absence of high ESR or other features of temporal arteritis.[9,14]

4. Histology and culture (for bacteria, mycobacteria and fungi) should be performed on all biopsy specimens.[2]

5. The diagnostic yield of blind (in the absence diagnostic clues) radiologic or endoscopic investigations of the gastrointestinal tract and sinus X-rays are very low; so these tests should not be performed as screening investigations in the hope that something important will come up.[8,20]

6. Misleading diagnostic clues[8,20]
   - Although looking for possible diagnostic clues is always very important in establishing diagnosis in FUO, in many cases, the potential clues (obtained from both clinical and investigation results) may be misleading, even abdominal or chest CT findings may be false positive in many cases. In one study, 28% of the abdominal and 17% of the chest CT results were false positive.[8] False positive findings may lead to subsequent unnecessary investigations.
   - Diagnostic yield of specific investigations including biopsies directed by only less specific diagnostic clues, such as nonspecific anemia (as an indication for bone marrow biopsy), abnormal liver enzymes (for liver biopsy), or inguinal lymphadenopathy (for lymph node biopsy), is low.

What can be done when there is no clue to the diagnosis after extensive investigations?

Consider the followings:

1. If the patient is stable: Watchful waiting is generally recommended.[8,9]
   - History should be repeated several times and physical examination should be repeated on regular basis, preferably daily. New features or previously overlooked features may be revealed through it.
   - Some investigations such as inflammatory markers, cultures are generally repeated regularly and some imaging such as CXR and abdominal ultrasound are usually repeated periodically looking for new findings.
   - Some experts suggest empiric therapy with NSAIDs in these patients, which may be helpful if the fever is due to an inflammatory disorder.[8,9]

- Rarely, when the patients deteriorate while on NSAIDs without presenting new diagnostic clues, further diagnostic workup and empiric treatment with antibiotics, steroids, or antituberculous agents should be considered.[20]

2. If the patient is unstable or deteriorating: Initiate empiric treatment with antibiotics, steroids, or antituberculous agents promptly and consider further diagnostic workup.[9]
3. Consultation with other specialists such as infectious disease specialist, rheumatologist, hematologist, or an oncologist should be considered.

[**Abbreviations:** ANA-Anti-nuclear antibodies; ANCA - Anti-neutrophil Cytoplasmic Antibody; AFB- Acid Fast Bacilli; CT- Computed Tomography; CMV- cytomegalovirus; CXR-Chest X-ray; EBV - Epstein-Barr virus; HIV- Human Immunodeficiency Virus; IGRA-Interferon-Gamma Release Assay; ICT- Immunochromatographic test; LDH- Lactate Dehydrogenase; RF- Rheumatoid factor; FDG-PET- Fluorodeoxyglucose – Positron Emission Tomography; NSAIDs- Nonsteroidal Anti-inflammatory Drugs]

Summary of the diagnostic approach to FUO

History & physical examination →no clue to the diagnosis → order step 1 investigations → no clue → consider step 2 investigations except any biopsies, CT scan and FDG-PET; if no clues → you have 2 options: consider either (a) CT chest and abdomen plus less invasive biopsies mentioned in step 2 (bone marrow and temporal artery biopsy), or (b) FDG-PET; some experts suggest to perform FDG- PET before CT and biopsies;[8] if you perform CT and the less invasive biopsies first, but they become unhelpful, order FDG-PET and vice versa; if FDG-PET, CT, and biopsies mentioned in step 2 all fail to reveal any clues → at this stage, decision usually depends on clinical state of the patient; if the patient is stable, there are three options: (a) watchful waiting,[8] (b) empiric NSAID[8], or (3) considering step 3 investigations if at least minimum diagnostic clues that justify their indications are present[2,9]; on the other hand for unstable or deteriorating patients, therapeutic trial and step 3 investigations are commonly suggested.

Notes:

1. If any diagnostic clues are found at any stage of evaluation, observation, or therapeutic trial, order specific tests to confirm the diagnosis.
2. ***Order FDG-PET only when ESR or CRP is elevated.***[9]

Some suggestions on investigation for health system with limited resources:

Following modifications to the above mentioned (three-step) approach can be considered:

1. Blind serologic tests for infectious diseases are generally low-yielding in the absence of possible diagnostic clues.[8,11,20] So these tests can be excluded from the list of 'step 1' investigations when no possible diagnostic clues justifying their indications are present. Possible diagnostic clues to an infectious disease may be living in or recent travel to the endemic area; characteristic symptoms or signs; or investigation results. For example, lymphadenopathy and/ or lymphocytosis may be possible diagnostic clue to EBV infection, CMV infection, or toxoplasmosis.

2. For abdominal imaging, ultrasound can be considered first and CT scan can be left for the later stage of investigation.

3. Blind chest CT (in the absence of any clues to chest disease) is generally not considered as yielding as blind abdominal CT. Therefore, during step 2 investigations when blind CT scan is considered, only abdominal CT can be ordered. When no clues are found, a stable patient can be observed for a period before ordering chest CT.

4. As FDG-PET may not be available in health systems with limited resources, ^{67}Ga-citrate scintigraphy can be considered when nuclear imaging is needed although the latter is less sensitive and less specific.

5. When the diagnosis remains uncertain after reasonable investigations (usually after selected tests of step 1&2) and the patient's condition is stable, watchful waiting with repeating some simple investigations can be considered with priority instead of ordering many expensive possibly low-yielding blind investigations.

Brief description of some investigations

Nuclear imaging in FUO

^{18}F FDG-PET/CT scan

- ^{18}F FDG-PET/CT scan may be helpful to pinpoint the origin of fever and is now the nuclear imaging of choice in FUO. However, FDG-PET/CT is not helpful if patient's ESR or CRP is not elevated.[9,21]
- FDG-PET scan is a form PET where '^{18}F (Fluorine) – FDG (fluorodeoxyglucose)' is used as the radiotracer.
- FDG is a glucose analogue; following intravenous injection, it is preferentially taken up by tissues with high glucose consumption.[22] Its uptake and accumulation in a part of the body depend on metabolic activity (glucose utilization) of that area.[23]
- FDG uptake and accumulation are increased in malignant cells and cells involved in inflammation and infection (eg, activated leukocytes, cells of granulation tissue and granuloma) because of their higher metabolic rate.[22,23] So FDG is detected at higher concentration in areas involved with these disease processes.
- FDG-PET scan may be helpful to differentiate between benign and malignant tumors. The rate of glycolysis is higher in malignant tissues; so the uptake of ^{18}F-FDG by malignant tumors is usually higher than that of benign lesions and normal tissues.[24]
- After the radio tracer (^{18}F-FDG) injection, Gamma Camera is used to take images of the whole body. The areas with higher metabolic activities (i.e. the site of lesion) can be identified by the increased uptake of ^{18}F-FDG.
- Currently incorporated computed tomography with this procedure has been very helpful in anatomic localization of the site of lesion.
- The result of this test can be obtained much earlier (usually within 24 hours) than any other nuclear scans (^{67}Ga- citrate scintigraphy takes 2- 3 days) used in FUO.
- ^{18}F FDG-PET/CT Scan is highly useful to detect the site of-
  - Malignancy
  - Inflammation

    - Infection
- Diagnostic yield of the test:
    - FDG-PET/CT may be helpful for diagnosis in 46% -77% of patients with FUO.[23]
    - When the results of ^{18}F FDG-PET/CT and ^{18}F FDG-PET of some studies are combined, the sensitivity of this nuclear imaging appears 50% to 93% and specificity 33% to 90% for detecting the cause of FUO.[24] Negative predictive values for FDG-PET/CT range from 50 to 100%.[9,23,24]
- When to order FDG – PET/CT in FUO:
    - This test can be considered when other commonly performed structural imaging such as plain x-ray, ultrasonography and CT scan fails to reveal any clues to the diagnosis.[24]
    - Some experts suggest early use of FDG-PET, before CT scan and any biopsies.[8]

Other nuclear scans used in FUO

^{67}Ga-citrate scintigraphy and ^{111}In labeled leukocytes scintigraphy are the two other nuclear techniques which can be used to localize the pathology in FUO. They are cheaper and more widely available than ^{18}F FDG-PET scan, but are less sensitive, less specific and more time consuming than FDG-PET; also, they cause high radiation burden to the patient.[9,23]

(1) ^{67}Ga-citrate scintigraphy [23]

- It can detect both acute and chronic infections, inflammations and some neoplasms. Until recently it was the most commonly used nuclear imaging in patients with FUO.
- It has several disadvantages:
    - In one study, only 29% of the total scans were helpful for diagnosis and about 49% of the abnormal scans were not useful to establish the diagnosis.
    - Its imaging characteristics are unfavorable and specificity is low.
    - It may take 2-3 days to finish the procedure.
    - It causes high radiation burden to the patient.

(2) ^{111}In labeled leukocytes scintigraphy

- It can detect infection and inflammation, but is usually not helpful in detecting neoplasm.[9]
- Its imaging characteristics are poor and it is helpful for diagnosis in only about 20% of cases of FUO.[23]
- It causes high radiation burden to the patient.[23]

Considering all the advantages and disadvantages, ***^{18}F FDG-PET/CT is considered as the nuclear imaging of choice in FUO, but if the test is not available, ^{67}Ga-citrate scintigraphy can be considered.***

Serum ferritin in FUO

- Serum ferritin may be elevated in a variety of disorders including infection, inflammation malignancy and chronic iron-overload syndromes.[25]
- Ferritin is an acute phase reactant and may be elevated in a wide range of infectious or noninfectious inflammatory conditions, but the elevation is generally < 2 times of upper limit of normal.[26]

- Some experts reported that, in FUO, highly elevated serum ferritin, roughly >2 times of upper limit of normal, is less likely due to infectious etiology; instead, it is more likely due to an underlying rheumatologic disorder or malignancy, particularly hematologic malignancy. They believe highly elevated serum ferritin may be used to differentiate between infectious and noninfectious etiologies of FUO;[27] and the likelihood of a malignancy is greatly reduced in a patient with normal serum ferritin level.[28] However, this area needs more studies.

Echocardiography (preferably transesophageal) may be helpful even in the absence of an audible heart murmur or positive blood culture. For the detection of endocardial vegetation, transesophageal echocardiography is more sensitive (sensitivity 95-100%) than transthoracic echocardiography (63%) and both the methods are 98% specific.[9]

Bone marrow biopsy (trephine biopsy, not simple aspiration) can contribute to the diagnosis in about 25% cases of FUO.[9] Although it is useful even in the absence of any features indicating possible bone marrow involvement, it is more useful when some clue such as thrombocytopenia or anemia (hemoglobin < 11 g/dl) is present.[2,9]

Liver biopsy

- Liver biopsy may be diagnostic in 14% to 17% cases of FUO. [8,11]
- In the absence of any specific clues to liver disease, generally liver biopsy is considered after unrevealing step 1&2 investigations if at least some nonspecific abnormalities in liver enzymes or imaging are present. However, blind liver biopsy may also be helpful even in the absence of any diagnostic clues to liver disease.[2,8]
- Although rare, granulomatous hepatitis may be diagnosed (with determination of its cause such as infectious, inflammatory, or neoplastic disease)[11] by liver biopsy in the absence of hepatic enzyme abnormalities or any other diagnostic clues to liver disease.[2,8] However, many experts do not suggest blind liver biopsy, considering its potential hazards.[8,10,14]

Interferon gamma release assay (IGRA)

- Interferon gamma release assays (IGRAs) are the newer immunological tests for the diagnosis of tuberculosis.
- Two widely used IGRAs are:
    - QuantiFERON–TB Gold In-Tube test (QFT-GIT)
    - T-SPOT. TB test (T-Spot)
- Basic methods of QFT-GIT and T-Spot:[29,30]
  Fresh blood samples from patients are mixed with antigens of *Mycobacterium tuberculosis* to stimulate the T lymphocytes with the *Mycobacterium tuberculosis* antigens. T lymphocytes of most *M. tuberculosis* infected persons will release gamma interferon with the stimulation.
    - In QFT-GIT, the released gamma interferon is measured by ELISA method.
    - In T-spot, the numbers of interferon gamma producing cells (Spots) are counted using enzyme-linked imunospot assay (ELISpot technique).

Sensitivity and specificity of three commonly used immunological tests for tuberculosis (QFT-GIT, T-spot and TST*):

- Generally, the sensitivities of QFT-GIT, TST and T-Spot are considered similar although the results of some published studies show wide variation.[29]
- In general, QFT-GIT and T-Spot are considered to be more specific than a TST as more specific *Mycobacterium tuberculosis* antigens are used in QFT-GIT and T-Spot.[29,31]

*TST: Tuberculin Skin Test

A comparison of sensitivities and specificities of QFT-GIT, T-spot and TST[29]

Test	*Sensitivity*	*Specificity*
QFT-GIT	81%	99%
T- spot	91%	88%
TST	89%	86%

Advantages of IGRAs compared to TST:

- IGRAs can be completed in a single patient visit and the test results may be available within 24 hours.[30]
- Previous BCG (Bacille Calmette-Guérin) vaccination does not cause a false-positive IGRA result.[30]
- IGRAs do not cause false positive results in patients with most nontuberculous mycobacterial infections since relatively specific *Mycobacterium tuberculosis* antigens are used in IGRA.[29]
- Unlike TST, IGRAs do not cause booster phenomenon on repeated testing.[29]

Limitations of IGRAs

- Blood sample must be fresh (preferably within a few hours of collection)
- Like TST, negative results of IGRAs do not rule out tuberculosis.[2]
- The cost for IGRAs may be substantially higher than that for TST.[30,31]

Indications for the use of IGRAs (QFT-GIT or T-Spot)

- Generally QFT-GIT or T-Spot can be used in all situations where TST is indicated for testing tuberculosis.[29] However, there are certain situations when QFT-GET or T-Spot is preferred to TST:[30]
  - Patients who have received Bacillus Calmette-Guerin (BCG) vaccine.
  - People who have a low-rate of returning for TST reading such as homeless people and drug-users.

*For children of less than 5 years old, TST is preferred to an IGRA.[30]

What is the possible best immunologic test (TST or an IGRA) for TB in immunocompromised individuals?

Limited data are available on this issue and the available information indicates that TST and IGRAs are almost equally useful.[29]

How about combined use of a TST and an IGRA?[29,30]

- Routine testing with both a TST and an IGRA is usually not recommended.

- In some special situations, when the initial test result (TST or IGRA) is negative, positive result of a second test increases the diagnostic sensitivity.
- When in some special circumstances, it appears that the result of combined testing (a TST and an IGRA) can make a useful contribution to the patient management then both the tests can be performed. For example, when the result of the initial test (a TST or an IGRA) is negative in an immunocompromised individual or children < 5 years old, the other test can be performed, as these individuals are at increased risk for tuberculosis and also at increased risk for TB progression.

Causes of false negative tuberculin skin test (Information from references 2,32,33)

- Overwhelming TB (including miliary tuberculosis)
- Sarcoidosis
- Hodgkin's disease
- Malnutrition
- Immunocompromised state (including AIDS and immunosuppressive therapy)
- Very early TB (within 8-10 weeks of exposure)
- Very old TB (many years)
- Age: < 6 months; or the elderly
- Recent live-virus vaccination (e.g., measles and smallpox)

Causes of false positive TST[29]

- Previous BCG vaccination
- Infection with nontuberculous mycobacteria

Habitual hyperthermia and low grade fever (LGF)

Habitual hyperthermia (Information from references 6,34,35)

There is no widely recognized definition of 'habitual hyperthermia.' Persistently elevated basal body temperatures up to 38.3°C (101°F) without any organic cause can be considered as habitual hyperthermia.

- Typically it affects young women.
- Temperature remains normal or subnormal during the first half of the menstrual cycle and usually begins to rise in the mid-cycle and remains elevated until the onset of menstruation.
- Temperature records show an exaggerated diurnal variation with generally relatively normal morning temperatures and intermittent evening rises.
- It may be associated with malaise, fatigue, body aches, headaches, insomnia and bowel disturbances.
- No organic cause is found with extensive investigations.
- The temperature is unresponsive to antipyretics.
- Observation for a prolonged period with temperature measuring is needed to confirm the diagnosis.

- Treatment is generally explanation and reassurance. However, there is a recent case report where fever was improved with oral treatment with synthetic estrogen and progesterone.[34]
- Habitual hyperthermia may persist for years.

Notes:

1. Habitual hyperthermia should not be considered when the temperature is ≥ 38.3 °C, because it is an exceptional event in habitual hyprthermia.[6]
2. Habitual hyperthermia can occur in male. A recent study on low-grade fever showed among individuals with habitual hyperthermia about one-third were men.[6]

Low-grade fever (LGF)

Body temperature from 99.5°F (37.5°C)/ 100°F to 101°F (38.3 °C) can be defined as low-grade fever.[6,7] Actually, mild elevation of body temperature within this range is not always pathological and does not fulfill the temperature requirement for FUO. Temperature elevation in habitual hyperthermia also falls in this range.

When the duration of the low- grade fever (LGF) is <3 weeks or when there is an obvious organic cause of the fever, usually it does not create diagnostic difficulty. In this category of patients, the cause of LGF may be minor infection, inflammation, trauma etc.; or the fever may be a manifestation of a major disorder such as a major infection, inflammation, or malignancy. Their management approach depends on suspicion about the cause. But diagnostic difficulty generally arises when the duration of the low- grade fever (LGF) is >3 weeks and there is no obvious organic cause.

Low-grade fever (LGF) for > 3 weeks (without any obvious organic cause):
This category of patients can be divided into two groups:[6]

1. Organic LGF (underlying organic pathology ultimately revealed) (46%)
2. Habitual hyperthermia (organic cause not found) (54%)

How the above mentioned two sub-groups of LGF, habitual hyperthermia and 'organic LGF', can be differentiated and managed?
Few study reports on low grade fever (LGF) have been published so far and more studies are needed for the better understanding of this entity. However, the following management approach may be considered:[6]

(1) If thorough clinical evaluation (history and/ or physical examination) indicates the presence of an underlying organic pathology → consider the fever as 'organic LGF' and proceed for diagnostic workup according to the clinical impression which is like classic FUO.

(2) When clinical evaluation (history and physical examination) does not points to the presence of an underlying organic disease → suspect habitual hyperthermia → order CBC, ESR, CRP and urinalysis. If results of the laboratory tests also do not indicate the presence of any organic pathology → the diagnosis is ***'probable habitual hyperthermia'*** which needs long term follow up for confirmation; but if the test results suggest any or-

ganic pathology → suspect 'organic LGF' and proceed for further diagnostic workup which is like classic FUO.

**The etiologies of 'organic LGF' are similar to those of classic FUO, so diagnostic workup also should be similar.*

Follow up for *'probable habitual hyperthermia'*
In a recent study, the following approach was found very useful.[6]

- Repeat clinical evaluation every 2 months and laboratory tests every six months for the initial two years.
- Then repeat clinical evaluation every 6 months and laboratory tests every 12 months.
- If any positive finding is found at reevaluation any time, proceed for further diagnostic workup according to the suspicion.

Treatment of classic FUO

- ***Treatment should be directed towards the underlying cause when found.***
- ***When no cause is found after extensive investigations, and the patient's condition is stable*** watchful waiting is generally recommended.[8,9] However, some experts suggest NSAIDs (eg, ibuprofen, naproxen) for these patients;[8,9] NSAIDs are helpful when the underlying cause of FUO is an inflammatory condition[9], and the response may be dramatic in some inflammatory disorders, such as rheumatic fever and Still's disease.[2]
- ***Generally, empiric therapy with antibiotics, steroids, or antituberculous drugs are considered only when the clinical condition is deteriorating.***[8,12]
- ***Therapeutic trial with antibiotics:***
  - Empiric use of antibiotics is usually discouraged if the patient's condition is stable.[11]
  - Some physicians give a trial of ***fluoroquinolone (eg, ciprofloxacin 500 mg twice daily)*** for several days in stable FUO patients when an infectious etiology is likely but no specific infection has been identified.[10] In areas where quinolone resistance is not high, quinolones are effective in UTI; enteric fever; and infections caused by Rickettsia, Chlamydia, Legionella etc.
  - Although there is no published data, some physicians in South Asia, who work in the regions where quinolone resistance seems high and standard investigations cannot be performed because of resource constraints, give a trial with ***oral cefuroxime 500 mg 12 hourly plus azithromycin 500 mg 12 hourly*** in stable and otherwise healthy FUO patients, in whom infection is a possibility but has not been confirmed. If there is improvement, cefuroxime is continued for 10-14 days and azithromycin for 5-7 days. ***Sometimes, a trial of only oral azithromycin 500 mg twice daily is given for 5 days.***
  - ***When patient's condition is deteriorating and no cause of FUO has been identified,*** a trial with Piperacillin-tazobactum plus a fluoroquinolone can be considered.[2]

- ***Trial with anti-tuberculosis drugs*** for up to six weeks[2] can be considered if there is a suspicion of tuberculosis.

- TB should be suspected if TST is positive or granuloma is detected on histology (granulomatous hepatitis or another entity) but sarcoidosis is not likely[2] (serum ACE and CXR are not suggestive of sarcoidosis). In sarcoidosis, serum ACE is elevated in 40-80% cases[10] and CXR is abnormal in about 95% cases.
- In TB endemic areas, anti-TB drugs may be considered for virtually all undiagnosed FUO patients who are unstable or deteriorating, and have not responded to trial with broad-spectrum antibiotics.

- **Colchicine** is very effective in preventing attacks of fever in Familial Mediterranean Fever (FMF) and can be considered when FMF is suspected.
- **Drug fever** usually resolves within 48 hours of discontinuing the offending drug.[17]
- **Rifampicin** can suppress fever of even noninfectious origin.[9]

Some indications for trial with glucocorticoids in FUO:

Glucocorticoids have anti-inflammatory effects, can suppress fever and improve debility; but they may favor the spread of infection, so should be used very cautiously only in selective cases. They can be considered in FUO in the following conditions:

1. ***In undiagnosed FUO patients***, a trial with these drugs is generally considered as a last resort when the patient's condition is deteriorating and infection has been largely excluded[2,8,12] (by clinical evaluation and the results of lab tests including urinalysis, sputum microscopy, cultures, serology for infections, and imaging). However, probably it is not an uncommon practice to give empiric antimicrobial therapy first in these undiagnosed FUO patients; and if unresponsive, then a trial with corticosteroids is considered.

2. ***Glucocorticoids can be considered in a probable inflammatory disorder*** which is debilitating or threatening, particularly where trial with NSAID was also unsuccessful. Glucocorticoids usually cause dramatic improvement in some inflammatory conditions such as temporal arteritis, polymyalgia rheumatica and granulomatous hepatitis.[2]

   However, when only some nonspecific markers of inflammation are present (eg, elevated ESR, CRP and WBC count) causes of which could not be established and the patient is deteriorating, some experts give antimicrobial trial first before initiating corticosteroid.[36]

3. ***To improve debilitating symptoms:*** Many cases of FUO remain undiagnosed despite adequate diagnostic workup and after long term follow-up (>6months). Debilitating symptoms of these patients can be treated with NSAIDs, and ***glucocorticoids can be considered as a last resort.***[2]

4. ***Addition of a glucocorticoid to the empiric antibiotic or anti-TB regimen*** may be considered in rapidly deteriorating patients, where no cause of FUO has been established.

****Trial with corticosteroid is probably more commonly considered in aged patients*** (age >55 years).

Antipyretic selection for different categories of adult patients:[37]

Clinical state	***Suggested antipyretic***

Patients with hypertension or diabetes	Acetaminophen (paracetamol)
Patients with dehydration/ hypotension	Acetaminophen (paracetamol)
Patients with renal disease	Acetaminophen (paracetamol)
Patients with liver disease (especially in acute liver disease)	NSAID (eg, ibuprofen) (avoid in volume depleted state)

Notes:

- Continuous paracetamol is better than prn (as needed) doses, which causes some fluctuations in temperature.[10]
- Use of adequate antipyretics can prevent further deterioration of the patient's condition, particularly in some clinical states, such as patients with cardiopulmonary disorders or CNS dysfunction. Oxygen consumption increases by about 13% for each degree of temperature elevation from 37°C.[2]
- Acetaminophen is safe at therapeutic doses in stable chronic liver disease. So it can be used as analgesic and antipyretic in this group of patients.[38]
- When oral therapy is not possible, parenteral acetaminophen (paracetamol) or NSAIDs, or rectal suppositories of antipyretics can be used.
- In hyperthermia, physical cooling is the most important measure and antipyretics are not useful.

Prognosis

The overall prognosis of undiagnosed FUO cases (despite appropriate evaluation) is favorable. Most patients' fever resolves without treatment.[13] In one study, mortality at five years was only about 3% in the undiagnosed group.[9,13]

References

1. 'Body temperature norms' in **Medline plus;** at https://www.nlm.nih.gov/medlineplus/ency/article/001982.htm

2. Relevant chapters of **Harrison's Principles of Internal Medicine**; 18th edition; Dan L Longo et al (Editors). New York, McGraw-Hill 2012.

3. Jill Waalen et al. Is Older Colder or Colder Older? The Association of Age With Body Temperature in 18,630 Individuals. **J Gerontol A Biol Sci Med Sci. 2011**; May;66A(5):487–492

4. Philip A. Mackowiak et al: A Critical Appraisal of 98.6°F, the Upper Limit of the Normal Body Temperature, and Other Legacies of Carl Reinhold August Wunderlich. **JAMA 1992**; 268 (12):1578-1580.

5. Fever: First aid; **Mayo Clinic**. At: http://www.mayoclinic.org/first-aid/first-aid-fever/basics/art-20056685

6. M. Affronti et al. Low-grade Fever: How to Distinguish Organic from Non-organic Forms. **Int J Clin Pract. 2010**; 64(3):316-321.

7. Fever in adult. **Emedicinehealth**. At: http:// www.emedicinehealth.com/fever_in_adults/article_em.htm#fever_in_adults_overview

8. Chantal P. Bleeker-Rovers et al. A Prospective Multicenter Study on Fever of Unknown Origin: the Yield of a Structured Diagnostic Protocol. **Medicine (Baltimore) 2007**; 86(1):26–38

9. George M Varghese et al. Investigating and managing pyrexia of unknown origin in adults. **BMJ 2010**; 341:c5470

10. Relevant chapters of **Current Medical Diagnosis and Treatment**; Maxine A. Papadakis et al (Editors). New York, McGraw-Hill, **2013**.

11. Elizabeth C. Hersch et al. Prolonged Febrile Illness and Fever of Unknown Origin in Adults. **Am Fam Physician 2014**; Jul 15; 90(2):91-96

12. D. C. Knockaert. Fever of unknown origin in adults: 40 years on. **Journal of Internal Medicine 2003**; 253: 263–275

13. Fergus To. Fever of Unknown Origin: A Clinical Approach. **University of British Columbia Medical Journal,** February **2013;** 4(2); at: http://www.ubcmj.com/pdf/ubcmj_4_2_2013_14-16.pdf

14. Relevant chapters of **Davidson's Principles and Practice of Medicine**, 21st edition, Nicki R. Colledge et al (editors). India, Elsevier, **2010**.

15. Relevant chapters of **Kumar &Clark's Clinical Medicine,** 8th edition; Parveen Kumar and Michael Clark (Editors). Edinburgh, Elsevier, **2012**.

16. Patel RA and Gallagher JC. Drug fever. **Pharmacotherapy 2010**; Jan; 30(1):57-69.

17. Benjamin A. Lipsky and Jan V. Hirschmann. Drug fever. **JAMA 1981**; 245(8):851-854

18. 'Familial-Mediterranean-Fever' on the website of **The American College of Rheumatology (ACR)**. At: http://www.rheumatology.org/I-Am-A/Patient-Caregiver/Diseases-Conditions/Familial-Mediterranean-Fever-Juvenile

19. Ji-Fang Sheng et al. Diagnostic value of fluorine-18 fluorodeoxyglucose positron emission tomography/computed tomography in patients with fever of unknown origin. **European Journal of Internal Medicine 2011;** 22: 112–116

20. de Kleijn EM et al. Fever of unknown origin (FUO). II. Diagnostic procedures in a prospective multicenter study of 167 patients. The Netherlands FUO Study Group. **Medicine (Baltimore) 1997**; 76(6):401-14.

21. Bleeker-Rovers CP et al. A prospective multi-centre study of the value of FDG-PET as part of a structured diagnostic protocol in patients with fever of unknown origin. **Eur J Nucl Med Mol Imaging 2007**; May; 34(5):694-70

22. Johannes Meller et al. 18F-FDG PET and PET/CT in Fever of Unknown Origin. **J Nucl Med 2007**; 48:35–45

23. H. Balink et al. A Rationale for the Use of F18-FDG PET/CT in Fever and Inflammation of Unknown Origin. **International Journal of Molecular Imaging 2012**. Article ID 165080;

24. Ji-Fang Sheng et al. Diagnostic value of fluorine-18 fluorodeoxyglucose positron emission tomography/computed tomography in patients with fever of unknown origin. **Eur J Intern Med. 2011**; Feb; 22(1):112-16

25. Charles Moore et al. Causes and Significance of Markedly Elevated Serum Ferritin Levels in an Academic Medical Center. **J Clin Rheumatol. 2013**;19(6):324-328

26. Burke A. Cunha. Highly Elevated Serum Ferritin Levels as a Diagnostic Marker for *Legionella* Pneumonia. Correspondence • **CID 2008:**46 (1 June) • 1791; at: http://cid.oxfordjournals.org/content/46/11/1789.2.full.pdf

27. Seong Eun Kima et al. Diagnostic use of serum ferritin levels to differentiate infectious and noninfectious diseases in patients with fever of unknown origin. **Disease Markers 2013**; 34: 211–218

28. Burke A. Cunha. Fever of unknown origin. (in) Clinical infectious disease published by **Cambridge University Press**. At: http://assets.cambridge.org/97805218/71129/excerpt/9780521871129_excerpt.pdf

29. Gerald H. Mazurek et al. Updated Guidelines for Using Interferon Gamma Release Assays to Detect *Mycobacterium tuberculosis* Infection — United States, 2010. **Centers for Disease Control and Prevention.** At: http://www.cdc.gov/mmwr/pdf/rr/rr5905.pdf

30. TB Elimination: Interferon-Gamma Release Assays (IGRAs) – Blood Tests for TB Infection. **Fact sheet 2011 by CDC (USA)**; at: http://www.cdc.gov/tb/publications/factsheets/testing/igra.pdf

31. TB Manual: Interferon Gamma Release Assay Testing Guideline for Diagnosis of Latent Tuberculosis Infection by Physicians. **British Columbia Centre for Disease control, Canada**. At: http://www.bccdc.ca/resource-gallery/Documents/Communicable-Disease-Manual/Chapter%204%20-%20TB/CPS_TB_Manual_IGRA_guidelines_20150624.pdf

32. 'Diagnosis of Latent Tuberculosis Infection' in **Canadian tuberculosis standards, 7th edition, 2014.** At: http://www.respiratoryguidelines.ca/sites/all/files/CTB_Standards_EN_Chapter%204.pdf

33. Surajit Nayak et al. Mantoux test and its interpretation. **Indian Dermatol Online J. 2012**; Jan-Apr; 3(1): 2–6.

34. Otto O. Yang et al. Reimann's "Habitual Hyperthermia" Responding to Hormone Therapy. **Open Forum Infectious Diseases 2016**; Volume 3, Issue 3

35. Hobart A. Reimann. Habitual Hyperthermia: Premenstrual "Fever"**. JAMA. 1946**; 132(3):144.

36. Suzuki A et al. Fever of unknown origin responding to steroid therapy. **Nihon Rinsho Meneki Gakkai Kaishi 1997**; 20(1): 21-9.

37. Karen I. Plaisance. Toxicities of Drugs Used in the Management of Fever. **Clinical Infectious Diseases 2000;** 31(Suppl 5):S219–23

38. Benson GD et al.The therapeutic use of acetaminophen in patients with liver disease. **Am J Ther. 2005** Mar-Apr;12(2):133-41.

Chapter 2
Acute phase reactants

Acute-phase reactants (APRs)

- Acute-phase reactants are a group of plasma proteins whose levels may increase or decrease by at least 25% in inflammatory disorders.[1] Conditions causing this type of changes in plasma concentration of acute phase reactants include infection, inflammation, trauma, tissue infarction and malignancy.[1,2]
- ***Most APRs are mainly synthesized by the liver,*** although other type cells such as macrophages, endothelial cells, fibroblasts, and adipocytes have also been implicated in their synthesis.[2] The synthesis of APRs involves a complex mechanism stimulated by cytokines.
- The blood levels of acute phase reactants are not only altered by acute conditions as their name implies but also influenced by the chronic state of the same illnesses.[1,3]
- Although high CRP and ESR may be important indicators of acute phase response, their normal values do not rule out active disease.[4]

Acute phase reactants whose plasma levels may increase in active disease (positive acute-phase proteins) include:(Information from references 1,2,4,5)

- C - reactive protein (CRP) (may increase rapidly up to five-to one thousand-fold)
- Ferritin
- Procalcitonin (PCT)
- Complements (C3; C4) (may increase 25-50%)
- Fibrinogen (may increase 2-to 3-fold)
- Haptoglobin (may increase 2-to 3-fold)
- α_1 AT
- Serum amyloid A (may increase up to one thousand-fold)
- Ceruloplasmin (may increase 25-50%)

*The ESR is an indirect estimation of plasma acute phase protein concentration.[1,2]

Acute phase reactants whose plasma levels may decrease in active disease (negative acute-phase proteins) include:(Information from references 1,2,4)

- Albumin
- Transferrin
- Transthyretin (Prealbumin)
- Retinol binding proteins

Among acute phase reactants CRP and ESR are most commonly measured; however, clinicians have great interest in procalcitonin (PCT).

C-reactive protein (CRP)

CRP is synthesized mainly by the liver. The rate of CRP synthesis is proportional to the intensity of the stimulus.[6] However, CRP responses may be reduced in severe hepatic insufficiency and its levels may be elevated in renal dysfunction.[5]

CRP Kinetics:

Usually CRP begins to rise within 4-6 hours of the stimulation, doubles every 8 hours and peaks within about 36- 48 hours;[3] its approximate half-life is 19 hours.[3] CRP falls back towards normal rapidly after resolution of the insult; following resolution of a single stimulus (eg, a trauma or surgery), it may return to normal within 3-7 days.[6]

Causes of elevated serum CRP levels include:[3,5]

- Acute or chronic inflammatory conditions
- Acute or chronic infection
- Tissue necrosis or tissue infarction (eg, myocardial infarction and acute pancreatitis)
- Tissue injury (eg, trauma, surgery and burn)
- Cancer (eg, lymphoma, sarcoma)

Interpretation of CRP values:

Normal serum concentration: <10 mg/L[7] (most normal individuals have <2mg/L, but some have up to 10mg/L)[1,2]

General interpretation of high CRP levels[3,5,6,8]

Serum CRP level (mg/L)	*More likely causes*
10-40	Mild inflammation; viral infection; bacterial infection (early stage)
40-200	More severe inflammation; bacterial infection
>200-300	Severe bacterial infection; severe inflammation or injury

Here inflammation includes that occur in connective tissue diseases.

Conditions cause no or minimal (10-20 mg/L) CRP elevation (even in active disease)[3,5]

- Systemic lupus erythematosus (SLE)
- Ulcerative colitis
- Systemic sclerosis
- Dermatomyositis
- Leukemia

However, intercurrent infection in any of these conditions can cause significant elevation of CRP.

Notes:

- When serum CRP level >100 mg/L, the possibility of having a bacterial infection is 80% to 85%.[1]
- In active SLE, serum CRP level is usually normal unless associated with serositis, chronic synovitis, or vasculitis with tissue infarction.[1,3] In the absence of these characteristics, increased CRP in SLE suggests superadded infection. However, ESR is often high in active SLE and should be used to assess the disease-activity.[3]

How can serum CRP level help clinicians?

1. Most commonly, CRP is elevated in inflammatory conditions (infectious or noninfectious), so when clinically an inflammatory condition is suspected, CRP can help to diffe-

rentiate it from noninflammatory conditions.[1,3] However, CRP and ESR are not useful to screen asymptomatic individuals for infection, inflammation or malignancy.[6]Also, none of these tests are generally useful for assessing patients with vague clinical presentation, although they are often used in this context.[3]

2. When an infection is suspected clinically, CRP level can help to differentiate viral from bacterial infection. In viral infection, usually CRP level is normal or mildly elevated[9] (often <40 mg/L), while a normal CRP is very unusual in significant bacterial infection; CRP values higher than 100 mg/L is a strong indication of bacterial rather than viral infection.[5]
3. Serum CRP level monitoring is useful to assess antibiotic response in infection, as CRP level falls rapidly with resolution of an infection.
4. In many connective tissue disorders, such as rheumatoid arthritis, disease activity and therapeutic response can be assessed with serum CRP monitoring.
5. It may help to differentiate ulcerative colitis from Crohn's disease, since in active ulcerative colitis usually CRP level is normal or minimally elevated, while in active Crohn's disease it is markedly elevated.[8]
6. In SLE, CRP is useful to distinguish between lupus flare and infection; CRP is usually normal in disease-flare but increased in infection. On the other hand, ESR is generally high in both the conditions.[6]
7. In postoperative patients, it can help to detect secondary bacterial infection; persistently elevated CRP about one week after the surgery or a second rise after coming down from the first postoperative peak may be an indication of secondary bacterial infection.[10]

It should be noted that CRP is a supportive test, not specific one; sometimes CRP elevation may be delayed,[3] so a clinician should not be over reliant on it. To make a clinical decision, CRP values should be considered along with clinical data and other laboratory test results.

How frequently should CRP be tested?

Daily (every 24 hour) measurement of CRP may be useful in:

- Hospitalized patients with suspected or confirmed systemic inflammatory or acute infectious diseases (eg, fever of unknown origin), unless the diagnosis has been established and the patient is improving with a falling trend in CRP. The daily CRP measurement is particularly important when the clinical condition is unstable or the diagnosis remains uncertain.
- Critically ill patients
- Seriously ill patients at high risk of acute infection such as patients with mechanical ventilation, central vascular catheter, or increased risk for aspiration.

Less frequent checking may be appropriate in other cases, including for outpatients with already diagnosed (acute or chronic) inflammatory or infectious diseases in whom periodic repetition of CRP (eg, at each outpatient visit) may be sufficient.

High-sensitivity CRP (hs-CRP)

The lowest level of serum CRP that can be detected by conventional methods is 3 mg/L,[8] but more recently available high-sensitivity CRP assays can detect much lower concentrations with lowest detectable level being 0.03 mg/L.[3]

- hs-CRP has cardiovascular importance, but there is no clear consensus on its optimal clinical use.
- hs-CRP is commonly ordered with other tests necessary for cardiovascular risk stratification such as a fasting lipid profile.

Cardiovascular importance of hs-CRP
Many investigators have suggested that minor CRP elevations within the reference range for inflammatory conditions (i.e., <10 mg/L) have some cardiovascular applications:

1. *In apparently healthy individuals, this minor CRP elevation is an independent risk factor for cardiovascular diseases* such as coronary artery disease and stroke; some prophylactic measures (eg, statin therapy, particularly rosuvastatin) can reduce the risk.[3,8]
2. The CRP elevation (even when this type of minor) may be a bad prognostic factor in stable coronary disease and acute coronary syndrome.[3]

Interpretation of the hs-CRP values in determining the risk for cardiovascular events:[11,12]

1. Levels < 1mg/L: low risk
2. Levels 1-3mg/L: Average risk
3. Levels >3mg/L: high risk

When CRP level > 10mg/L in an apparently healthy individual (tested for cardiovascular risk stratification):
In these individuals, the CRP levels >10mg/L may be to be due to acute phase response resulting from minor infection or inflammation. The test should be repeated after 2 to 3 weeks, the time by which the level should come down to normal if it is due to acute phase response. But on repeat testing, if the CRP level remains high, the patient is most likely in the high-risk group.[12]

The relative risk for the high-risk group is estimated to be double of that for the low-risk group.[11]

CRP in metabolic syndrome:

- Minor CRP elevation (1-10 mg/L) may be found in metabolic syndrome, the condition which is known to predispose diabetes and heart disease.[12]
- Metabolic syndrome has five commonly measured components, namely: abdominal obesity, arterial hypertension, hyperglycemia, low HDL cholesterol and high triglyceride. At least three of the five components should be present for the diagnosis of metabolic syndrome.[12,13]
- CRP levels increase with the increase in the number of components of the metabolic syndrome.[12,13]
- Individuals with CRP levels >3 mg/L have 4 to 6 times higher risk of developing diabetes than those with lower CRP levels.[12]

Minor CRP elevations in other conditions:

- Minor CRP elevation (1-10 mg/L) may also be seen in smoking, uremia and myocardial ischemia.[2]
- CRP levels between 2-10 mg/L may be found in patients with osteoarthritis, especially those with progressive joint damage, which supports the association of inflammation in this disorder.[1]

Can I get any additional advantages if I test hs-CRP instead of conventional CRP for routine uses?

- No; for routine uses, conventional CRP measurement is enough. High-sensitivity CRP assays detect the same CRP up to a much lower concentrations than conventional methods do. But that lower concentration of CRP falls within the normal reference range of CRP for routine uses, so it does not provide additional information in the management of a patient with infection, inflammation or malignancy.
- In some labs, the cost of hs-CRP measurement is about five times higher than that of conventional CRP measurement. Therefore, ordering hs-CRP instead of conventional CRP for routine uses would be an unnecessary expense.[3]

Erythrocyte sedimentation rate (ESR)

- ESR is an indirect estimation of plasma acute phase proteins.[1]
- Like CRP, ESR is not the measurement of a single plasma protein concentration; instead, it is influenced by the concentration of several plasma proteins and some other factors as well.

Factors influencing ESR

1. ***Plasma protein concentration***
   - Normally the negative charges on the red cell surface repel the red cells each other, thus inhibiting their aggregation. Positively charged plasma proteins neutralize some of the negative charges on the red cell surface, favoring the aggregation of red cells and formation of RBC clumps or stacks (rouleaux formation). Increased levels of some plasma proteins accelerate rouleaux formation. The rouleau (pleural of rouleaux) are heavier than single RBCs and sediment at a faster rate resulting in increased ESR.
   - The plasma proteins that have an important role in rouleaux formation include fibrinogen, beta globulin, alpha globulin, gamma globulins and albumin. Of these, fibrinogen has the highest red cell aggregating power while globulins' power is roughly half of that of fibrinogen with albumin's ability being the lowest.[8]

2. ***Red cell number and morphology***
   - The ESR is high in anemia and low in polycythemia. <u>In conditions associated with moderate to severe anemia, ESR has little significance</u>.[6]
   - Abnormal red cell morphology interferes with rouleaux formation which causes low ESR in spherocytosis and sickle cell anemia.

3. ***Age, sex, pregnancy, obesity and end stage renal disease***
   - Fibrinogen level is increased in old age, pregnancy and end stage renal disease causing up to a moderately increased ESR. ESR may be elevated up to 60 mm/hr in patients with chronic kidney disease and nephrotic syndrome.[2]
   - Female sex and obesity are also associated with higher ESR.[14]

4. ***Drugs*** can affect ESR; for example, oral contraceptive pill and heparin can increase ESR.[8]

The mechanisms of ESR rise

(a) *In acute phase response*: synthesis of acute phase proteins → ↑level of some plasma proteins →↑rouleaux formation (particularly due to ↑ fibrinogen) → ↑ ESR (with concomitant increase in CRP);
In acute phase response, acute phase protein fibrinogen accounts for about 60-70% of the rise in ESR.[8]

(b) *In the absence of acute phase response:* High ESR can occur in conditions associated with increased levels of polyclonal or monoclonal immunoglobulins (eg, multiple myeloma).
Hypergammaglobulinemia → ↑rouleaux formation → ↑ ESR
As there is no acute phase response, CRP often remains normal in these cases.

Reference range of ESR for adults:

In general, for males: < 10mm/hr; **for females** <20mm/hr;

However, it may be more accurate if the normal value of ESR is calculated considering individuals' age and sex; the calculation is as follows:

ESR for males: age divided by 2; **for females**: age +10 divided by 2;[2,15]

Most common causes of very high ESR (> 100 mm/hour):[16]

- Infection (eg, Tuberculosis; osteomyelitis)
- Malignancy (eg, lymphoma; multiple myeloma; metastatic cancer)
- Collagen vascular disease (eg, Rheumatoid arthritis; SLE; Giant cell arteritis; polymyalgia rheumatica)

When ESR is higher than 100 mm/hr, an underlying significant cause is found in more than 90% of cases; so a prompt search for the underlying disorder should be made.[2]

Causes of low ESR[1,2]

1. Polycythemia
2. Disorders affecting RBC morphology- eg, sickle cell disease and hereditary spherocytosis
3. Low fibrinogen levels
4. Severe liver disease

Which one is the better marker of inflammation, CRP or ESR?

Generally CRP is considered superior to ESR as a marker of inflammation and the estimation of the ESR has been largely replaced by CRP measurement these days, because:

1. ESR response is slow
   Usually ESR begins to rise within 24–48 hours of the onset of inflammation,[2] may take a week to peak, then falls back slowly with resolution of the inflammation, and normalization may take weeks to months.[14] On the other hand, CRP changes are rapid; it begins to

rise within 6 hours of the stimulation, peaks within 48 hours, and then falls back to normal rapidly over days after resolution of the stimulus.

2. ESR is influenced by multiple factors (stated above); therefore, it is a less specific marker of inflammation than CRP and its interpretation is also more difficult in some situations.

   For these reasons, in most clinical conditions, CRP is more useful than ESR for both diagnostic and monitoring purposes. However, there are some exceptional situations where ESR is more useful than CRP.

Conditions in which ESR is more useful than CRP include:

1. SLE: In active SLE, CRP level is often normal or minimally elevated (10-20 mg/L) unless associated with serositis, chronic synovitis or vasculitis with tissue infarction,[3] but ESR is raised. Therefore, ESR is better than CRP in monitoring disease activity in SLE.
2. Paraproteinemia: In paraproteinaemias, usually ESR is elevated but not the CRP, as they often do not induce an acute phase response.[5]

Procalcitonin (PCT):

Procalcitonin is a promising diagnostic marker of bacterial infection. It is a precursor of calcitonin and normally produced mainly by thyroid C cells (Parafollicular cells). But in response to bacterial infection and inflammation, it is produced by many non-thyroid tissues. However, in these pathological conditions, serum calcitonin level remains normal despite the elevation of procalcitonin level.[17] For PCT measurement, either serum or plasma can be used.

PCT kinetics:(Information from references 17-19)

In response to triggering stimuli, PCT becomes detectable in plasma usually within 2 to 4 hours and peaks within 6 to 24 hours; after cessation of the stimuli, the elimination half-life of this peptide is 25-30 hours.

Causes elevated serum/ plasma PCT level(Information from references 17,20,21)

Most common cause: bacterial infection (including sepsis and septic shock)

Other causes include:

- Severe viral infection
- Severe fungal infection
- Massive stress such as severe trauma, surgery or shock state
- Some neoplasms- eg, medullary carcinoma of the thyroid, small cell carcinoma of the lung and carcinoid syndrome;
- Some autoimmune diseases such as Kawasaki disease or various types of vasculitis
- Some noninfectious inflammatory conditions: Pulmonary aspiration, pancreatitis, heat stroke, acute graft-versus-host disease etc. However, noninfectious inflammatory stimuli usually need to be very severe to cause PCT elevations.
- PCT levels may be elevated in untreated end-stage renal disease in the absence of infection or inflammation.

How PCT can help clinicians?

1. Procalcitonin is a more specific biomarker of bacterial infection than others, such as CRP and leukocyte count with differential.[22] PCT is useful to differentiate bacterial infection from viral infection, particularly in community acquired pneumonia and meningitis; also, it is useful to distinguish bacterial infection from noninfectious causes of inflammation. So PCT may be a supportive evidence for the clinical decision of initiation or discontinuation of antibiotic therapy, particularly in acute exacerbation of COPD, community acquired pneumonia and sepsis.[20]
2. In fever of unknown origin (FUO), PCT may be useful to narrow the differential diagnoses. PCT levels generally remain normal or <0.5 ng/ml in viral infections and inflammatory causes of FUO such as Still's disease, SLE and inflammatory bowel disease.[17,20]
3. PCT level may be helpful to monitor the disease progression and response to antibiotic therapy in bacterial infection.
4. PCT levels usually remain unaffected by the use of nonsteroidal anti-inflammatory drugs or corticosteroid. So in inflammatory conditions, PCT levels may be a valuable marker of the host inflammatory status even when other markers of inflammation such as CRP and WBC count with differential have been altered with the use of these drugs.[20]
5. PCT values are not affected by neutropenia, so helpful for the diagnosis of bacterial infection in neutropenic patient.[17]
6. The addition of procalcitonin testing to standard clinical practice can reduce the frequency and duration of antibiotic therapy.[22]

Limitations of PCT[20,21]

- Although increased levels of PCT help clinicians to differentiate bacterial from viral infections, PCT is not increased in all bacterial infections; for example, it may remain low in subacute bacterial endocarditis and mycoplasma infection;
- PCT levels may be elevated in many conditions other than bacterial infection (stated above) such as severe viral or fungal infection; major trauma; autoimmune diseases; and some noninfectious inflammatory conditions.

Interpretation of PCT values(Information from references 7,17,18,20-23)

- Interpretation of PCT values is still unclear and more studies are needed to determine its optimal use.
- Clinical context should be taken into account during the interpretation. Some general interpretation of PCT values have been given below. However, the decision of starting or stopping antibiotic treatment in patients with suspected significant bacterial infection should not be taken based mainly on PCT values.

Clinical state	*PCT level*	*Clinical impression*
Normal person	<0.10 ng/ml	Significant bacterial infection unlikely; (consider to repeat within 6-24 hours if bacterial infection is suspected clinical-

		ly)
Suspected lower respiratory tract infection	(a) 0.1-0.25 ng/ml (b) >0.25 ng/ml	(a) Low possibility of bacterial infection; despite this antibiotics may be needed in some cases, particularly when severe respiratory infection is suspected clinically or the patient has preexisting lung disease. (b) Increased possibility of bacterial infection; Antibiotics recommended;
Suspected systemic bacterial infection or generalized sepsis	(a) 0.1 – 0.5 ng/ml (b) ≥ 0.5– < 2 ng/ml (c) ≥ 2 ng/ml (d) ≥ 10 ng/ml	(a) Low possibility systemic bacterial infection; antibiotics usually discouraged; (b) Increased possibility of systemic bacterial infection; antibiotics encouraged; (c) High possibility of sepsis; antibiotics strongly indicated; (d) Severe sepsis or septic shock; antibiotics strongly indicated;
Suspected bacterial meningitis	Usually >0.5 ng/ml; in many cases >5 ng/ml	
Autoimmune diseases; viral infections; localized mild bacterial infections; chronic inflammatory conditions	Usually <0.5 ng/ml	

Notes:

1. In the emergency department, to rule out bacteremia in a febrile patient, PCT value < 0.1ng/ml as the cutoff has a 96% negative predictive value; and some experts believe blood culture may not be necessary for these patients (with PCT < 0.1ng/ml).[24]
2. In ward setting, PCT levels can be repeated daily or less frequently for monitoring the response to antibiotic therapy in a diagnosed patient of bacterial infection.
3. Although procalcitonin test shows promise, its routine use is not recommended currently because of insufficient evidence.[22]

References

1. Cem Gabay and Irving Kushner. Acute-phase proteins and other systemic responses to inflammation. **N Engl J Med. 1999**; Feb 11;340(6):448-54

2. Anurag Markanday. Acute phase reactants in infections: evidence-based review and a guide for clinicians. **Open Forum Infectious Diseases 2015**; at: http://ofid.oxfordjournals.org/content/2/3/ofv098.full

3. Francisco J.B. Aguiar et al. C-reactive protein: clinical applications and proposals for a rational use. **REV ASSOC MED BRAS. 2013**; 59(1):85-92

4. Acute phase reactants. **RCPA (The Royal College of Pathologists of Australia) manual**. At: https://www.rcpa.edu.au/Library/Practising-Pathology/RCPA-Manual/Items/Pathology-Tests/A/Acute-phase-reactants

5. Glenn Reeves. C-reactive protein. **Aust Prescr 2007**;30 (3):74–6

6. CRP vs ESR: assessing and measuring the inflammatory response. **The Best Practice Advocacy Centre New Zealand** (bpac^{nz}); 2005. At: http://www.bpac.org.nz/resources/campaign/crp_esr/bpac_crp_vs_esr_poem_2005_wv.pdf

7. 'Reference intervals for commonly used tests' in the appendix of **Current Medical Diagnosis and Treatment**; Maxine A. Papadakis et al (Editors). New York, McGraw-Hill, 2013

8. Stephen Adelstein and Alan Baker. 'Making sense of inflammatory markers (2014)' on the website of the **Royal College of Pathologists of Australasia**. At: https://www.rcpa.edu.au/getattachment/7d8d8036-473e-4e15-8756-bf07e597de43/Making-Sense-of-Inflammatory-Markers.aspx

9. Sasaki K et al. Differentiating between bacterial and viral infection by measuring both C-reactive protein and 2'-5'-oligoadenylate synthetase as inflammatory markers. **J Infect Chemother. 2002** Mar;8(1):76-80.

10. Man Kyu Choi et al. Sequential Changes of Plasma C-Reactive Protein, Erythrocyte Sedimentation Rate and White Blood Cell Count in Spine Surgery: Comparison between Lumbar Open Discectomy and Posterior Lumbar Interbody Fusion. **J Korean Neurosurg Soc 2014**; 56 (3):218-223

11. 'High-sensitivity C-reactive protein' in **Emedicine**. At: http://emedicine.medscape.com/article/2094831-overview#showall

12. Paul M Ridker. C-reactive protein: a simple test to help predict risk of heart attack and stroke. **Circulation 2003;**108:e81-e85

13. Genel SUR et al. The Relevance of Inflammatory Markers in Metabolic Syndrome. **MAEDICA – A Journal of Clinical Medicine 2014**; 9(1): 15-18

14. Erythrocyte sedimentation rate and C-reactive protein. **Australian prescriber**. volume 38: number 3: June 2015

15. 'Laboratory values (ESR)' in **GP note book**; at: http://www.gpnotebook.com/simplepage.cfm?ID=-966066110

16. Muhammad Yousuf et al. Extremely elevated erythrocyte sedimentation rate: etiology at a tertiary care center in Saudi Arabia. **Saudi Med J. 2010**; 31(11):1227-31

17. 'PCT'. **Mayo Clinic (Mayo Medical Laboratories)**. At: http://www.mayomedicallaboratories.com/test-catalog/Clinical+and+Interpretive/83169

18. 'Procalcitonin (PCT) Guidance' on the website of **Nebraska Medical Center, USA.** At: http://www.nebraskamed.com/careers/education-programs/asp/procalcitonin-pct-guidance

19. William Shomali et al. Can procalcitonin distinguish infectious fever from tumor-related fever in non-neutropenic cancer patients? **Cancer 2012**; 118:5823-29.

20. Hyuck Lee. Procalcitonin as a biomarker of infectious diseases. **Korean J Intern Med 2013**; 28:285-291

21. 'Procalcitonin **(2013)'** on the website of **Association for Clinical Biochemistry, UK.** At: http://www.acb.org.uk/Nat%20Lab%20Med%20Hbk/Procalcitonin.pdf

22. Procalcitonin testing for diagnosing and monitoring sepsis (ADVIA Centaur BRAHMS PCT assay, BRAHMS PCT Sensitive Kryptor assay, Elecsys BRAHMS PCT assay, LIAISON BRAHMS PCT assay and VIDAS BRAHMS PCT assay). **NICE (UK) guideline 2015**. At: https://www.nice.org.uk/guidance/dg18

23. 'Procalcitonin' on the website of the department of pathology and laboratory medicine, **UCDAVIS Health system (USA)**. At: https://www.ucdmc.ucdavis.edu/pathology/services/clinical/change_of_service/CP/2014/Procalcitonin_Test_Notification_12182014.pdf

24. Stefan Riedel et al. Procalcitonin as a marker for the detection of bacteremia and sepsis in the emergency department. **Am J Clin Pathol 2011**;135:182-189

Chapter 3

Community acquired pneumonia (CAP)

Pneumonia

Definition

- There is no universally accepted definition of pneumonia.
- Simply pneumonia can be defined as the acute inflammation of the lung parenchyma due to infection.
- Most physicians use the term 'pneumonitis' to refer inflammation of the lung tissue due to non-infectious causes such as airborne irritants, drugs, radiotherapy etc.

Classification of pneumonia

Traditional Classification:

- Traditionally pneumonia has been classified clinically as 'typical' and 'atypical'.[1]
- 'Typical' pneumonia is usually caused by *Streptococcus pneumoniae*, while 'atypical pneumonia' is commonly caused by common atypical bacteria (mycoplasma, Chlamydia and Legionella) and respiratory viruses. However, the differentiation between 'typical' and 'atypical' pneumonia is often not possible only on clinical ground.[1]

Now the traditional classification has been largely replaced by a clinically more useful classification based on the context in which the pneumonia has developed.

New classification: (Information from references 2,3)

A. Community Acquired Pneumonia (CAP)
B. Nosocomial pneumonia (NP) [Include: Hospital-Acquired, Ventilator-Associated and Health Care- Associated Pneumonia]
C. Aspiration Pneumonia (AP)
D. Pneumonia in the immunocompromised hosts

In this chapter, only community acquired pneumonia (CAP) has been discussed; however, immunocompromised patients has not been included.

Community acquired pneumonia (CAP)

Community acquired pneumonia (CAP) is the deadliest infectious disease in the USA and the eighth leading cause of death. It occurs in about 4 to 5 million people in the United States each year, 25% of whom need hospitalization.[3]

Microbiology of CAP

- Although myriads of organisms can cause CAP, a few pathogens are responsible for most cases.[4]
- *Streptococcus pneumoniae* is the most commonly identified pathogen.
- The pathogens can be divided into two groups: typical and atypical.[4]
- The term 'atypical' is used to indicate the organisms which are neither detectable on Gram-stain nor cultivatable on standard bacteriologic media.[4]
- <u>Common typical organisms:</u>

    - *Streptococcus pneumoniae*
    - *Haemophilus influenzae*
    - *Staphylococcus aureus*
    - Gram-negative enteric bacteria (eg, *Klebsiella pneumoniae* and *Pseudomonas aeruginosa*)
- Common atypical organisms:
    - *Mycoplasma pneumoniae*
    - *Chlamydia pneumoniae*
    - *Legionella species*
    - Respiratory viruses (eg, influenza A&B, adenovirus, respiratory syncytial virus and parainfluenza)

  *Influenza is the predominant viral cause of CAP in adults.[4]

One British study of hospitalized adult patients showed following representation of common agents causing CAP:[5]

- *Streptococcus pneumoniae 48%*
- Influenza A virus 19%
- *Chlamydia pneumoniae 13%,*
- *Haemophilus influenzae 7%,*
- *Mycoplasma pneumoniae 3%*
- *Legionella pneumophilia* 3%

*Overall, the causative organism(s) of CAP remains unknown in about 40% cases,[1] more commonly among outpatients.

Polymicrobial CAP

- A combination of two or more organisms may be present in CAP.[6]
- The reported percentage of polymicobial CAP is very variable, 5% - 38%.[7]
- The combination often includes typical and atypical organisms with most common being the combination of *S. pneumoniae* and a respiratory virus.[6]
- Polymicrobial CAP is more common in the elderly and severely ill patients.[8]

Anaerobic pneumonia

- It is more common in the elderly and in patients with increased risk of aspiration (eg, alcoholism, stroke, epilepsy)[8]
- In CAP, anaerobic infection is usually suspected when an episode of aspiration possibly has occurred in the preceding weeks of presentation, particularly in patients with gingival disease or esophageal motility disorders.
- Abscess formation, empyema, or parapneumonic effusion is frequent complication of anaerobic pneumonia.[4]

Methicillin-Resistant Staph. aureus (MRSA) and Risk factors for CA-MRSA

MRSA: Basic information

- About one-third of the normal people have *Staphylococcus aureus* on their skin or in the nose. They are usually harmless unless they enter the body through a cut or other wound, and even then they generally cause only minor skin and soft tissue infections in healthy individuals.[9]

- MRSA is a particular sub-set of *Staphylococcus aureus* which is resistant to many antibiotics and difficult to treat.
- There are two types of MRSA: Community-Acquired MRSA (CA-MRSA) and Health Care Associated MRSA (HA- MRSA).
- CA-MRSA strains are epidemiologically, genotypically, and phenotypically distinct from HA-MRSA.[4] Although CA-MRSA strains can cause severe infections in otherwise healthy individuals, they are resistant to fewer antibiotics than Health Care Associated MRSA (HA-MRSA) strains.[4]
- In community, 2% of the population carries MRSA.[10]

Risk factors for CA-MRSA

- Participation in contact sports- the bacteria can spread easily through frequent skin-to-skin contact.
- Living in overcrowded conditions- dormitories, military training camps, day-care centers, prisons etc.
- Touching contaminated objects (eg, sharing towels, razors etc.)
- Broken skin (i.e., cuts or abrasions)
- Lack of cleanliness
- Homosexuality

CA- MRSA CAP

- Although CA-MRSA CAP remains rare in most communities, it is an emerging problem.
- CA-MRSA CAP has following characteristics which are helpful for diagnosis:
    - CA-MRSA pneumonia is often associated with preceding influenza.
    - Most strains of CA-MRSA can produce the toxin Panton- Valentine leukocidin which can cause severe necrotizing pneumonia as well as abscess and empyema formation. Therefore, CA-MRSA infection should also be suspected in necrotizing pneumonia; pneumonia with cavitary lesions or empyema, without risk factors for anaerobic aspiration pneumonia.
- In its characteristic clinical scenario, diagnosis of CA-MRSA pneumonia can often be established with sputum and blood cultures.[4]

Commonly isolated pathogen(s) in some specific categories of CAP patients:[4,11]

Patient categories	***Commonly identified pathogen(s)***
Aspiration	Oral anaerobes; Gram-negative enteric bacilli
Alcoholism	Aspiration more common; *Pneumococcus;* Gram-negative enteric bacilli; oral anaerobes; *M. tuberculosis*
COPD	Study reports variable; *Haemophilus influenzae* and *Moraxella cararrhalis* may be more frequent; other common isolates: *Streptococcus pneumoniae; Pseudomonas aeruginosa; Legionella* spp.; enterobacteriaceae; mixed infections more common.

Structural lung disease (such as bronchiectasis)	*P. aeruginosa; Burkholderia cepacia; S. aureus*
Influenza season in the area	Influenza virus; *Pneumococcus; Staph. aureus; S. aureus pneumonia is a recognized complication of influenza.*
Endobronchial obstruction *(eg, by tumor)*	Anaerobes; *Pneumococcus; H. influenzae; S. aureus*
Injection drug use	*Staph. aureus*; anaerobes; *Mycobacterium tuberculosis; Pneumococcus*
Staying in hotel or on cruise ship in previous 2 weeks	*Legionella* spp.

Clinical features of CAP

Presentation is usually acute or subacute and severity varies from mild to fatal disease.

Symptoms:

- Usual minimal initial symptoms: fever and cough.
  - Fever may be associated with chills and rigors. Fever may be absent in immunocompromised and in the elderly. Hypothermia can occur in severe sepsis.
  - Cough is often initially dry and later accompanied by mucopurulent sputum. Hemoptysis occurs occasionally. Rust-colored sputum may be seen in streptococcus pneumoniae infection.[2,12]
- Pleuritic chest pain which may be referred to the anterior abdominal wall or shoulder;[2]
- Breathlessness
- Anorexia, fatigue, myalgia, arthralgia and headache;
- Gastrointestinal symptoms such as nausea, vomiting, abdominal pain, or diarrhea may be present in up to 20% cases.[13]

Signs:

Signs vary depending on the extent of lung consolidation and the presence or absence of pleural effusion.

- At the early stage, chest examination may not reveal any signs; fever and tachycardia may be the only physical signs.
- Tachypnea and arterial oxygen desatuartion are common.
- Inspiratory crackles and signs of consolidation, such as bronchial breath sounds and increased vocal resonance, are also often found.
- Percussion note may be dull over a consolidation or a parapneumonic pleural effusion.
- Pleural rub is heard in some cases.
- Upper abdominal tenderness may be present in lower lobe pneumonia or if there is associated hepatitis.[2]

*If symptoms have been present for several weeks or unresponsive to standard antibiotic therapy, tuberculosis should be considered in the differential diagnosis.[12]

Atypical presentations of infectious diseases (including pneumonia) in the elderly:

Fever and leukocytosis may not be present, and only symptom(s) may be one or more of the followings:

(1) Confusion (new-onset or worsening)
(2) Falls (new-onset or worsening)
(3) Decreased appetite
(4) Change in functional status

Notes:

(1) Pneumonia is most frequently missed diagnosed in the elderly as atypical presentation is common.[14]
(2) In unexplained sickness in the elderly, infection (including CAP) should always be suspected.[12]

CAP due to typical versus atypical pathogens: Is it possible to differentiate clinically?

Reliable differentiation between the two groups is often not possible solely on clinical grounds. However, pneumonia due to atypical pathogens has some characteristic clinical features which may be helpful to distinguish them from pneumonia caused by typical pathogens:

(1) The presence of extrapulmonary feature(s) is the main characteristic feature feature(s) of CAP due to atypical pathogens which helps differentiate it from CAP caused by typical pathogens.[15]
(2) Atypical pathogens often cause slower onset less severe disease, except Legionella spp.

Is it possible to identify clinically the specific atypical pathogen causing the pneumonia?
Although not always, a particular atypical bacterium can produce a relatively specific pattern of extrapulmonary involvement which may be helpful to identify that organism. For example:

- Relative bradycardia in CAP is characteristic of legionnaire's disease, Psittacosis and Q fever. Psittacosis and Q fever are zoonotic diseases and are less likely in the absence of positive contact history.[15]
- Acute abdominal pain usually does not occur in CAP other than legionnaire's disease.[15]
- In the presence of otherwise unexplained loose stools or diarrhea, most likely pathogens are *Legionella spp.* or *M. pneumoniae*. However, relative bradycardia, acute abdominal pain and CNS involvement usually do not occur in mycoplasma pneumonia, but are characteristics of legionnaire's disease.[15]
- Relative bradycardia, gastrointestinal manifestations-such as loose stool or non-bloody watery diarrhea, nausea, vomiting and abdominal pain- and neurologic symptoms- like headache, lethargy and disorientation- are common features of legionnaire's disease.

Clinical features of CAP due to specific atypical organisms:

1. *Mycoplasma pneumoniae*[2,12,1617]

- Affects mainly children and young adults.
- Occurs in epidemics every 3-4 years.
- Usually causes milder disease (Fever usually <101^0F) and patients usually does not look toxic.
- Gradual onset over days to weeks (1 to 4 weeks)[16,17] with prominent extrapulmonary symptoms (headache, malaise, myalgia etc). However, dry to mildly productive cough is

always present, without it mycoplasma pneumonia is unlikely;[16] sore throat is also common.[16,17]

- Rarely causes hemolytic anemia, erythema multiforme (Stevens-Johnson syndrome) or other type of rashes, erythema nodosum, hepatitis and meningoencephalitis, myocarditis, pericarditis etc.
- Immunocompetent young adults are usually recovered after several weeks without antibiotics[16] but cough may persist for weeks or months.[17] Antibiotics may speed recovery.

2. <u>*Chlamydia pneumoniae*</u>[2,12,16-18]

- Can occur at any age; most common among school-age children
- Subclinical infection is common; in the USA, about 50% of the young adults (age <20 years) have serologic evidence of this infection. Reinfection can occur throughout life.[17]
- Often causes mild, self-limiting disease with prolonged prodrome.
- Typical symptoms: gradual onset of unproductive cough with low-grade fever which may be preceded by upper respiratory tract symptoms such as sore throat and hoarseness. Physical examination often shows no abnormalities.
- Fever is usually present in the first several days, but some symptoms such as cough and malaise may persist for weeks to months despite antibiotic therapy.[16,18]
- Some investigators *reported that C. pneumoniae* infection may be related to atherosclerotic vascular disease.[17]

3. <u>*Chlamydia psittaci*</u>[2,3,12.16-18]

- Acquired from birds; so exposure to birds is a clue to the diagnosis of *C psittaci* pneumonia. Poultry worker, pet shop employees are particularly at risk. However, only 20% of the affected individuals have a positive history of bird exposure and person to person spread can occur.[12]
- Usually causes milder disease; typically low-grade fever, headache, myalgia, and a dry cough; however, severe illness with high fever may occur.
- May present with culture-negative endocarditis[3,16] or pyrexia of unknown origin.
- *Physical signs that point to psittacosis include relative bradycardia, rash, splenomegaly or hepatosplenomegaly.*
- Chest signs may be absent initially;[16] however, pneumonia is often detectable on chest x-ray.[17]

4. <u>*Legionellosis*</u>

Legionellosis includes two distinct clinical syndromes:

a) Legionnaire's disease: manifest as pneumonia
b) Pontiac fever: acute, febrile, self-limiting illness like mild influenza. Usually persist less than one week.

<u>Legionnaire's disease</u>[2,3,12,16,17,19]

- Usually caused by *Legionella pneumophila* but other species are involved in about 10% of cases.[12]
- Incubation period is usually 2-10 days, may be up to 2 weeks.[17]
- Legionella can cause more severe disease than other atypical bacteria requiring early intensive care and rarely lung abscess may develop.
- Older adults, smokers, patients with preexisting lung disease and immunocompromised individuals are particularly susceptible to Legionnaires' disease.

- The disease is usually acquired by inhalation of contaminated water mist, which could be from the air conditioning system; humidifier; or spray from a shower, faucet, whirlpool or the water dispersed through the ventilation system in large buildings such as hotels, hospitals etc. Contaminated water source related local outbreaks have occurred. Person to person transmission is uncommon.[2]
- Many features of Legionnaire's disease are like typical pneumonia, such as high fever, toxic appearance and pleuritic chest pain. The Cough is initially non-productive, but by the second or third day becomes productive with mucopurulent sputum like typical pneumonia.
- Common extrapulmonary features: Relative bradycardia; gastrointestinal symptoms (in 20-40% cases)[19] such as non-bloody watery diarrhea, nausea, vomiting and abdominal pain; neurologic symptoms like headache, lethargy and disorientation.
- Hyponatremia, elevated liver enzymes, elevated creatine kinase and microscopic hematuria may be found.

5. *Viral CAP*

Clinical features of viral pneumonia have many similarities with those of bacterial pneumonia, especially atypical bacterial pneumonia. So the differentiation between viral and bacterial pneumonia, particularly atypical bacterial pneumonia, on clinical ground is often difficult. However, presence of some epidemiologic and clinical clues increases the possibility of viral pneumonia:[20]

- Viral pneumonia more common in young children and older adults.
- Commonly occurs during flu season.
- Onset of viral pneumonia is usually less abrupt than typical bacterial pneumonia.
- In viral pneumonia, initial flu-like symptoms (fever, headache, myalgia, fatigue, dry cough etc) are followed by more prominent chest symptoms (such as more severe cough, breathlessness etc.) developed over several days. However, viral pneumonia due to some unusual viruses (Avian Flu, SARS etc) may follow an aggressive course of rapid deterioration.
- In viral pneumonia, chills are often present, but rigors and chest pain are less common.
- At the early stage, patients look less sick than in typical bacterial pneumonia, and the toxic look which is common in typical bacterial pneumonia is usually not seen.
- On examination, the signs of lobar consolidation which are frequently found in typical bacterial pneumonia are often absent in viral pneumonia;[1] instead, crackles and wheezes are commonly found.
- Pleural effusion or cavitation is usually do not develop.
- Viral pneumonia is unresponsive to antibiotic therapy.
- Secondary bacterial pneumonia is common and may manifest as the relapse of the fever, cough after an initial improvement.

Differential diagnoses of pneumonia

- Acute bronchitis
- Acute exacerbation of COPD
- Pulmonary edema (may be unilateral)
- Pulmonary embolism
- Pulmonary tuberculosis
- Pulmonary eosinophilia
- Lung cancer

- Radiation pneumonitis
- Drug induced pneumonitis (eg, anticancer drugs, antibiotics, analgesics etc)
- Cryptogenic organizing pneumonia or bronchiolitis obliterans organizing pneumonia) (COP /BOOP)

Diagnosis of CAP

- ***Diagnosis of pneumonia usually needs clinical and radiological evidence.***
- For the diagnosis of pneumonia, clinical findings are about 50% sensitive and 67% specific compared to chest imaging.[3,13] Therefore, in most cases, a pulmonary opacity on chest x-ray (or CT scan) is needed to confirm the diagnosis of pneumonia and to differentiate pneumonia from other common causes of cough and fever, such as acute bronchitis.[1,3,4]

Investigations of CAP

For out-patients:

- Etiologic diagnosis by microbiological tests is usually not necessary for the treatment mild CAP, as empiric antibiotic therapy is almost always successful.[3,12] However, in most cases of suspected CAP, a chest radiograph is needed to establish the diagnosis of CAP.[3] Therefore, for outpatient-treatment of mild CAP, chest x-ray may be the only specific investigation needed for management.
- Tests for etiologic diagnosis should be considered even in ambulatory patients with mild disease if the patient's presentation suggests a possible pathogen that is not covered by standard empiric therapy or if there is a public health concern.

For hospitalized patients: (Information from references 1-4,11,12,21)

1. Complete Blood Count (CBC), ESR, CRP
2. Blood urea, creatinine and electrolyte
3. Blood sugar
4. Chest radiograph
5. Urinalysis (microscopic hematuria may be present in Legionnaire's disease)
6. Sputum tests: Sputum for Gram-stain and culture (preferably pre-antibiotic) for all admitted patients; in some cases, sputum special stain for acid fast bacilli and fungi; Legionella culture in severe CAP;
7. Blood culture (preferably pre-antibiotic) is indicated in all moderate to severe CAP patients.
8. Liver function tests (ALT/AST, Serum Bilirubin, ALP) - for all hospitalized patients
9. HIV testing (for all adult pneumonia patients)
10. Pulse Oxymetry (for all)
11. Arterial Blood Gas analysis (if SaO2 <93% or features of severe pneumonia present).[2]
12. Rapid antigen detection test for influenza (in severe CAP or when influenza is suspected clinically)
13. Urinary antigen tests for *Streptococcus pneumoniae and Legionella species* (in moderate to severe pneumonia, particularly in severe disease or unresponsive to standard empiric antibiotics)
14. CT scan of the chest: rarely needed; usually considered in severe or antibiotic unresponsive cases, especially when bronchial obstruction by a tumor is suspected.

Notes:

- *WBC count*
  - Although a WBC count >10,400 per mm^3 and a CRP level of ≥5.0 mg per dl are modestly helpful when positive, normal values do not rule out pneumonia.[1]
  - Very high (>20,000 per mm^3) or low (<4,000 per mm^3) indicates severe pneumonia.[2]
  - A Neutrophilic leukocytosis of >15,000 per mm^3 is more suggestive of bacterial etiology[2] where as leucopenia and lymphocytosis favor a viral cause.
- *Serum or plasma procalcitonin* measurement can help physician to differentiate viral from bacterial pneumonia.[1]
- *Tests for tuberculosis* should be considered in CAP with unknown etiology when the disease is severe or unresponsive to empiric antibiotics (particularly in TB endemic areas).
- In severe CAP, if the etiologic agent is unknown, full diagnostic evaluation should be considered.

More information on some tests:

Chest Radiograph

For clinical purposes, chest radiographic features of pneumonia can be grouped as follows:

1. <u>Lobar pneumonia pattern</u>
   - Lobar or segmental consolidation commonly involving one lobe; more than one lobe involvement is an indication of severe disease;
   - Most commonly caused by streptococcus pneumoniae;

2. <u>Bronchopneumonia pattern</u>
   - Patchy consolidations and or interstitial infiltrate; usually multiple and bilateral more commonly involving lower zone;
   - Confluent patches may appear as lobar consolidation, and extensive interstitial infiltrate may give rise to a ground glass appearance;
   - More common in pneumonia caused by 'atypical' pathogens.

3. <u>Features of complication</u>
   - Pleural effusion, cavitation, atelectasis etc.
   - Usually develop in bacterial pneumonia;

Some facts about radiographic findings of CAP:

- Radiological abnormalities can never establish etiologic diagnosis in pneumonia,[22] even some noninfectious conditions which may mimic pneumonia (eg, pulmonary infarction, contusion etc.) cannot be differentiated reliably from pneumonia on the basis of radiographic findings alone.
- Previously, it was considered that Streptococcus pneumoniae produce only lobar pneumonia pattern, but actually bronchopneumonia pattern is also common in pneumonia with this organism. In fact, almost any bacteria causing CAP ('typical' or 'atypical') can produce either lobar pneumonia or bronchopneumonia patterns. Despite this limitation, <u>radiographic findings may be helpful for etiologic diagnosis of pneumonia in some cases:</u>
  - Lobar consolidation, cavitation, or pleural effusions is usually caused by a bacterial pathogen.[1]

- Cavitary lesion in the upper lobe is generally suggestive of tuberculosis.
- Pneumatoceles are generally suggestive of Staph aureus infection.
- Viruses usually give rise to bronchopneumonia pattern.
- The typical findings of Pneumocystis jiroveci Pneumonia (PJP) include bilateral diffuse symmetrical interstitial infiltrates, most marked in the perihilar regions.[23]

Evolution of CXR changes

- In lobar pneumonia, a homogenous opacity of the affected lobe or segment generally appears within 12-18 hours of the onset of symptoms.[2] However, it may be delayed, especially in immunocompromised individuals including patients with diabetes or uremia.
- For hospitalized with suspected CAP, who have negative chest radiograph at presentation, it may be justified to treat their condition presumptively with antibiotics and the x-ray should be repeated in 24–48 hours.[4]
- It may take six weeks or longer to clear the pulmonary opacities on CXR in CAP.[3] The clearance may be delayed further if host defenses are weak and in bacteremic pneumonia.

Gram-stain and culture of sputum

Sputum for Gram-stain and culture (preferably pre-antibiotic) should be performed in all hospitalized patients.[12]

What are the purposes of Gram-stain of sputum?

- One important purpose of Gram-stain of sputum is to ensure that the sample is suitable for culture. A sputum specimen is suitable for culture if leukocytes are >25 and squamous epithelial cells are <10 per low power field.[24,25] In about 40% cases, patients cannot produce evaluable sputum.[4]
- Gram-stain is also helpful to identify certain pathogens:
  (1) Streptococcus pneumoniae- Gram-positive diplococci;
  (2) Staphylococcus aureus- Gram-positive cocci in clusters;
  (3) Gram-negative bacteria including Haemophilus influenzae and M. catarrhalis.

Sensitivity and specificity of Gram-stain and culture

- The sensitivity and specificity of Gram-stain and culture of sputum are very variable.
- Sputum culture grows *Streptococcus pneumoniae* in only 40%-- 50% cases of proven bacteremic pneumococcal pneumonia.[4] False positive results are also common. So many physicians now want to use sputum culture for more specific indications such as severe disease; unresponsive to empiric antibiotics; alcohol abuse; severe obstructive pulmonary disease; or positive pneumococcal or Legionella urine antigen test results.

*Sometimes, other specific stains and cultures of sputum, such as for Mycobacterium tuberculosis and fungus, are also considered.

Blood Culture

- Blood culture (preferably pre-antibiotic) is indicated in all moderate to severe CAP patients.[12] However, blood culture is positive in only 5%-14% of hospitalized CAP patients,[4] and false positive results are also common.[3]
- Most commonly, the culture grows pneumococcus which is covered by all empiric antibiotic regimens used in CAP and the empiric therapy is highly effective. As a result, the overall impact of blood culture on patient outcome is unclear.[4] In addition, false-positive

blood culture results may lead to inappropriate antibiotic use, particularly significantly higher vancomycin use.[4] For these reasons, some authorities are in favor of using blood culture for more specific indications such as severe CAP, alcohol abuse, leukopenia, asplenia, chronic liver disease, or positive pneumococcal urine antigen test result.[4]

- In pneumococcal pneumonia, positive blood culture indicates more severe disease with higher mortality.[12]

Antigen tests and tests for viruses

There are three widely available rapid antigen tests for CAP.

1. Urine test for Pneumococcal antigen:[4]

- Sensitivity 50% to 80%; specificity >90%;
- Although false positive results can occur, the test is generally reliable; in adults, false positive results can occur mainly in patients with an episode of CAP within the last 3 months.

2. Urine test for Legionella antigen:

- Sensitivity 70% -- 90%; specificity >99%;[4]
- The test may be positive one day after the onset of symptoms and remains positive for weeks;[4,26]
- Although several urinary antigen tests are available for Legionella, all detect only antigen of Legionella pneumophila serogroup 1; however, this serogroup accounts for 80-95% cases of community acquired Legionnaire's disease worldwide except in some parts of North America where other species and serogroups predominate.[4]

Indications for pneumococcal and Legionella urine antigen tests:

- Moderate to severe pneumonia[21] or CAP unresponsive to standard empiric antibiotics, particularly in severe disease or 'unresponsive to empiric antibiotics' category.
- Antigen test for Legionella should also be considered in other cases of CAP if Legionnaires disease is suspected.

IDSA/ATS (USA) guidelines recommend pneumococcal and Legionella urine antigen tests for more specific indications:[4]

- Indications for both pneumococcal and Legionella urine antigen tests:
  - Severe CAP
  - Outpatient therapy is ineffective
  - Alcohol abuse
  - Pleural effusion
- Additionally, pneumococcal antigen should be tested in leucopenia, asplenia and chronic severe liver disease; and Legionella antigen should be tested if there is history of a recent travel.

Notes:

- Both the urine antigen test results (Pneumococcus and Legionella) are available immediately and not affected by prior initiation of antibiotic therapy.[1,3,13]
- A negative urine antigen test result does not rule out infection with that particular pathogen.[1]

3. Rapid antigen detection tests for influenza virus A&B [Rapid influenza diagnostic tests (RIDTs)]

- Rapid influenza diagnostic tests (RIDTs) are immunoassays that can identify the antigens of influenza A and B virus in respiratory specimens.[27] RIDTs are screening tests.[27] There are several commercially available RIDTs.
- *Indication:* An RIDT is not routinely recommended in CAP; instead, it is performed in severe CAP or when viral pneumonia is suspected.
- *Generally used specimen*: Nasopharyngeal swab, throat swab, nasal wash or aspirate;
- *Time required*: <30 min
- *Sensitivity and specificity* are variable. False negative results are common and false positive results can occur. For seasonal influenza: generally sensitivity 50--70% (reported range: 10%--80%); specificity 90--95% when compared to viral culture or reverse transcriptase polymerase chain reaction (RT-PCR).
- Because of limited sensitivities and predictive values of RIDTs, **negative result of any RIDT does not rule out influenza virus infection when clinically suggestive**. Therefore, when RIDT is negative but influenza virus infection is suspected clinically, a confirmatory test (eg, RT-PCR) should be considered. At the same time, if clinically indicated, initiation of antiviral treatment should not be delayed pending test results. Also, already started antiviral treatment should not be withheld based on only negative RIDT result in a patient with suspected influenza virus infection.

Other tests for influenza virus A and B[27]

Test	*Required specimen*	*Time requirement*
Viral tissue cell culture (conventional)	Nasopharyngeal swab; throat swab; bronchial wash; nasal or endotracheal aspirate; or sputum	3-10 days
Rapid cell culture	As above	1-3 days
Immunofluorescence test: Direct (DFA) or Indirect (IFA) Florescent Antibody Staining [antigen detection]	Nasopharyngeal swab or wash; bronchial wash; nasal or endotracheal aspirate	1-4 hours
RT-PCR	Nasopharyngeal swab or wash; throat swab; bronchial wash; nasal or endotracheal aspirate; sputum	Variable; usually 1-6 hours

Notes:

- Confirmatory ("Gold standard") test for influenza virus infection: RT-PCR or viral culture
- Tests for avian influenza (H5N1): H5N1 is a subtype of influenza-A. Rapid antigen detection tests (not optimally sensitive and specific) and RT-PCR can be used for their diagnosis.[3]
- Diagnostic test for non-influenza viruses:
    - PCR on respiratory specimen;
    - This test can be performed in severe CAP when testing for non-influenza viruses is considered.

Polymerase Chain Reaction (PCR)

- PCR is available for Streptococcus pneumoniae, all respiratory viruses, atypical bacteria (Mycoplasma, Chlamydia and Legionella) and Mycobacterium tuberculosis.
- Respiratory specimens such as sputum, throat swab, or bronchoalveolar lavage fluid are used for the test.
- PCR is expensive and mainly used in severe CAP and research purposes.

Liver Function Tests in CAP

- Abnormal LFTs are common findings in CAP and have prognostic value.
- Low albumin or raised ALT is associated with significantly higher mortality or longer hospital stay. Other LFTs including alkaline phosphatase and gamma-glutamyl transferase (GGT) have less value in predicting prognosis.[28]

Pleural fluid studies

- Pleural fluid should be aspirated when present in more than trivial amount, preferably under ultrasound guidance.[2,3]
- The aspirated fluid should be studied for:
    - Biochemistry: Protein; glucose; lactate dehydrogenase; pH etc.
    - Blood cells and cytology: WBC count with differential; RBC; malignant cells etc.
    - Microbiologic studies: Gram-stain; Acid Fast Stain; cultures etc.

- Serum protein, glucose and LDH levels are also needed to interpret the pleural fluid study results.

Diagnostic tests for specific atypical bacteria

Pathogen	***Diagnostic tests*** (required specimen)	***Sensitivity and specificity***
Mycoplasma pneumoniae[12,13]	Serology (acute and convalescent phase serum samples; 10-14 days apart); PCR (Respiratory specimen: nasopharyngeal/ oropharyngeal/ lower respiratory secretions) *Combination of serology and PCR are most useful.	Sensitivity: 55-100% Specificity: 55-100% Sensitivity: 65-90% Specificity: 90-100%
Chlamydia pneumoniae	Serology (acute and convalescent phase serum samples; 10-14 days apart); microimmunofluorescence (MIF) test is the gold standard serologic test;[12,13] complement fixation test (CFT) only weekly positive; PCR (Respiratory specimen)	
Chlamydia psittaci	Serology (acute and convalescent phase serum samples; 10-14 days apart); MIF is the gold standard serologic test; complement fixation test (CFT) is also useful.[12,13]	
Coxiella burnetii (Q fever)	Serology: indirect immunofluorescence assay (IFA) is the serologic method of choice; a fourfold rise in antibody titer between acute and convalescent sera (10-14 days apart) is diagnostic.[3,12]	

	PCR (on blood- only in the first 2 weeks of onset of symptoms[3] ; or on tissue sample may be helpful)	
Legionella Spp. For most situations, combination urinary antigen test plus sputum culture is the best approach.[26]	Urinary antigen test: The test may be positive one day after onset of symptoms and continues to be positive for weeks;[4,26] Culture of lower respiratory specimen (usually sputum or bronchoscopy samples) on special media; in most cases, growth detectable in 3-5 days; sometimes takes up to two weeks)[26,29] Serology: (acute and convalescent phase serum samples taken 3 weeks after the onset of symptoms); [26] not useful for clinical decision making but useful for epidemiological purposes ; serology is not commonly used now.[29] Direct fluorescent antibody (DFA) staining of bacteria (in pleural fluid, sputum, bronchial washing, or other infected materials); rapid test, can be finished < 4 hours; but less sensitive than culture and technically difficult; rarely used these days;[29]	Sensitivity: 70 - 90% Specificity >99%; Sensitivity highly variable: <10 - 80%; Specificity: 100% For serology: Sensitivity: 60 - 80% Specificity: >95% DFA: Sensitivity: 25--70% Specificity: >95%.

Notes:

- As Mycoplasma pneumoniae and Chlamydia pneumoniae usually cause milder disease where empiric treatment is very effective, laboratory confirmation is often not considered in CAP is likely due to these organisms.
- Acute- and convalescent-phase serologic testing that has been used traditionally for the laboratory diagnosis of most atypical causes of CAP allows virtually a retrospective diagnosis which often does not have any direct impact on the patient management.

Severity assessment:

There are several scoring systems for assessing severity of CAP of which CURB 65 and PSI (Pneumonia Severity Index) are probably most widely used. CURB-65 has five variables whereas PSI has twenty variables. Therefore, PSI is less practical to use in busy emergency room setting.

CURB-65 (Information from references1,4,11)
(One point for each feature below)

Confusion
Urea >7 mmol/L
Respiration rate≥30/min
Blood pressure (Systolic<90 mm of Hg or Diastolic ≤60 mm of Hg)
Age ≥65 years

Score 0 or 1 (mortality <3%): usually suitable for outpatient treatment. However, the decision should be individualized considering patient's comorbidity and home support system.

Score 2 (mortality: about 9%): should be admitted to hospital ward.
Score 3 or more (mortality: 15-40%): should be managed in hospital as severe pneumonia and often needs intensive care.

Treatment of CAP

General measures:

- *Maintain adequate hydration*; if necessary give IV fluid.
- *Oxygen:*
    - Give Oxygen to all patients with tachypnea, hypoxemia, hypotension or acidosis.
    - Maintain SO2 between 94% and 98% if there is no risk of CO2 retention. Humidified oxygen at high concentration is preferable unless the patient has hypercapnia due to COPD.
    - Maintain SO2 between 88% and 92% if the patient has COPD.[12]
    - Consider assisted ventilation early if hypoxemia persists despite adequate oxygen therapy.
- *Analgesic for pleuritic chest pain:* usually paracetamol (acetaminophen), cocodamol (paracetamol plus codeine) or NSAIDs are sufficient.
- *Physiotherapy* to assist expectoration if there is copious sputum production;

Empiric antibiotic therapy

Empiric antibiotic therapy for CAP somewhat varies among different parts of the world. You should follow your local guidelines. Empiric antibiotic(s) must cover pneumococcus. North American guidelines also advocate 'atypical bacteria' coverage in their empiric antibiotic treatment in all cases. In contrast, some European countries (eg, United Kingdom and Sweden) do not recommend 'atypical coverage' so widely.[1,30]

How 'atypical bacteria' coverage can be given?
Generally the following drugs are effective against atypical bacteria:

1. Macrolides: Clarithromycin, Azithromycin
2. Respiratory fluoroquinolones: Moxifloxacin, Gemifloxacin, Levofloxacin
3. Doxycycline

All the above mentioned drugs also cover pneumococcus.

Empiric antibiotic regimens for CAP: (Information from references 1,4,11,21,31,32)

1. For outpatient treatment: (Mild CAP; CURB 65 score= 0-1)

a) *Otherwise healthy person and no antibiotic taken in the last three months*[4]

i. A macrolide: Clarithromycin (500 mg PO bid) or azithromycin; **Or**
ii. Doxycycline 100 mg PO bid

b) *Patients with comorbidities* or antibiotic taken in the last three months* (select an alternative agent from a different class):[4]

i. Two-drug combination: *An oral β-lactam antibiotic* (amoxycillin 1g tid, co-amoxyclav 2g bid, or cefuroxime 500 mg bid) **Plus** *a macrolide* (clarithromycin 500 mg bid PO or azithromycin); **Or**

ii. Monotherapy with a respiratory fluoroquinolone (Moxifloxacin 400 mg od PO, Gemifloxacin 320 mg od PO, or Levofloxacin 750 mg od PO)

*Comorbidities include: chronic heart, lung, liver or kidney disease; diabetes mellitus; alcoholism; and malignancies.[4]

In areas with high (>25%) or unknown pneumococcal macrolide resistance rate, only the above regimen 1(b) should be used in all outpatients (irrespective of comorbidities and recent antibiotic exposure).

In developing countries, where pneumococcal macrolide resistance rate is not known, the above regimen 1(b) may be the only out-patient based treatment option for CAP.

In some European countries (eg, UK), generally amoxycillin (500 mg PO tid) is considered the first line agent for both outpatient and inpatient treatment in all patients with mild CAP (CURB 65 score 0—1), while clarithromycin (500 mg bid) or doxycycline (200 mg once then 100mg daily from the next day) is considered as an alternative to amoxycillin for penicillin allergic patients.[11]

Notes

- Comorbidities or recent antibiotic exposure increase the likelihood of infection with drug resistant *Streptococcus pneumoniae* and enteric gram-negative bacteria, so the above regimen 1(b) is justified in such cases.
- Therapy with an antibiotic within the last three months increases the likelihood of resistance to that drug. Therefore, an alternative agent from a different class should be selected in such cases when the pneumonia is mild. However, these patients with recent antibiotic exposure are also at increased risk of Pseudomonas infection. Therefore, when they present with severe pneumonia, adequate Pseudomonas coverage (described in the treatment of severe pneumonia) should be considered.
- Because of increased risk of hepatic adverse effects with moxifloxacin use, the European Medicines Agency recommends that moxifloxacin should only be given in CAP when other antibiotics cannot be used.[11]
- Macrolides have immunomodulatory effects which may help to eradicate the infections; additionally, they have anti-inflammatory effect.

2. For hospitalized non-ICU patients (Moderate CAP; CURB 65 score= 2)

Any of the following two regimens (a or b):

a) ***Combination of a β-lactam antibiotic Plus a macrolide*:** Preferred combination may be:

i. *Ceftriaxone (1-2 gm) IV daily Plus a macrolide* (clarithromycin/azithromycin PO as mentioned above for outpatients); Macrolides can also be given IV (IV Clarithromycin 500mg bid or IV Azithromycin 1 gm first dose then 500 mg od from the next day). **Or**

ii. *Amoxycillin (500mg—1g tid PO or IV) Plus clarithromycin* (500mg bid PO or IV) (**Preferred regimen in the UK;** oral route is preferable when possible)[11]

Or

b) ***Monotherapy with a respiratory fluoroquinolone*** (Levofloxacin 750 mg od PO/ IV, Gemifloxacin 320 mg od PO, or Moxifloxacin 400 mg od PO/ IV). This regimen is suitable for penicillin allergic patients.

In mild penicillin allergy, when limited to skin rash, usually a cephalosporin can be given.

3. For hospitalized ICU patients (Severe CAP; CURB 65 score ≥3):

(All antibiotics should be administered intravenously)[11]

A β-lactam IV [eg, Ceftriaxone 2 gm od (or bid) or Co-amoxyclav 1.2g IV tid]
Plus
A macrolide IV (Azithromycin/ Clarithromycin) **or *a respiratory fluoroquinolone*** IV

For patients with β-lactam allergy: Aztreonam (1-2g, 6-12 hourly) **Plus** a respiratory fluoroquinolone

Preferred regimen in the USA:[4] A potent antipneumococcal cephalosporin such as ceftriaxone **plus** either azithromycin **or** a respiratory fluoroquinolone;

Preferred regimen in the UK for these ICU patients:[11]
Co-amoxyclav 1.2g tid IV Plus clarithromycin 500 mg bid IV;*
**Consider adding levofloxacin with this regimen, if Legionella is strongly suspected; however, the combination of macrolide and fluoroquinolone increases the risk of QT prolongation.*

Some physicians prefer broader antibiotic coverage for this category of severe CAP patients with the following regimen:[31]
Piperacillin-tazobactam 4.5 g tid + clarithromycin 500mg bid intravenously;

****IDSA recommends all severe CAP patients requiring intensive care should receive empiric MRSA coverage, so addition of MRSA coverage to the above empiric regimens should be considered.***[32]

In severe CAP, IDSA/ ATS guidelines recommend antibiotic regimens with additional coverage in some special situations, such as:[4,32]

(i) When pseudomonas infection is a concern:
A β-lactam with both antipneumococcal and antipseudomonal activity [eg, ***Piperacillin-tazobactum*** (Piptazo) / imipenem/ meropenem], **Plus *levofloxacin*** (750mg od).

Another regimen may be:
Piperacillin-tazobactum (Piptazo) **Plus an *aminoglycoside*** (eg, amikacin 15 mg/kg daily) **Plus *azithromycin*.**
[i.e. Piptazo + Amikacin +Azithromycin]

*The principle behind the above regimens: The regimen should include two drugs effective against pseudomonas with at least one of them covering pneumococcus as well; the regimen should also include one drug covering atypical bacteria. Piperacillin-tazobactam covers both Pseudomonas and Pneumococcus. Levofloxacin covers pneumococcus, atypical bacteria as well as Pseudomonas. Aminoglycosides cover Pseudomonas.

Indications for Pseudomonas coverage in severe CAP include:[4]
(1) A consistent Gram-stain result (numerous and predominant gram-negative bacilli) of adequate sputum or other respiratory specimen (the best indication)
(2) Structural lung disease such as bronchiectasis or COPD, particularly severe COPD requiring frequent steroid and or antibiotic therapy.
(3) Alcoholism
(4) Antibiotic therapy within the last three months

These patients do not always need ICU admission for their CAP, so *Pseudomonas* infection remains a concern for them even when they are admitted on a general ward.[4]

(ii) When CA-MRSA is a concern:[4,32]
Add Vancomycin (1 gm IV 12 hourly) or Linezolid (600mg IV 12 hourly) to the antibiotic regimen.

When to consider CA-MRSA coverage in CAP
CA-MRSA induced CAP is rare in most communities. Probably there is no consensus about when to add CA-MRSA coverage in empiric treatment of CAP. However, such coverage may be justified in severe CAP possibly caused by Staph aureus until culture and sensitivity results are known. Therefore, in severe CAP, empiric CA-MRSA coverage can be considered in any of the following conditions:[4,32]

- If Gram-stain of an adequate sputum sample or another respiratory sample is suggestive of *Staph aureus* (best indication);
- If any clinical risk factor for *S. aureus* CAP is present; clinical risk factors for *S. aureus* CAP include recent influenza, end-stage renal disease, injection drug use and recent antibiotic therapy (particularly fluoroquinolones).
- CAP patients requiring intensive care[32]
- All CAP patients with necrotizing pneumonia or cavitary lesion[32]
- All CAP patients with empyema[32]

According to IDSA, hospitalized CAP patients with any one of the following: (1) requirement intensive care, (2) necrotizing or cavitary lesion, or (3) empyema should be considered as having severe community acquired pneumonia where empiric MRSA coverage should be provided.[32]

* During periods of high influenza activity in the community, some physicians consider empiric CA-MRSA coverage for all severe CAP patients, irrespective of risk factors for CA-MRSA CAP.

When can empiric antibiotic coverage for Pseudomonas aeruginosa or MRSA be withheld or discontinued?

- For Pseudomonas: Negative Gram-stain and culture results for gram-negative bacilli of a good-quality respiratory specimen are usually adequate to withhold or stop empiric antibiotic coverage for Pseudomonas.[4]

- For MRSA: Negative Gram-stain and culture results for S. aureus of a good-quality respiratory specimen are generally sufficient to withhold or discontinue empiric antibiotic coverage for MRSA.[4]

*All specimens should be preantibiotic; Gram-stain and culture results of a specimen collected after starting antibiotic are difficult to interpret.[4]

Notes:

- If gram-stain of a respiratory specimen (sputum, endotracheal aspirates etc) shows Staph aureus or Gram-negative organisms, adequate empiric antibiotic coverage for these organisms should be considered.[4]
- Usually empiric coverage for Pseudomonas also covers other enteric Gram-negative bacilli.[4]

Antiviral therapy:[33]

- According to CDC, antiviral treatment (oseltamivir or zanamivir) should be given as soon as possible to all hospitalized patients with suspected or confirmed influenza, irrespective of their previous health or immunization status.
- Although early initiation of treatment (within 48 hours of onset of symptoms) has greater benefit, treatment initiated within 5 days after the onset is also associated with reduced morbidity and mortality in severe illness.
- In severely ill patients, empiric antiviral treatment should not be delayed while awaiting confirmatory test results.
- Patients with suspected influenza should complete a full course of antiviral treatment, even when the initial test results are negative unless an alternative diagnosis is established and clinical judgment rules out influenza.

Use of steroid in CAP

- Because of their immunomodulatory properties, glucocorticoids have been used as an adjunctive therapy in serious infections.
- There is growing evidence that in pneumonia an excessive inflammatory response may have deleterious effects and may contribute to the lung injury. But trial results of corticosteroid therapy to prevent it are controversial, particularly in noncritical care setting.
- Some studies have demonstrated steroid has marginal benefit and can reduce hospital stay marginally, but others didn't find significant advantages with its use. However, corticosteroid therapy may have value in CAP patients with persistent shock despite adequate volume replacement and vasopressor support. Testing for confirmation of cortisol deficiency, such as random cortisol level and the ACTH stimulation test, may be misleading in these patients.[34] ***For details please see Chapter 10, 'septic shock'***.

*Another immunomodulatory agent, activated drotrecogin alfa (a recombinant human activated protein C) can be considered within 24 hours of admission in some cases of CAP with persistent shock despite adequate fluid resuscitation.[4] Protein C is a natural anticoagulant and may have significant anti-inflammatory effects when activated.

Antibiotic changing on obtaining microbial test results

- Switching the antibiotic from empiric to specific ones after obtaining the culture and sensitivity result is not always straightforward.

- A Significant proportion of CAP patients have 'atypical' co- infection with 'typical' bacterial infection. These atypical pathogens do not grow in the ordinary culture media. Moreover, bacteremic pneumococcal pneumonia (a subgroup of CAP with high mortality rate) when treated with combined therapy (particularly β-lactam + macrolide) is associated with significantly lower mortality compared to monotherapy; the reason is unclear, but antibiotic resistance is not the cause.[35]
- During antibiotic changing, the probability of a particular pathogen considering clinical presentation and various risk factors, and response to the already started empiric antibiotics should be taken into account; the decision should be individualized. Consultation with an infectious disease specialist or a pulmonologist may be needed in some cases.

Route of antibiotic administration

- Traditionally almost all hospitalized patients are initially treated with intravenous antibiotics and are switched to oral drugs when they are showing overall improvement. However, no studies have established superiority of intravenous route over oral therapy in hospitalized CAP patients when they can tolerate oral therapy and the drug is well absorbed.[3]
- Some drugs, particularly the fluoroquinolones, are usually very well absorbed and can be given orally from the beginning.[4.11] However, parenteral therapy should always be considered:[2,11]
  - In severe CAP or
  - If there is any contraindication to oral therapy such as depressed level of consciousness, dysphagia, vomiting, or gastrointestinal absorption problem.

When can initial parenteral therapy be switched to oral form?

Generally, parenteral therapy can be switched to oral form when the following conditions are met:[11]

- Afebrile for >24 hours
- All vital signs such as pulse, blood pressure and respiration rate are normal and stable;
- The patient is fully conscious and no other contraindications to oral therapy;
- The infection is non-bacteremic and no microbiological evidence of Legionella, Staphylococcal or enteric Gram-negative bacilli infection;

Suitable agents for oral switching:

- If the same agent used for intravenous therapy is available in oral form, it is generally used.[4,11]
- When the same agent is not available in oral form, one from the same class can be selected,[4] but not always; for example, for switching from a parenteral cephalosporin, oral co-amoxiclav (625 mg tid) is usually considered better than an oral cephalosporin.[11]
- Sometimes, oral monotherapy can be used replacing combined intravenous therapy; for example:
  - From intravenous benzylpenicillin + levofloxacin to oral levofloxacin with or without oral amoxicillin (500 mg–1.0 g tid) can be considered.[11]
  - From intravenous β-lactam+macrolide to an oral macrolide alone may be safe for those who do not have drug resistant pneumococcal or gram-negative enteric bacterial infection (culture and sensitivity proven).[4]

Response to antibiotic therapy

- In hospitalized CAP patients with appropriate antibiotic therapy, some improvement in the clinical course is usually evident within 2-3 days.[11] In general, most patients become stable clinically within 3–7 days.[4]
- In uncomplicated CAP, fever often resolves after 2-4 days, but physical signs may persist longer.[13] In pneumococcal pneumonia, generally cough resolves within 8 days and crackles clear within 3 weeks. However, resolution of the clinical and the chest radiographic features is considerably slower in the elderly and in patients with comorbidity.[8]
- Antibiotics are usually not changed within the first 72 hours unless there is deterioration, or new culture data or epidemiologic clues make it justified.[4]
- Young patients with uncomplicated CAP usually recover fully in two weeks. Older patients and those with comorbidities can take several weeks or longer to recover completely.[13]

Failure to improve with antibiotic therapy

Failure to improve with initial management is not uncommon (6–24%).[11] Nonresponding patients have several-fold increased mortality compared to responding patients.[4]

Causes of failure to improve: (Information from references 4,8,11)

1. Incorrect diagnosis (Pulmonary embolism; lung carcinoma; aspiration; ARDS*; heart failure; pulmonary eosinophilia; pulmonary involvement in connective tissue diseases; cryptogenic organizing pneumonia etc may appear as pneumonia)
2. Inappropriate antibiotic therapy (inappropriate drug or dose, or both; resistant organism; multiple organisms, not covered by the empiric antibiotics)
3. Unsuspected organism (CA-MRSA; Mycobacteria; fungus; virus; Pneumocystis jirovecii etc)
4. Complications of CAP (pleural effusion/ empyema; lung abscess; ARDS*; drug fever etc)
5. Underlying bronchial obstruction
6. Nosocomial superinfection (Nosocomial pneumonia; extrapulmonary infection including IV cannula site infection)
7. Exacerbation of comorbid illness
8. Overwhelming infection
9. Improvement expected too early (eg, elderly patients or patients with comorbidity)

[*ARDS=Acute respiratory distress syndrome]

What can be done for nonresponding CAP patients?

Consider the followings:

1. *Further careful diagnostic evaluation*
   - History and physical examination should be repeated.
   - Some of the tests including initial microbiological tests may need to be repeated. Other tests to identify specific pathogens such as urine antigen tests for Pneumococcus and Legionella; tests for viruses and tuberculosis (in TB endemic areas) should be considered if not already done.
   - Some patients may need to undergo chest CT, bronchoscopy etc.
2. *Review antibiotic therapy*
   - For an oral regimen, patient's compliance with and adequate absorption of the drug(s) should be evaluated first.[11]

- Initial empiric antibiotic coverage may need to be broadened until the results of diagnostic tests are available if any risk factor for or evidence of a potentially uncovered pathogen is found during reevaluation.[4]
- British Thoracic Society guidelines recommend the addition of a macrolide in hospitalized patients with mild or moderate pneumonia who are on amoxicillin alone.[11]
- British Thoracic Society guidelines also recommend the addition of levofloxacin in patients with severe pneumonia who are already on empiric β-lactam plus clarithromycin regimen. A pulmonologist should also be consulted urgently.[11]

Duration of antibiotic treatment

- The optimal duration of antibiotic therapy in CAP is still unclear.
- Although traditionally patients have been treated for 10-14 days, recent studies showed that shorter courses may be adequate for many cases of uncomplicated CAP.[1]
- The duration should be based on clinical judgment considering disease severity, causative agent, speed of recovery etc.[11]
- <u>The minimum duration should be 5 days</u> and the patient should be afebrile for 48-72 hours before stopping the antibiotic(s).[4]
- <u>For most cases of uncomplicated CAP, 7-10 days</u> <u>of antibiotic therapy</u> is adequate.[2]
- A course of 14 to 21 days is usually considered when pneumonia due to more virulent organisms, such as Legionella, S aureus, or Gram-negative enteric bacilli, is suspected or confirmed.[11,21]
- A longer course, decided mainly on clinical judgment, is also considered in some other conditions such as pneumonia with metastatic infection (eg, meningitis or endocarditis) or complications (eg, empyema or lung abscess).[4]

Complications of CAP

- Parapneumonic effusion
- Empyema
- Lung abscess
- Respiratory failure
- Septic shock
- Multiorgan failure (eg, ARDS, renal failure, adrenal insufficiency)
- Coagulopathy (DVT, pulmonary embolism, DIC etc.)
- Collapse due to retained sputum
- Metastatic infection (eg, brain abscess, endocarditis)
- Exacerbation of comorbid illness

Parapneumonic effusion and empyema:

- Pleural effusion develops in 36-57% hospitalized patients with bacterial pneumonia.[11]
- Pleural fluid should always be aspirated for both diagnostic and therapeutic purposes when present in more than trivial amounts, preferably under ultrasound guidance.[2]
- <u>Pleural space drainage</u> is needed in:[11]
    - Empyema (cloudy fluid, pus, or organisms on Gram stain or culture)
    - Clear pleural fluid but pH <7.2

Follow-up

- Recommendations for follow-up vary among different authorities.
- In uncomplicated CAP, a clinical follow up can be performed about six weeks after discharge from the hospital.
- A follow-up chest radiograph should be considered if:
    - Symptoms or signs persist at the time of follow up evaluation;
    - Age > 50 years or smoker;
    - Any suspicion of underlying bronchial malignancy;

Prevention

- Smoking increases the risk of recurrent pneumonia, so smoking should be stopped.
- Patients should receive pneumococcus and influenza vaccines before leaving the hospital when indicated. These vaccines can be given simultaneously even immediately after an episode of pneumonia.[3]
- Common indications for pneumococcal vaccinations are: Age ≥65 years; patients with cardio-pulmonary disorders or any other conditions that increase the risk of pneumococcal pneumonia.

Summary of the empiric antibiotic therapy for CAP

1. For outpatient treatment: (Mild CAP; CURB 65 score= 0-1)

a) *Otherwise healthy person and no antibiotic taken in the last three months*

i. A macrolide: Clarithromycin (500 mg PO bid) or azithromycin; **Or**

ii. Doxycycline 100 mg PO bid;

b) *Patients with comorbidities or antibiotic taken in the last three months*

i. Two-drug combination: *An oral β-lactam antibiotic* (amoxycillin 1g tid, co-amoxyclav 2g bid, or cefuroxime 500 mg bid) **Plus** *a macrolide* (clarithromycin 500 mg bid PO or azithromycin); **Or**

ii. Monotherapy with a respiratory fluoroquinolone (Levofloxacin 750 mg od PO, Gemifloxacin 320 mg od PO, or Moxifloxacin 400 mg od PO)

In some European countries (eg. UK), generally *amoxycillin (500 mg PO tid)* is considered as the first line agent for both outpatient and inpatient treatment of all patients with mild CAP (CURB 65 score 0—1), while *clarithromycin (500 mg bid) or doxycycline (200 mg once then 100mg daily from the next day)* is considered as an alternative to amoxycillin for penicillin allergic patients.

2. For hospitalized non-ICU patients (Moderate CAP; CURB 65 score= 2)

a) Combination of a β-lactam antibiotic Plus a macrolide

i. *Ceftriaxone (1-2 gm) IV daily* Plus a macrolide *(clarithromycin/azithromycin PO or IV)* **Or**

ii. *Amoxycillin (500mg—1g tid PO or IV)* Plus *clarithromycin (500mg bid PO or IV)* (**Preferred regimen in the UK**; oral route is preferable when possible)

b) *Monotherapy with a respiratory fluoroquinolone* *(Levofloxacin 750 mg od PO/ IV, Gemifloxacin 320 mg od PO, or Moxifloxacin 400 mg od PO/IV)*

3. For hospitalized ICU patients (Severe CAP; CURB 65 score ≥3)
(All antibiotics should be administered intravenously)
A β-lactam [eg, Ceftriaxone 2 gm od (or bid) or Co-amoxyclav 1.2g tid]
Plus
A macrolide (Azithromycin/ Clarithromycin) **or *a respiratory fluoroquinolone***

Preferred regimen in the UK for hospitalized ICU patients:
Co-amoxyclav 1.2g tid IV Plus *clarithromycin 500 mg bid IV*;
Consider adding levofloxacin with this regimen, if Legionella is strongly suspected; however, the combination of macrolide and fluoroquinolone increases the risk of QT prolongation.

Some physicians prefer broader antibiotic coverage for this category of CAP patients (in ICU) with:
Piperacillin-tazobactam (4.5 g tid) + clarithromycin (500mg bid IV)

*IDSA recommends all severe CAP patients requiring intensive care should receive empiric MRSA coverage, so addition of MRSA coverage to the above empiric regimens should be considered.

*Some patients may need additional coverage for Pseudomonas, MRSA, or viral pneumonia. *For details please see the text.*

References

1. Richard R. Watkins et al. Diagnosis and Management of Community Acquired Pneumonia in Adults. **Am Fam Physician. 2011**; 83(11):1299-1306

2. Relevant chapters of **Davidson's Principles and Practice of Medicine**, 21 edition, Nicki R. Colledge et al (editors). India, Elsevier, 2010.

3. Relevant chapters of **Current Medical Diagnosis and Treatment**; Maxine A. Papadakis et al (Editors). New York, McGraw-Hill, 2013

4. Lionel A. Mandell et al. **Infectious Diseases Society of America/American Thoracic Society** Consensus Guidelines on the Management of Community-Acquired Pneumonia in Adults. Supplement Article. **Clinical Infectious Diseases 2007**; 44:S27–72

5. W S Lim et al. Study of community acquired pneumonia aetiology (SCAPA) in adults admitted to hospital: implications for management guidelines. **Thorax 2001**;56:296–301

6. Niclas Johansson et al. Etiology of Community-Acquired Pneumonia: Increased Microbiological Yield with New Diagnostic Methods. **Clinical Infectious Diseases 2010;** 50:202–9

7. Catia Cillóniz et al. Community-acquired polymicrobial pneumonia in the intensive care unit: aetiology and prognosis. **Critical Care 2011**, 15:R209

8. Management of community-acquired pneumonia in adults by Working Group of the **South African Thoracic Society**. **South Afr J Epidemiol Infect 2008**;23(2):31-34, 36-38, 40-42

9. 'MRSA infection: Causes' on the website of **Mayo Clinic (USA)**. At: http://www.mayoclinic.org/diseases-conditions/mrsa/basics/causes/con-20024479

10. 'General Information about MRSA in the Community' on the website of CDC (USA). At: http://www.cdc.gov/mrsa/community/index.html

11. W S Lim et al. **British Thoracic Society guidelines** for the management of community acquired pneumonia in adults: update 2009. **Thorax 2009**; 64(Suppl III):iii1–iii55

12. Relevant chapters of **Kumar &Clark's Clinical Medicine**, 8th edition; Parveen Kumar and Michael Clark (Editors). Edinburgh, Elsevier, 2012

13. Relevant chapters of **Harrison's Principles of Internal Medicine**; 18 th edition; Dan L Longo et al (Editors). New York, McGraw-Hill 2012.

14. Fox RA. Atypical presentation of geriatric infections. **Geriatrics 1988**; May;43(5):58-9, 63-4, 68

15. B. A. Cunha. The atypical pneumonias: clinical diagnosis and importance. **Clin Microbiol Infect 2006;** 12 (Suppl. 3): 12–24

16. Relevant topics in **Emedicine;** at: http://emedicine.medscape.com

17. 'Pneumonia' on **CDC (USA) website**; at: http://www.cdc.gov/pneumonia/

18. Relevant topics in 'Antimicrobe'. At: antimicrobe.org

19. Kristopher P. Thibodeau et al. Atypical Pathogens and Challenges in Community-Acquired Pneumonia. **Am Fam Physician 2004**;69:1699-706.

20. Ann R. Falsey et al. Viral Pneumonia in Older Adults. **Clinical Infectious Diseases 2006;** 42:518–24

21. 'Guideline for the management of community acquired pneumonia in adults (2014)' in clinical guidelines (Clinical support: pathology-microbiology) on the website of **Nottingham University Hospital (NHS trust, UK)**. AT: https://www.nuh.nhs.uk/healthcare-professionals/clinical-guidelines

22. T. Franquet. Imaging of pneumonia: trends and algorithms. **Eur Respir J 2001**; 18: 196–208.

23. Xiangpeng Zheng et al. Imaging pulmonary infectious diseases in immunocompromised patients. Radiology of Infectious Diseases 2014; 1(1): 37—41

24. Beatriz Roson et al. Prospective Study of the Usefulness of Sputum Gram Stain in the Initial Approach to Community-Acquired Pneumonia Requiring Hospitalization. **Clinical Infectious Diseases 2000;**31:869–74

25. Joon Young Song et al. Diagnosis of Pneumococcal Pneumonia: Current Pitfalls and the Way Forward. **Infect Chemother 2013**;45(4):351-366

26. David R. Murdoch. Diagnosis of *Legionella* Infection. **Clinical Infectious Diseases 2003**; 36:64–9

27. Rapid Diagnostic Testing for Influenza: Information for Clinical Laboratory Directors on the website of **CDC (USA).** At: http://www.cdc.gov/flu/professionals/diagnosis/rapidlab.htm

28. Jinks MF et al. The pattern and significance of abnormal liver function tests in community-acquired pneumonia. Eur J Intern Med. **2004**. Nov;15(7):436-440.

29. Jeffrey W. Mercante et al. Current and Emerging Legionella Diagnostics for Laboratory and Outbreak Investigations. ***Clin. Microbiol. Rev.*** **2015;** 28 (1): 95-133

30. Daniel M. Musher et al. Community-Acquired Pneumonia. **N Engl J Med 2014;**371:1619-28.

31. Clinical guideline for hospital management of community acquired pneumonia' on the website of **Royal Cornwall Hospitals (NHS trust, UK);** at: www.rcht.nhs.uk/GET/d10159534

32. Catherine Liu et al. Clinical Practice Guidelines by the Infectious Diseases Society of America for the Treatment of Methicillin-Resistant Staphylococcus Aureus Infections in Adults and Children. **Clinical Infectious Diseases 2011**;1–38

33. 'Seasonal Influenza (Flu): Use of antivirals' on the website of **CDC (USA)**: At: http://www.cdc.gov/flu/professionals/antivirals/antiviral-use-influenza.htm

34. R. Phillip Dellinger et al. Surviving Sepsis Campaign: International Guidelines for Management of Severe Sepsis and Septic Shock: 2012. Crit Care Med. **2013**. 41(2): 580-637

35. Weiss K et al. Clinical characteristics at initial presentation and impact of dual therapy on the outcome of bacteremic Streptococcus pneumoniae pneumonia in adults. **Can Respir J. 2004**;11(8):589-93.

Chapter 4

Nosocomial pneumonia

Nosocomial pneumonia

Nosocomial pneumonia includes two entities -- Hospital-acquired Pneumonia (HAP) and Ventilator-associated pneumonia (VAP). Previously Healthcare -Associated Pneumonia (HCAP) was also included in nosocomial pneumonia, but it has not been included in the recent (2016) IDSA/ATS guidelines.[1] Healthcare-associated Pneumonia (HCAP) has been described at the end of this chapter.

1. <u>Hospital-acquired pneumonia (HAP)</u>
   HAP is defined as a newly developed pneumonia occurring at least 48 hours after hospital admission. HAP is the second most common hospital acquired infection (after urinary tract infection).[2]

2. <u>Ventilator-associated pneumonia (VAP)</u>
   VAP is defined as a newly developed pneumonia occurring at least 48 hours after endotracheal intubation.

Microbiology of HAP and VAP (Information from references 1-10)

- The causative pathogens of hospital-acquired pneumonia (HAP) differ from those of community-acquired pneumonia (CAP).
- Limited data are available about the microbiology of non-intubated HAP, since lower respiratory tract sample adequate for culture is difficult to obtain.
- Although a wide range of organisms are associated with HAP and VAP, ***the causative organisms of HAP and VAP are mostly similar and as follows:***[2,5,6]
  - *<u>Gram-negative bacilli (35 – 80%):</u>* Pseudomonas aeruginosa (17—30%), Klebsiella pneumoniae, E coli, Enterobacter species, Proteus species, Acinetobacter species (2—10%) etc.
  - *<u>Gram-positive cocci</u>:* Staphylococcus aureus (20--30%, of which >50% MRSA), Streptococcus pneumoniae (0—10%) etc.
  - *<u>Anaerobes (0–54%)</u>:* Bacteroides, anaerobic streptococci, fusobacterium etc.
- *<u>Most commonly isolated organisms from respiratory specimens:</u>* P. aeruginosa, S. aureus and Enterobacteriaceae (particularly Klebsiella, E. coli and Enterobacter spp.)[6]
- The infection is polymicrobial in 9–80% cases.[5]
- Anaerobic infection in nosocomial pneumonia is usually a part of polymicrobial pneumonia.
- Viruses, Chlamydia, Mycobacteria, fungi etc. are uncommon causes of nosocomial pneumonias.
- S. aureus pneumonia is more common in patients with diabetes mellitus, head injury and those admitted in ICUs.[7]

Pseudomonas

- Pseudomonas is a ubiquitous Gram-negative bacillus, commonly found in water, soil, plants, and animals; it is also commonly isolated from hospital environment and healthcare personnel.

- *P. aeruginosa* is the most common species of Pseudomonas causing infections in humans.
- It is a relatively low virulence opportunistic pathogen and rarely causes disease in healthy individuals. However, it can cause life-threatening disease when host defense is seriously compromised.
- This organism may be resistant to many antibiotics used for empiric therapy of pneumonia and new resistance may develop quickly during antibiotic treatment making an initially effective therapy ultimately ineffective.

*Among other gram-negative bacilli which can cause nosocomial pneumonia, Acinetobacter spp., Stenotrophomonas maltophilia and Burkholderia cepacia may also be resistant to many empirically used antibiotics in pneumonia.

Risk Factors for Nosocomial Pneumonia due to MDR Pathogens

Traditionally considered risk factors for MDR pathogens include:

- Previous antibiotic therapy within the last 90 days
- History of hospitalization for two or more days in the last three months
- Current hospitalization for 5 days or longer
- Immunosuppressed state due to disease or drugs
- Chronic dialysis or home infusion therapy (in the last 30 days)
- Residence in a nursing home or any other long-term care facilities
- Local high prevalence of MDR organisms
- Family member with MDR pathogen

Actually, for most of the above risk factors, evidence regarding their relevance to MDR nosocomial pneumonia is insufficient.

Risk factors for MDR Pseudomonas aeruginosa nosocomial pneumonia[1,8]

Potential risk factors for MDR *P. aeruginosa* pneumonia include:

- Prior use of antibiotics within the last 90 days
- Recent ICU admission
- Structural lung diseases: COPD, cystic fibrosis, bronchiectasis etc
- Immunosuppressed state due to disease or drugs

Although the above mentioned conditions are potential risk factors for MDR Pseudomonas pneumonia, the published evidence is limited and of low quality. Based on the limited data, ***the prior use of intravenous antibiotic(s) within the last 90 days is the most clearly known risk factor for MDR Pseudomonas pneumonia.***[1]

Risk factors for MRSA nosocomial pneumonia[1,8,9]

Traditionally considered risk factors for MRSA nosocomial pneumonia include:

- Prior antibiotic therapy within the last 90 days
- Late-onset nosocomial pneumonia (≥5 days after admission)
- History of recent hospitalization, particularly recent admission to a high risk clinical area (e.g. intensive care unit, high-dependency unit, burn unit etc)
- Use of invasive devices such as an IV line (Cannula or catheter), urinary catheter, or endotracheal tube for a long period (currently or in the recent past)
- The presence of chronic wounds without healing, especially in diabetic patients

- Undergoing chronic dialysis
- Residence in a nursing home or other long term care facilities (particularly patients with long term break in the skin)
- Patients with past history of MRSA infection
- MRSA colonization

Although the above mentioned conditions are potential risk factors for MRSA pneumonia, the published evidence is limited and of low quality. Based on the limited data, ***the prior use of intravenous antibiotic(s) within the last 90 days is the most clearly known risk factor for MRSA HAP/ VAP.***[1]

Note:

Various definitions of 'multidrug resistance' have been used for gram-negative bacilli in different studies. Some experts have considered all P. aeruginosa, Acinetobacter spp. and Stenotrophomonas maltophilia as possible drug resistant pathogen until their sensitivity pattern is known.[10] However, for P. aeruginosa, more stringent definition of multidrug resistance is resistance to multiple classes of antipseudomonal antibiotics.[1]

Pathogenesis of nosocomial pneumonia

In most cases, the pathogenesis can be divided into three steps:[2,5,11]

Step1: Change in the upper respiratory tract flora: Hospital environment has some different types of organisms (predominantly gram-negative bacilli and S. aureus) than usual home environment in the community. The upper airway of 75% seriously ill hospitalized patients becomes colonized with organisms from the hospital environment within 48 hours of admission.[2] Therefore, hospitalized patients carry different flora with different antibiotic resistance pattern than healthy individuals in the community.

Step 2: Entrance of the new flora into the lower respiratory tract: In most cases, new floras (hospital organisms) enter the lower respiratory tract through micro or macro aspiration. Factors favor such aspiration include reduced level of consciousness, vomiting, dysphagia, achalasia, severe reflux, endotracheal or nasogastric intubation.

Step 3: Settling down and colonization of the aspirated bacteria leading to pneumonia:
Reduced host defense mechanisms favor settling down and colonization of the aspirated bacteria in the lower respiratory tract leading to pneumonia.
Factors reducing host defense mechanisms include:

- Immunosuppression due to drug or the disease itself (eg, Diabetes, malignancy, AIDS, cytotoxic drugs and steroids)
- Reduced mucociliary function of the respiratory tract due to depressed level of consciousness or intubation.
- Mechanical obstruction by the endotracheal or nasogastric tube affecting natural clearance;
- Reduced cough reflex

Other potential routes of infection in nosocomial pneumonia:

- Nosocomial pneumonia can also occur due to hematogenous spread of infections from a distant source (eg, abdominal sepsis, IV cannula site infection or infected emboli).
- Use of contaminated respiratory equipments or inhalation of contaminated air originating from infected humidifier, air conditioning system etc. can cause direct introduction of the organisms into the lower respiratory tract leading to pneumonia.

*Some studies have demonstrated that use of gastric acid suppressants can facilitate overgrowth of bacteria including gram-negative bacilli in the stomach. Subsequently, the bacteria may colonize tracheobronchial tree leading to nosocomial pneumonia.[12] But there is controversy regarding the role of stomach pathogens in nosocomial pneumonia.[7]

Clinical features of nosocomial pneumonia (HAP/VAP)

- Clinical features of HAP and VAP are mostly similar to those of community acquired pneumonia (for details please see 'community acquired pneumonia').
- There are no universally accepted diagnostic criteria for HAP or VAP.
- Like other forms of pneumonia, both clinical and radiographic evidence of pneumonia are needed for the diagnosis of nosocomial pneumonia (HAP/VAP).
- In a hospitalized patient admitted with other problem, additional pneumonia (which may be HAP or VAP) should be considered if a new or progressive opacity is found on the chest radiograph along with clinical evidence which suggest that the opacity is infectious in origin;[7] the clinical evidence of infection in this regard include newly developed: [5-7,11]
    (a) Fever [core temperature greater than 38.3°C (101^0F)]
    (b) Purulent sputum (or tracheal secretion)
    (c) Leukocytosis (>10 X 10^9/L) or leucopenia (<4 X 10^9/L)[6]
    (d) Decreased oxygenation[5]

Some experts suggest additional (i.e., newly developed after hospitalization) pneumonia should be suspected and chest radiograph should be ordered if two or more of the above four findings are present, in the absence of an alternative focus of infection.[5]

Investigations

- Laboratory tests are mostly similar to those considered for hospitalized community-acquired pneumonia (CAP); however, unlike CAP, microbiological confirmation is usually sought in nosocomial pneumonia whenever possible.
- The microbial diagnosis of HAP/VAP usually requires a lower respiratory specimen culture, but rarely can be made from blood or pleural fluid cultures.[7]
- <u>Lower respiratory specimens:</u>
    - *Obtained noninvasively* – eg, adequate sputum; endotracheal aspirates (can be collected at bedside using a sterile suction catheter)
    - *Obtained invasively* – eg, bronchoscopy-directed protected specimen brush (PSB) sample; bronchoalveolar lavage (BAL) sample;

    In nonintubated HAP patients, sputum is cultured most commonly, while in intubated patients with HAP/VAP endotracheal aspirates are often used as a respiratory specimen for culture.

- As in CAP, sensitivity and specificity of Gram-stain and culture of sputum is low in nosocomial pneumonia. Moreover, identification of an organism by sputum culture does not confirm that it is a lower respiratory tract pathogen.
- Blood culture should be considered in all patients with suspected VAP and HAP. However, overall sensitivity of blood cultures is <25% and in a large percentage of patients, the organism isolated from blood culture may be of extrapulmonary source.[7]
- Despite these limitations the culture results may be helpful to identify antibiotic sensitivity pattern and to adjust empiric antibiotic therapy.
- Measurement of serum procalcitonin levels may be helpful in differentiating bacterial pneumonia from pneumonia like syndrome due to non-infectious causes.
- Respiratory virus PCR (usually on sputum or throat swab sample) should be considered if features are suggestive of influenza during influenza season.[8]

Respiratory specimen culture: IDSA/ATS guidelines:[1]

- Recent IDSA/ATS guidelines (2016) recommend noninvasive respiratory sampling (endotracheal aspiration) with semiquantitative cultures for the microbial diagnosis of VAP, as these are simple, quick and can be performed with limited resources and expertise.
- There is no evidence that invasive bacteriological sampling with quantitative cultures improves patient outcomes compared to noninvasive sampling with either semiquantitative or quantitative cultures.

Some interpretations of respiratory culture results:[7]

- Although an etiologic diagnosis in nosocomial pneumonia is usually made from the culture of a respiratory specimen, a positive culture cannot always distinguish infection from colonization. Colonization of the trachea often precedes the development of pneumonia in VAP.
- In the absence of a recent change in antibiotic treatment, a sterile culture from the lower respiratory tract of an intubated patient is strongly against the pneumonia diagnosis. So the need for antibiotic therapy in these patients should be reviewed.
- In the absence of a recent change in antibiotics (within the last 72 hours), the absence of MDR pathogens in any lower respiratory specimen from intubated patients strongly suggest that MDR pathogens are not the causative agents.

Treatment of HAP/VAP

Treatment of nosocomial pneumonia (HAP/VAP) is usually empiric. However, there is no consensus on the best empiric antibiotic regimen because-

- Host factors vary from patient to patient
- Local flora and antibiotic resistance patterns also vary from place to place.

A doctor should follow his or her local guidelines.

<u>Factors need to consider during selecting an empiric antibiotic regimen:</u>

- Local flora and resistance patterns
- Risk factors for multi-drug resistant pathogens (particularly recent administration of antibiotics)
- Co-morbidities

- Severity of the infection
- The pneumonia is early onset (within 4-5 days of hospitalization) or late-onset

Empiric antibiotic regimens for HAP/VAP

Empiric antibiotic therapy for HAP and VAP are mostly similar.

A. In all patients with HAP or VAP empiric antibiotic should cover the following pathogens:

- Pseudomonas aeruginosa and other gram-negative bacilli
- Staph. aureus (MSSA)
- Streptococcus pneumoniae

Monotherapy with anyone of the following agents can be used for that coverage:[1]

1) Piperacillin-tazobactam 4.5g 6-8 hourly IV *(probably most commonly used regimen)* or
2) Cefepime 2g 8 hourly IV or
3) Imipenem-cilastatin or
4) Meropenem 1g 8 hourly IV or
5) Levofloxacin 750 mg IV daily

The above empiric antibiotic regimen containing single drug is generally sufficient for all HAP or VAP patients who neither have any risk factors for MDR pathogens nor at high risk of mortality. High risk of mortality in HAP/VAP includes septic shock, rapid deterioration and endorgan dysfunction; additionally, all HAP patients requiring ventilatory support for their pneumonia are also at high risk of mortality.

Consider atypical coverage (eg, by adding clarithromycin 500 mg bid) if the pneumonia develops within 4-5 days of hospitalization.[13]

****Some experts generally avoid the use of carbapenems (eg, Imipenem, meropenem) and fluoroquinolones as first-line agents in patients without MDR risk factors.***[13,14] Carbapenem (particularly meropenem) is reserved for patients with risk factor for MDR pathogen or relatively severe pneumonia; fluoroquinolone therapy is associated with increased risk of Clostridium difficile infection and quinolone resistance rates in many hospitals in the USA are >10% for common Gram-negative bacilli (e.g. E. coli).[14]

B. Additional coverage that should be considered for HAP/VAP patients with risk factors for MDR pathogens or at high risk of mortality:

1. MRSA coverage (Information from references 1,5,8,13,14)
Indications for MRSA coverage:
(a) Presence of anyone of the following risk factors for MRSA infection:

- Antibiotic (particularly IV) taken within the last 90 days;
- Local prevalence of MRSA among S. aureus isolates is high (> 10 -- 20%) or unknown;
- ≥4 or 5 days of hospitalization before the onset of pneumonia;
- Known or past history of MRSA infection/colonization;

Or

(b) <u>HAP or VAP Patients at high risk of mortality</u> (eg, septic shock, rapid deterioration, or endorgan dysfunction); additionally, all HAP patients requiring ventilatory support for their pneumonia are also at high risk of mortality and should receive MRSA coverage.

**Intravenous antibiotic therapy within the last 90 days is the most clearly known risk factor for MRSA nosocomial pneumonia.*[1]

Commonly used drugs for MRSA coverage:
Vancomycin 15mg/Kg (usual maximum1g/dose) 12 hourly IV or linezolid 600mg 12 hourly IV;

2. <u>Double antipseudomonal coverage</u> (Information from references 1,5,8,14)
Double antipseudomonal coverage is given by selecting two antipseudomonal agents from different classes such as a β-lactam (eg, piperacillin-tazobactam) plus either a fluoroquinolone (eg, levofloxacin/ ciprofloxacin) or an aminoglycoside.
Indications for double antipseudomonal coverage:
(a) <u>Presence of anyone of the following risk factors for Pseudomonas and other gram-negative infections:</u>

- Antibiotic (particularly IV) taken within the last 90 days;
- Patients with structural lung disease (eg, Bronchiectasis, COPD, or cystic fibrosis);
- Local prevalence of drug resistant gram-negative bacilli (i.e. resistant to an agent being considered for monotherapy) among gram-negative isolates is high (> 10%) or unknown;
- ≥4 or 5 days of hospitalization before the onset of pneumonia;

Or

(b) <u>HAP or VAP Patients at high risk of mortality</u> (eg, septic shock; rapid deterioration; or endorgan dysfunction); additionally, all HAP patients requiring ventilatory support for their pneumonia are also at high risk of mortality and should receive double antipseudomonal coverage.

**If Gram-stain of a high-quality respiratory specimen shows numerous and predominant gram-negative bacilli, it is another supportive evidence for the diagnosis of a gram-negative pneumonia.*[1]

**Like the risk for MRSA nosocomial pneumonia, intravenous antibiotic therapy within the last 90 days is the most clearly known risk factor for MDR Pseudomonas nosocomial pneumonia.*[1]

Drugs that can be used for additional antipseudomonal coverage:
A Fluoroquinolone (Ciprofloxacin 400 mg 8-12 hourly IV or Levofloxacin 750 mg IV 24 hourly)
Or
An Aminoglycoside (Amikacin 15–20 mg/kg IV daily or Gentamicin 5–7 mg/kg IV daily)

*Recent IDSA/ATS guidelines (2016) suggest avoiding aminoglycoside when possible because of aminoglycosides' poor lung penetration; increased risk of nephrotoxicity and ototoxicity; and poorer clinical response.[1]

Example of a commonly considered empiric antibiotic regimen for HAP or VAP patients when both MRSA and double antipseudomonal coverage is needed:

Piperacillin-tazobactam

Plus
A fluoroquinolone (Levofloxacin/ Ciprofloxacin) or an aminoglycoside
Plus
Vancomycin/ Linezolid

This regimen is applicable for HAP/VAP patients with high risk of mortality or who have received IV antibiotics within 3 months, as these patients need both MRSA and double antipseudomonal coverage.

Notes:

- For all HAP or VAP patients with high risk of mortality, both MRSA coverage and double antipseudomonal coverage should be considered. [1,5,14]
- Some physicians are in favor of giving single antipseudomonal antibiotic (instead of double antipseudomonal agents) in HAP patients with increased risk of Pseudomonas and other gram-negative infections but not at high risk of mortality.[5]
- Expected trough levels (pre-dose):[7]
  Gentamicin and tobramycin < 1 mg/L
  Amikacin < 4–5 mg/L
  Vancomycin 15–20 mg/ L
- Penicillin allergy:[15]
  - Manifestations of severe penicillin allergy (usually symptoms start within one hour of taking the drug, may be delayed up to 12 hours): anaphylaxis, urticaria/pruritus, angioedema, wheezing, stridor etc.
  - Manifestations of nonsevere penicillin allergy (symptoms often develop 24 hours after the administration of the drug): maculopapular or morbillifofrm rash; serum sickness (fever, arthralgia, rash, glomerulonephritis etc.)
  - In nonsevere penicillin allergy, usually other β-lactam antibiotics such as a cephalosporin or carbapenem can be used instead of penicillin.

De-escalation of empiric antibiotic therapy

De-escalation means changing of an empiric broad-spectrum antibiotic regimen to a narrower spectrum regimen; it can be done in two ways:[1]

1) Pre-existing monotherapy with a broad spectrum antibiotic can be changed to monotherapy with a narrower spectrum antibiotic.
2) Pre-existing combination therapy can be changed to monotherapy.

Empiric de-escalation in culture negative HAP patients:[1]

In HAP patients who are not at risk for MDR infections, have a reliable negative sputum culture and are clinically improving, it is reasonable to de-escalate the antibiotic regimen empirically.

- A single broad-spectrum antibiotic which is appropriate according to local HAP antibiogram should be selected.
- If local antibiogram is not available, an antibiotic with adequate activity against enteric Gram-negatives and MSSA can be considered.

De-escalation may not be appropriate for patients who are at high risk of MDR infection or do not have reliable sputum culture (eg, sputum culture not performed, poor-quality sample or antibiotic taken before obtaining the sample).

De-escalation in culture positive HAP/VAP patients:

- In patients with positive culture results, antibiotic therapy can be tailored according to the sensitivity results.[8,14]
- Patients with HAP/VAP caused by P. aeruginosa, who are not in septic shock or at high risk of mortality, do not need to continue double antipseudomonal coverage; instead, monotherapy using an antibiotic to which the isolate is susceptible can be used. However, when these patients are in septic shock or at high risk of mortality, double antipseudomonal coverage using two antibiotics to which the isolate is susceptible is generally suggested.[1]

In many cases of HAP/VAP, the de-escalation of empiric antibiotic therapy is a complex issue, and needs consultation with a medical microbiologist.

Oral antibiotic therapy in HAP

Switching to oral drugs from parenteral

- Most patients with HAP are not suitable for oral antibiotic therapy, so the therapy remains parenteral throughout. However, oral switching may be possible in selected HAP patients.
- Most quinolones and linezolid have excellent oral bioavailability.[7,16] If an intravenous quinolone or linezolid is used in the initial empiric antibiotic regimen, it can be changed to oral form when the patient achieves clinical stability and is fit for oral therapy.[7]
- For oral switching from initial intravenous piperacillin-tazobactam, some British hospitals' guidelines suggest that oral co-amoxyclav (625 mg tid) can be used instead of piperacillin-tazobactam in clinically improved patients with negative microbiological results.[13,17]

Treatment of HAP with oral antibiotics from the beginning (in some British hospitals):
According to guidelines from some British hospitals, nonsevere HAP patients who are clinically stable and do not have any risk factor for resistant pathogens may be treated with oral antibiotics from the beginning. For such patients, suggested monotherapy with an oral agent include:

- Levofloxacin (500mg OD[8]; or 500 mg BID initially then upon improvement 500mg OD[17])
  Or
- Doxycycline (100mg BID[8] ; or 200mg 12 hourly for 48 hours then 200mg daily[18])
  Or
- Co-amoxyclav 625 mg tid[17]

*Doxycycline has some MRSA coverage.

Duration of antibiotic therapy in nosocomial pneumonia:[1,8]

- For most cases of HAP or VAP irrespective of microbial etiology, a 7-day course of antibiotic therapy is adequate.[1]
- In some cases, the duration may be shorter or longer depending on the rate of improvement of clinical and laboratory parameters.
- Previously pneumonia due to non-glucose-fermenting gram-negative bacilli such as Pseudomonas and Acinetobacter was commonly treated with a longer course (10 to 14-

day) of antibiotic therapy to prevent recurrence, but recent data show that such a longer therapy is not beneficial unless the therapeutic response is slow.

Supportive treatment

- The type and extent of supportive treatment needed in nosocomial pneumonia depends mainly on the severity of the pneumonia and comorbidities.
- Most commonly needed supportive treatments are fluid support and oxygen therapy.
- Physiotherapy is important for the elderly or immobile patients.

Prognosis:[1]

- The mortality among HAP and VAP patients is difficult to estimate, as many patients die of their underlying disease rather than pneumonia.
- Crude mortality among VAP patients (i.e. mortality among all patients who develop VAP) range from 20 – 50%, whereas a recent meta-analysis showed that attributable mortality in VAP (i.e. mortality directly related to VAP) is 13%.
- HAP is generally considered less severe than VAP although serious complications develop in about 50% of HAP patients.

Summary of the empiric antibiotic therapy for HAP/VAP

A doctor should follow his or her local guidelines if any.
Empiric antibiotic therapy for HAP and VAP are mostly similar.
Empiric antibiotic regimens:
A. HAP/VAP patients who neither have any risk factors for MDR pathogens (eg, MRSA/ Pseudomonas) nor at high risk of mortality[a]

Piperacillin-tazobactam 4.5g 8 hourly IV

Consider additional atypical coverage (eg, by adding clarithromycin 500 mg bid) if the pneumonia develops within 4-5 days of hospitalization.

B. Empiric regimens for HAP/VAP patients who need additional coverage:

1) HAP/VAP patients who need additional MRSA coverage[b]
   Piperacillin-tazobactam 4.5g 6-8 hourly IV
   Plus
   Vancomycin 15mg/Kg (usual maximum1g/dose) BID IV or linezolid 600mg BID IV;

2) HAP/VAP patients who need additional double antipseudomonal coverage[c] but do not need MRSA coverage:
   Piperacillin-tazobactam 4.5g 6-8 hourly IV
   Plus
   A Fluoroquinolone (Ciprofloxacin /Levofloxacin) or an Aminoglycoside

3) HAP/VAP patients who need both MRSA coverage and double antipseudomonal coverage:
   Piperacillin-tazobactam
   Plus
   A fluoroquinolone (Levofloxacin/ Ciprofloxacin) or an aminoglycoside
   Plus
   Vancomycin/ Linezolid

Duration of antibiotic therapy is 7 days for most cases of HAP or VAP irrespective of microbial etiology. Longer duration should be considered if the therapeutic response is slow.

[a]*High risk of mortality in HAP/VAP* include septic shock, rapid deterioration, or endorgan dysfunction; additionally, all HAP patients requiring ventilatory support for their pneumonia are also at high risk of mortality.

[b]*Indications for MRSA coverage include:*
(a) Presence of anyone of the following risk factors for MRSA infection:
- Antibiotic (particularly IV) taken within the last 90 days;
- Local prevalence of MRSA among S. aureus isolates is high (> 10 -- 20%) or unknown;
- ≥4 or 5 days of hospitalization before the onset of pneumonia;
- Known or past history of MRSA infection/colonization;

Or
(b) HAP or VAP Patients at high risk of mortality;

[c]Indications for double antipseudomonal coverage include:
(a) Presence of anyone of the following risk factors for Pseudomonas and other gram-negative infections:
- Antibiotic (particularly IV) taken within the last 90 days;
- Patients with structural lung disease (eg, Bronchiectasis, COPD, or cystic fibrosis);
- Local prevalence of drug resistant gram-negative bacilli among gram-negative isolates is high (> 10%) or unknown;
- ≥4 or 5 days of hospitalization before the onset of pneumonia;

Or
(b) HAP or VAP Patients at high risk of mortality

Intravenous antibiotic therapy within the last 90 days is the most clearly known risk factor for MRSA or MDR Pseudomonas nosocomial pneumonia.

Healthcare-associated pneumonia

Definition and risk factors for HCAP

Previously multidrug-resistant (MDR) pathogen induced pneumonia generally used to occur only in hospitalized patients. But over the past several decades, with diffusion of healthcare services outside the hospitals, MDR pathogens have been detected in pneumonia patients presented as outpatients with history of recent contact with healthcare environment. To describe this new category of pneumonia, many experts used the term 'healthcare-associated pneumonia' (HCAP).[7]

There is considerable variation in the definition of HCAP used in different studies.

Definition of HCAP according to the 2005 ATS/IDSA guidelines:
According to the 2005 ATS/IDSA guidelines for nosocomial pneumonia,[7] pneumonia of outpatients that develops in the presence of one or more healthcare related risk factors for multidrug-resistant (MDR) pathogens can be considered as healthcare-associated pneumonia (HCAP).[7] The healthcare-related risk factors for MDR pathogens (i.e., risk factors for health care associated pneumonia) include:[7]

- Hospitalization for at least two days in an acute care hospital within the last 90 days;
- Residence in a nursing home or long-term care facility;
- Recent home infusion therapy (including IV antibiotic therapy)
- Home wound care within the last 30 days
- Long-term dialysis (hemodialysis or peritoneal dialysis) (within 30 days)
- Exposure to family member with MDR pathogen

All the risk factors for HCAP are also risk factors for MDR pathogens, but there are other risk factors for MDR pathogens as well which are not related to healthcare, so they are not included in the risk factors for HCAP.

Epidemiology of HCAP

HCAP constitutes a significant proportion of pneumonia patients. In a recent meta-analysis (conducted from Europe) of >22,000 patients with CAP and HCAP, the frequency of HCAP ranged from 14% to 67%.[19] In another recent retrospective review of >43,000 patients with pneumonia admitted to 491 U.S. hospitals, about 34% had HCAP.[20]

Patient characteristics and outcomes:

- In general, HCAP patients are older and have more comorbidities compared to those with CAP. Also, HCAP patients need intensive care more frequently and have significantly higher mortality rate than CAP patients.[19.20]
- In a recent large-scale meta-analysis, some European experts found that the higher mortality of HCAP patients is due to their age and comorbidities, not due to a higher frequency of resistant pathogens.[19] But another large-scale retrospective review conducted by US experts showed that the mortality rate remained greater for HCAP group than CAP group even after adjusting for age and comorbidities, which may be due to resistant pathogens or the criteria for HCAP patient selection.[20] According to that American review, patients with multiple risk factors for HCAP appear to be at higher risk of death and may benefit most from empiric broad spectrum antibiotic therapy. [20]

What is the most conflicting area of HCAP currently?

The most conflicting area of HCAP is now its empiric antibiotic coverage.

The ATS/IDSA guidelines (2005) recommended that empiric antibiotic therapy for HCAP patients should be similar to that of HAP/VAP patients with risk factor for MDR pathogens, i.e.

dual antipseudomonal antibiotics plus MRSA coverage with either vancomycin or linezolid.[7]

But recent data show that many patients who should be diagnosed as HCAP according to the definition of HCAP in ATS/IDSA guidelines 2005 are actually not at high risk for MDR pathogens.[1] So all patients with HCAP (according to that definition) do not need MDR therapy. In fact, many patients with risk factors for MDR pathogens may develop pneumonia due to usual community-acquired pneumonia pathogens.

Microbiology: HCAP versus CAP

In general, S. aureus (including MRSA), gram-negative bacilli (including P. aeruginosa) are more common pathogens in HCAP, while Streptococcus pneumoniae and the atypical bacteria (Legionella, Mycoplasma and Chlamydia) are less common compared to CAP.[19,21]

MDR pathogens in HCAP include MRSA, Pseudomonas aeruginosa and extended-spectrum β-lactamase producing (MDR) enterobacteriaceae.[21]

Prevalence of MDR pathogens: HCAP versus CAP[19]

There is a large variation in the reported prevalence of MDR pathogens among both the HCAP and CAP patients.

MDR Pathogen	*HCAP*	*CAP*
MRSA	0.7%–30%	0%–12%
P. aeruginosa	0.7%–23%	0%–8%
Enterobacteriaceae	2%–46%	0%–28%

Who are really at risk of pneumonia due to MDR pathogens among pneumonia outpatients?

- It is difficult to determine.
- The most appropriate criteria to identify the outpatients at real risk of pneumonia due to MDR pathogen because of their recent contact with healthcare environment remain unclear. The HCAP criteria specified in the ATS–IDSA guidelines (2005) do not reliably identify the patients who need empiric antibiotic coverage for drug resistant pathogens.[22]

Some important facts about the risk stratification in HCAP

1) Although interaction with healthcare environment is a potential risk factor for MDR pathogen infection, underlying host characteristics are also important determinants in this regard.[1] For example, all nursing home residents are not at high risk of MDR pathogen infection. Among nursing home residents who are ambulant and mostly independent in maintaining their activities of daily living have a low risk for MDR infection; pneumonia in this group is more commonly caused by usual CAP pathogens than HAP pathogens. In contrast, nonambulant and functionally mostly incapacitated residents are at high risk of MDR infection.[23]
2) All risk factors for MDR pathogens do not increase the risk of infection with all MDR pathogens. For example, patients receiving home infusion therapy or undergoing long term dialysis are at higher risk for MRSA pneumonia, but they may not be at higher risk for pseudomonas or other MDR pathogens than patients with CAP.[4,23] Patients with structur-

al lung disease such as bronchiectasis, cystic fibrosis, or COPD are at increased risk for infection with pseudomonas species, but not with MRSA.[23]

3) Severity of the pneumonia is also important to determine whether MDR therapy would be beneficial. A recent meta-analysis (by European experts) showed that in nonsevere HCAP, outcomes are not better when treated with MDR therapy according to ATS–IDSA guidelines (2005) compared to treating in accordance with CAP guidelines.[19]

Until recently, the overall quality of published studies on HCAP was poor, and various definition of HCAP had been used. In most studies, 'pneumonia in the immunocompromised' was included in the HCAP, although it was not included in IDSA/ATS (2005) introduced definition.[19]

Empiric antibiotic therapy for HCAP

Following factors should be taken into account during empiric antibiotic selection for HCAP patients:

(Each patient should be considered individually)

- Local prevalence of MDR pathogens
- Disease severity
- Presence or absence of more recognized risk factors for MDR pathogen* such as recent antibiotic use; recent hospitalization; patients from a long term care facility with poor functional status;
- Risk factors for HCAP are single or multiple
- Gram-stain results of an adequate sputum or other respiratory specimen
- Atypical bacteria coverage may be needed in many patients.

*Although immunosuppressed state is also a widely recognized risk factor for MDR pathogen, it is probably better to consider pneumonia in the immunocompromised host as a separate entity.

One recent study with successful categorization of HCAP patients for empiric antibiotic therapy[24]

In a multicenter prospective study of 445 pneumonia patients (CAP = 124 and HCAP = 321) in Japan, HCAP patients were divided into four groups depending on severity of their pneumonia and how many risk factors for MDR pathogen were present. However, all the risk factors for HCAP according to IDSA/ATS 2005 guidelines[7] were not considered as risk factor for MDR pathogens in this study; instead, the following <u>four factors were considered as risk factors for MDR pathogens:</u>

1) Recent hospitalization
2) Recent antibiotic therapy
3) Poor functional status (for patients from long term care facilities)
4) Immunosuppression

Empiric antibiotic regimens:[24]

A. *<u>MDR therapy</u> [(a) an antipseudomonal β-lactam* **plus** *(b) a quinolone or an aminoglycoside ± (c) linezolid/ vancomycin) was given to two groups of patients:*

- Severe HCAP with at least one of the above four risk factors for MDR pathogens
- Nonsevere HCAP with at least two of the above four risk factors for MDR pathogens

B. *Antibiotic regimen as for CAP (Quinolone monotherapy or β-lactam plus macrolide) was given to the remaining two groups of HCAP patients:*

- Severe HCAP without any of the above four risk factors for MDR pathogens
- Nonsevere HCAP with no or only one of the above four risk factors for MDR pathogens

This categorization of patients for empiric antibiotic therapy was effective. However, in that study the frequency of MRSA was low with 6.9% in HCAP group and 0% in CAP group. Countries with higher rates of drug resistant pathogens (eg, USA) may need a modified approach.[24]

Some experts have proposed scoring system allocating specific points for each risk factor for HCAP depending on their importance.[22] Actually this area needs more studies to determine more appropriate guidelines for empiric antibiotic therapy.

IDSA/ATS guidelines for the management of CAP (2007)[23] include recommendations on empiric antibiotic therapy for patients at risk of MRSA and Pseudomonas infection, but according to the definition of HCAP (in ATS/IDSA guidelines for nosocomial pneumonia 2005)[7], some of these patients fulfill the criteria for HCAP diagnosis. *For details please see the management of severe CAP in the chapter 'Community acquired pneumonia.'*

References

1. Andre C. Kalil et al. Management of Adults With Hospital-acquired and Ventilator-associated Pneumonia: 2016 Clinical Practice Guidelines by the Infectious Diseases Society of America and the American Thoracic Society. Clin Infect Dis. **2016;** 63(5):e61-e111
2. Relevant chapters of **Current Medical Diagnosis and Treatment**; Maxine A. Papadakis et al (Editors). New York, McGraw-Hill, **2013**
3. Relevant chapters of **Kumar &Clark's Clinical Medicine**, 8th edition; Parveen Kumar and Michael Clark (Editors). Edinburgh, Elsevier, 2012
4. Relevant chapters of **Harrison's Principles of Internal Medicine**; 18 th edition; Dan L Longo et al (Editors). New York, McGraw-Hill 2012.
5. Coleman Rotstein et al. Clinical practice guidelines for hospital-acquired pneumonia and ventilator-associated pneumonia in adults. Can J Infect Dis Med Microbiol**. 2008**; 19(1): 19–53.
6. R. G. Masterton1et al. Guidelines for the management of hospital-acquired pneumonia in the UK: Report of the Working Party on Hospital-Acquired Pneumonia of the British Society for Antimicrobial Chemotherapy. **Journal of Antimicrobial Chemotherapy (2008);** 62(1): 5–34
7. Guidelines for the Management of Adults with Hospital-acquired, Ventilator-associated, and Healthcare-associated Pneumonia. **Official statement of the American Thoracic**

Society and the Infectious Diseases Society of America. Am J Respir Crit Care Med 2005; Vol 171. pp 388–416

8. 'Guidelines for the Management of Hospital Acquired Pneumonia (HAP) in Adults' in the antibiotic guidelines of **Nottingham University hospitals, NHS trust, UK**. At: https://www.nuh.nhs.uk/staff-area/clinical-guidelines/; (Clinical guideline ⟶ Clinical supports ⟶ Pathology - microbiology)

9. 'Guideline for the Management of Patients with Methicillin-resistant *Staphylococcus aureus* (MRSA) (2013)' approved by **South Australian Health Safety & Quality Strategic Governance Committee**. At: http://www.sahealth.sa.gov.au/wps/wcm/connect/bd32928042372b299e5bfeef0dac2aff/Clinical+Guideline_MRSA_April2014.pdf?MOD=AJPERES

10. O. Leroy et al. Hospital-acquired pneumonia: microbiological data and potential adequacy of antimicrobial regimens. **Eur Respir J 2002**; 20: 432–439

11. Relevant chapters of **Davidson's Principles and Practice of Medicine**, 21 edition, Nicki R. Colledge et al (editors). India, Elsevier, **2010**

12. Daren Heyland et al. Gastric Colonization by Gram-Negative Bacilli and Nosocomial Pneumonia in the Intensive Care Unit Patient: Evidence for Causation. **Chest 1992**; 101(1): 187–193

13. 'Hospital acquired pneumonia' in '**The Royal Liverpool and Broadgreen University Hospitals**: antimicrobial prescribing guidelines 2013-2015', **NHS trust UK.** At: http://www.rlbuht.nhs.uk/Education%20and%20Learning/Documents/Emergency%20Medicine%20Handbook%20Trust%20Policies/Antimicrobial%20Formulary%202015%20Final.pdf

14. 'Review of the 2016 IDSA/ATS Practice Guidelines for the Management of Adults with Hospital-acquired (HAP) and Ventilator-associated Pneumonia (VAP)' on the website of The Duke Antimicrobial Stewardship Outreach Network (DASON), **Duke University School of Medicine (USA)**. At: https://dason.medicine.duke.edu/sites/dason.medicine.duke.edu/files/2016-8_dason_nl.pdf

15. 'Antibiotics and Penicillin Allergy' on the website of **Gloucestershire hospital, NHS Trust UK**. At: http://www.gloshospitals.nhs.uk/SharePoint110/Antibiotics%20Web%20Documents/Penicillin%20Poster.pdf

16. Matthew S. Dryden. Linezolid pharmacokinetics and pharmacodynamics in clinical treatment. **J Antimicrob Chemother 2011**; 66 Suppl 4: iv7–iv15

17. 'Hospital acquired Pneumonia (excluding Critical Care)' in the antibiotic guidelines of **Gloucestershire Hospitals, NHS trust UK**. At:

http://www.gloshospitals.nhs.uk/en/Trust-Staff/Antibiotic-Guidelines/Chest-Infections/Pneumonia-/Hospital-acquired-Pneumonia-excluding-Critical-Care/

18. 'Respiratory Infection - Hospital Acquired Pneumonia' on the website of **Salisbury Hospital, NHS trust UK**. At: http://www.icid.salisbury.nhs.uk/MedicinesManagement/Guidance/AntimicrobialMedicine/Pages/ChestInfection-HospitalAcquiredPneumonia.aspx

19. James D. Chalmers et al. Healthcare-Associated Pneumonia Does Not Accurately Identify Potentially Resistant Pathogens: A Systematic Review and Meta-Analysis. **Clinical Infectious Diseases 2014;**58(3):330–9

20. Michael B. Rothberg et al. Outcomes of Patients with Healthcare-associated Pneumonia: Worse disease or sicker patients? **Infect Control Hosp Epidemiol. 2014** October ; 35(0 3): S107–S115.

21. Gil Myung Seong et al. Healthcare-Associated Pneumonia among Hospitalized Patients: Is It Different from Community Acquired Pneumonia? **Tuberc Respir Dis 2014**;76:66-74

22. Michelle Peahota et al. Healthcare-associated pneumonia: Who is truly at risk for multi-drug-resistant pathogens? **Am J Health-Syst Pharm. 2015**; 72:e65-72

23. Lionel A. Mandell et al. Infectious Diseases Society of America/American Thoracic Society Consensus Guidelines on the Management of Community-Acquired Pneumonia in Adults. Supplement Article. **Clinical Infectious Diseases 2007**; 44:S27–72

24. Takaya Maruyama et al. A New Strategy for Healthcare-Associated Pneumonia: A 2-Year Prospective Multicenter Cohort Study Using Risk Factors for Multidrug-Resistant Pathogens to Select Initial Empiric Therapy. **Clinical Infectious Diseases 2013**;57(10):1373–83

Chapter 5

Pneumonia in the immunocompromised patient

Pneumonia in the immunocompromised patient

Pneumonia is a common infection in immunocompromised individuals.

Microbiology[(1-6)]

- In most cases, the same organisms that cause pneumonia in immunocompetent individuals can cause pneumonia in the immunocompromised patients. However, other organisms which are normally considered non-pathogenic or low-virulence can also cause infection (opportunistic infection) in immunocompromised patients, particularly when the immunosuppression is severe.
- Polymicrobial infection is common in immunocompromised hosts.

Pathogens associated with pulmonary infections in immunocompromised hosts include:

1) Organisms that commonly cause community acquired pneumonia in immunocompetents;
2) Gram negative bacteria (including Pseudomonas aeruginosa)
3) Staph aureus (including MRSA)
4) Viruses (eg, Cytomegalovirus, Herpes simplex virus, Varicella- zoster virus and Adenovirus)
5) Fungi [eg, Pneumocystis jiroveci (former carinii), Aspergillus, Candida spp, Cryptococcus neoformans, Coccidioides spp and Histoplasma capsulatum]
6) Mycobacteria (Mycobacterium tuberculosis and nontuberculous mycobacteria)
7) Nocardia
8) Protozoa (eg, *Toxoplasma gondii)*
9) Helminths (eg, Strongyloides stercoralis can cause symptoms like pneumonia)

Although almost any organisms can cause pneumonia in immunocompromised patients two clinical factors are useful to narrow the differential diagnoses:[1]

1. Type of immunodeficiency and
2. Clinical course of the pneumonia

1. Relationship between the type of immunodeficiency and the most likely pathogens[4,6]

Individuals with a specific type of immunodeficiency are more likely to be infected with particular types of organisms. A table below showing the relationship:

Type of immunodeficiency	*Causes*	*Infecting pathogens*
Neutropenia (Risk of serious infection is high when absolute neutrophil count <500/mcL)	Acute leukemia; lymphoma; aplastic anemia; agranulocytosis; cytotoxic drugs etc.	Gram-positive and gram-negative bacteria; fungi etc.
Impaired cell-mediated immunity	HIV-AIDS; hematological malignancy; diabetes mellitus; renal failure; use of immunosuppressive drugs, steroids, anticancer drugs, biological preparations (eg, anti-TNF-α therapy) etc.	Viruses; fungi; mycobacteria; protozoa etc.

Type of immunodeficiency	*Causes*	*Infecting pathogens*
Humoral immunodeficiency	Multiple myeloma; chronic lymphocytic leukemia; congenital hypogammaglobulinemia; splenectomy etc.	Bacterial infections, particularly with encapsulated bacteria such as Streptococcus pneumoniae and Haemophilus influenzae

2) Clinical course of the pneumonia: Rapidly progressive pneumonia is commonly caused by bacterial infection, whereas insidious pneumonia is more likely to be caused by viral, fungal, mycobacterial, or protozoal infection.

Notes:

- Neutrophil dysfunction in the presence of normal neutrophil count can increase the risk of infection with the pathogens that cause infection in neutropenic patients by causing impaired phagocytosis. Neutrophil dysfunction may occur in diabetes mellitus, uremia, malignant neoplasm, steroid therapy etc.

- In many patients, more than one type of immunodeficiency may be present simultaneously; for example, patients who have received cancer chemotherapy may develop neutropenia as well lymphopenia causing impaired cell mediated immunity.

- In certain types of immunosuppression, some particular organisms are more likely to cause infection during specific periods of the immunosuppression[4]. For example, in post-transplant patients, pneumonia developing within 2-4 weeks of organ transplantation is usually bacterial, but when it occurs several months or more after transplantation, more likely pathogens are Pneumocystis jiroveci, viruses or fungi.[1]

- Immunodeficiency due to corticosteroid therapy: Corticosteroid therapy can cause impaired cell mediated immunity and impaired phagocytosis resulting from neutrophil dysfunction. Almost any type of pathogens including gram-positive and gram-negative bacteria, viruses, fungi, protozoa etc can cause infection in these patients.

- Nocardia species are Gram-positive aerobic bacteria. They are ubiquitous saprophytes, typically found in dead organic matter in soil, standing water and decaying plants. Nocardia can cause severe infection including pneumonia in immunocompromised individuals. However, up to one-third of patients with nocardiosis are not immunodeficient.[5] Patients with depressed cell-mediated immunity are particularly at high risk of infection with this bacteria.[5]

Clinical features

- Clinical features may be like community acquired pneumonia (Fever, cough, breathlessness etc.) or more nonspecific.[2]
- Patients may be febrile or have only a low-grade fever because of inadequate immune response.[6] Neutropenic patients are less likely to have purulent sputum.
- Respiratory signs also may be absent in pneumonia in immunocompromised patients.
- Pneumonia in a neutropenic patient following chemotherapy may suddenly become obvious and severe when the neutrophil count improves.[6]

Clinical presentation of Pneumocystis jiroveci pneumonia (PJP)

- In HIV infected person, a common presentation of PJP is subacute onset (over days to weeks) of progressive breathlessness (95%), nonproductive cough (95%) and low-grade fever (>80%).[7,8]
- Although physical examination generally reveals tachycardia and tachypnea, lung auscultation may be normal in about 50%, while in others only some nonspecific signs such as crackles and or ronchi may be present.[7.8]
- PJP when occurs in immunocompromised states other than HIV-AIDS, usually it manifests as a faster onset and more severe disease.

Investigations

Approach to investigation depends on the clinical context, severity of the pneumonia and in some cases response to initial empiric antimicrobial regimen. Although routine investigations are usually performed, they often cannot detect the causative organism.

HRCT (High Resolution Computed Tomography) and examination of the induced sputum are the most yielding and easy to perform investigations for majority of the patients.

- **HRCT:** In immunocompromised individuals, HRCT is a commonly considered investigation when pneumonia is suspected, as HRCT is more sensitive than plain chest radiograph for early diagnosis of pneumonia in these patients.[9] Moreover, many organisms causing pneumonia in the immunocompromised hosts produce characteristic CT features which are helpful in estimating the causative pathogen and selecting an appropriate empiric antimicrobial regimen. Also, HRCT findings may be a guide for the invasive procedures such as bronchoscopic biopsy or transthoracic needle aspiration. CT features in some of cases of pneumonia:
    1) The most common radiographic features of pneumocystis pneumonia are the bilateral interstitial and alveolar infiltrates (found in 65–70% cases), initially prominent in perihilar regions and lower lung lobes.[10]
    2) Characteristic halo sign (single or multiple pulmonary nodules surrounded by ground-glass opacity) is most commonly associated with invasive pulmonary aspergillosis.[11] Although many other infections and noninfectious conditions may be associated with halo sign, this sign may be useful to initiate empiric of antifungal therapy when present in immunocompromised patients with suspected pneumonia.[11]
    3) CT features of bacterial pneumonia in immunocompromised patients are similar to those of pneumonia in immunocompetent individuals[4], such as lobar or segmental consolidation, cavitation, pleural effusion etc.
- **Sputum induction:** Sputum induction is usually considered when sputum production is not sufficient. Hypertonic saline inhalation may be useful to increase sputum production. The sputum should be examined for bacteria, fungi, mycobacteria, Legionella, Pneumocystis jiroveci etc.
- **Serum tests for fungi:** The use of two serum fungal tests, the b-(1-3)-D glucan test and the galactomannan test, may be helpful in the detection of common invasive fungal infections[12] particularly combined use of both the tests.[13]
- **Invasive tests:** When examination of the adequate sputum, HRCT and other noninvasive tests fail to reveal the causative pathogen(s) and the patient remain unresponsive to empiric

antimicrobial treatment, invasive tests such as bronchoscopy with bronchoalveolar lavage (BAL) or transbronchial lung biopsy; transthoracic needle aspiration; or even surgical lung biopsy may be considered. However, many patients are not fit for such an invasive procedure; also, the obtained information may not alter patient outcomes in many cases.

Adequate sputum in neutropenic patient:
In immunocompetent patients with pneumonia, a sputum specimen is considered adequate for culture if leukocytes are >25 and squamous epithelial cells are <10 per low power field. But in neutropenic patients, a sputum specimen can be considered adequate even when almost no neutrophils are found if the epithelial cell count is low.

Treatment

Empiric antimicrobial therapy

- Empiric antimicrobial therapy should be started as soon as possible and the empiric antimicrobial regimen should be individualized.
- Many factors need to be taken into account during selecting an antimicrobial regimen such as the type of immunodeficiency and the underlying cause; clinical course and severity of the pneumonia; and the risk of empiric antimicrobial therapy.
- Empiric antimicrobial regimen may include various combinations of antibiotics, antifungal and antiviral drugs.
- Consult infectious disease or respiratory medicine specialists as well as the team caring for the primary illness.

Empiric antimicrobial regimen for neutropenia-associated pneumonia:
The initial antimicrobial regimen should cover gram-positive and gram-negative bacteria including Pseudomonas aeruginosa and may be: [12,14]

Piperacillin-tazobactam 4.5g TID IV (first line agent) or Meropenem 1g TID IV
+
An aminoglycoside [eg, gentamicin 5mg/kg (maximum 450mg) OD IV] or a fluoroquinolone
±
Vancomycin (IV)

Consider early addition of anti-MRSA drugs (Vancomycin/ linezolid) if the patient is at risk for MRSA infection or the patient's clinical condition is unstable. Risk factors for MRSA include recent intravenous antibiotic therapy; previous infection or colonization with MRSA; and high prevalence of MRSA in the hospital where the patient is receiving treatment.

Some patients may need additional antifungal coverage particularly unresponsive cases.

Empiric antimicrobial therapy may be tailored according to the results of microbiological tests.

In suspected or confirmed Pneumocystis jiroveci pneumonia cotrimoxazole is the most commonly used antibiotic.

Appropriate supportive care should be provided when required. For artificial ventilation in immunocompromised patients with respiratory failure, noninvasive ventilation should be preferred instead of traditional mechanical ventilation.[10] Mechanical ventilation is associated with increased risk of nosocomial pneumonia and higher mortality rate.

References

1. Relevant chapters of **Current Medical Diagnosis and Treatment**; Maxine A. Papadakis et al (Editors). New York, McGraw-Hill, **2013**

2. Relevant chapters of **Kumar &Clark's Clinical Medicine**, 8th edition; Parveen Kumar and Michael Clark (Editors). Edinburgh, Elsevier, **2012**

3. Relevant chapters of **Davidson's Principles and Practice of Medicine**, 21 edition, Nicki R. Colledge et al (editors). India, Elsevier, **2010**

4. Jitesh Ahuja et al. Thoracic Infections in Immunocompromised Patients. **Radiol Clin N Am 2014;** 52(1): 121–136

5. John W. Wilson. Nocardiosis: Updates and Clinical Overview. **Mayo Clin Proc. 2012;** 87(4):403-407

6. Japanese Respiratory Society. Pneumonia in immunocompromised patients. **Respirology 2009;** 14 (Suppl. 2): S44 – S50

7. Nicholas John Bennett. Pneumocystis jiroveci Pneumonia. **Emedicine, October 2016**; at: http://emedicine.medscape.com/article/225976-overview#a6

8. Charles F. Thomas, Jr. et al. Pneumocystis Pneumonia. **N Engl J Med 2004**; 350:2487-98

9. Figen Başaran Demirkazık et al. CT findings in immunocompromised patients with pulmonary infections**. Diagn Interv Radiol 2008**; 14:75-82

10. Corti M et al. Respiratory infections in immunocompromised patients. Curr Opin Pulm Med. **2009**; May;15(3):209-17

11. Sarah P. Georgiadou et al. The Diagnostic Value of Halo and Reversed Halo Signs for Invasive Mold Infections in Compromised Hosts. **Clinical Infectious Diseases 2011**; 52(9):1144–1155

12. Alison G. Freifeld et al. Clinical Practice Guideline for the Use of Antimicrobial Agents in Neutropenic Patients with Cancer: 2010 Update by the Infectious Diseases Society of America. **Clinical Infectious Diseases 2011**;52(4):e56–e93

13. C. Fontana et al. (1-3)-β-D-Glucan vs Galactomannan Antigen in Diagnosing Invasive Fungal Infections (IFIs). **The Open Microbiology Journal 2012**; 6: 70-73

14. 'Neutropenia-associated pneumonia' in Antibiotic guidelines (2015) of The **Royal Liverpool and Broadgreen university hospitals,** NHS trust, UK. At: http://www.rlbuht.nhs.uk/Education%20and%20Learning/Documents/Emergency%20Medicine%20Handbook%20Trust%20Policies/Antimicrobial%20Formulary%202015%20Final.pdf

Chapter 6
Aspiration pneumonia and lung abscess

Aspiration pneumonitis and aspiration pneumonia

The two major aspiration syndromes are aspiration pneumonitis and aspiration pneumonia.

Aspiration pneumonitis
Aspiration pneumonitis (also called chemical pneumonia/ chemical pneumonitis) can be defined as the acute chemical injury of the lung caused by aspiration of sterile acidic gastric content.

Aspiration pneumonia
Aspiration pneumonia is an infectious process; there are two types of aspiration pneumonia:

1. Primary bacterial aspiration pneumonia is caused by aspiration of pathogenic bacteria form the colonies of the upper airway or stomach.
2. Secondary bacterial aspiration pneumonia occurs due to secondary bacterial infection of aspiration (chemical) pneumonitis.

Aspiration pneumonia

Aspiration of small amount of oropharyngeal secretions occurs in about 50% of normal persons during sleep which usually does not cause any problem.[1] Host defense mechanisms such as cough reflex, mucociliary clearance, humoral and cellular immunities prevent the development of infection. But if these host defense mechanisms are impaired, or aspiration of large volume of materials or materials with high bacterial load occurs aspiration pneumonia may develop.[2]

How common is aspiration pneumonia?

- It is difficult to estimate the real incidence of aspiration pneumonia. However, aspiration pneumonia may account for 5-15% of community acquired pneumonia cases[1]
- Primary bacterial aspiration pneumonia may be the commonest form of aspiration syndromes.

Factors predispose to aspiration pneumonia

The predisposing factors can be divided into two groups:

(a) Factors that increase the risk of aspiration (i.e. risk factors for aspiration)

- Depressed level of consciousness (due to drug or disease: stroke; seizures; intoxication with alcohol or other drugs; general anesthesia etc)
- Dysphagia due to any cause (eg, neuromuscular disorders)
- Mechanical disruption of normal defenses of the airways (eg, nasogastric or tracheal tube; tracheostomy; and bronchoscopy)
- Esophageal disorders: Achalasia of the esophagus, stricture, tumor, gastro- esophageal reflux disease etc.
- Others: Constant supine position, general debility, dementia, critical illness etc.

(b) Factors that increase the bacterial load of potential aspirate:
Increased bacterial load of the aspirate increases the risk of pulmonary infection if aspiration occurs.

- *Gastric acid suppression:* Under normal circumstances gastric contents are sterile, as gastric acid prevents bacterial growth in the stomach. Use of gastric acid suppressants favors bacterial colonization of the stomach. Also, gastric colonization with gram-negative bacteria may occur in patients with gastroparesis, small-bowel obstruction, or who are receiving enteral feedings.

- *Poor oral and dental hygiene:* Poor oral hygiene and periodontal disease favor growth of anaerobes in the oral cavity.

Commonly affected part of the lung in aspiration pneumonia and aspiration pneumonitis

Dependent part of the lung at the time of aspiration is usually affected initially. Therefore, the affected part depends on patients' posture at the time of aspiration:

Most frequently affected parts are-

1. Apical and basal segments of the lower lobe and or
2. Posterior segment of the upper lobe

Right lung is more commonly affected than the left, as the *right main bronchus* is *shorter, wider* and more vertical than the *left main bronchus.*

If the patient is supine at the time of aspiration, usually the posterior segments of upper or apical segments of lower lobes are involved. But if the patient is upright or semirecumbent during the event of aspiration, the basal segments of lower lobes are generally involved.

Microbiology of aspiration pneumonia

There are conflicting evidences about the range of bacteria involved in aspiration pneumonia. According to recent studies, anaerobes are not as frequently involved as was previously thought. ***The organisms involved in aspiration pneumonia mainly depend on the circumstance in which aspiration has occurred:***

(1) Community-acquired aspiration pneumonia (without any risk factors for multidrug resistant pathogen such as history of recent hospitalization or recent antibiotic use):

- Predominant organisms are *S. pneumoniae*, *H. influenzae*, *Staphylococcus aureus* and Enterobacteriaceae.[2,3]

(2) Hospital-acquired aspiration pneumonia:

- The most commonly identified pathogens are gram negative bacteria such as *Pseudomonas aeruginosa, Klebsiella pneumoniae and Escherichia coli. S. aureus* is also an important causative organism in these cases. [2-4]

Anaerobes are rarely identified in aspiration pneumonia.[2]

Commonly isolated anaerobes in aspiration pneumonia[3,5]

- Peptostreptococci
- Fusobacterium
- Bacteroides
- Prevotella

Clinical features of aspiration pneumonia

- Aspiration pneumonia typically occurs in elderly patients with dysphagia and the episode of aspiration is usually not witnessed.

- The symptoms and signs of aspiration pneumonia are mostly similar to those of other forms of pneumonia such as cough, fever, breathlessness and signs of consolidation. However, aspiration pneumonia commonly follow a more indolent clinical course, evolving over days to weeks instead of hours although patients may present with a sudden onset disease like pneumococcal pneumonia.[5]
- Some patients may present with complications such as lung abscess or empyema.
- In hospitalized debilitated patients, dominating features of aspiration pneumonia may be new onset or worsening shortness of breath and crackles with or without wheezes, or recent desatuartion only.

When to suspect aspiration pneumonia:

Suspect aspiration pneumonia in the following conditions:

1. Symptoms and signs of pneumonia in a patient with risk factor(s) for aspiration;
2. Symptoms and signs of pneumonia plus radiographic opacity in the dependent lung segments; (look for risk factors for aspiration);
3. Recurrent pneumonia in the elderly; (look for risk factors for aspiration, particularly dysphagia, and consider formal swallowing test by a speech therapist);

When to suspect anaerobic pneumonia

1. Aspiration pneumonia in a patient with poor oral hygiene, alcoholism or severe periodontal disease;
2. Foul smelling breath, sputum or empyema fluid in a patient with pneumonia;
3. Necrotizing pneumonia (multiple small cavities in contiguous areas of the lung on chest radiograph), lung abscess or empyema in aspiration patients.

Confirmation of the diagnosis of primary bacterial aspiration pneumonia is often difficult, since the episode of aspiration is usually not witnessed and the patients with risk factors for aspiration may develop pneumonia unrelated to aspiration. However, when a patient with risk factor for aspiration develops pneumonia with radiographic evidence of involving characteristic (dependent) bronchopulmonary segment, it is highly suggestive of aspiration pneumonia.

Investigations

- Investigations for aspiration pneumonia are mostly similar to those for community-acquired pneumonia or hospital-acquired pneumonia depending on the circumstance in which the aspiration pneumonia has developed.
- A comprehensive swallowing test by a speech therapist should be considered in some cases with suspected dysphagia, particularly in the elderly with recurrent pneumonia.

Treatment of aspiration pneumonia

Empiric antibiotic treatment of bacterial aspiration pneumonia

Initial empiric antibiotic therapy depends on the circumstance in which the aspiration has occurred, severity of the condition, presence or absence of risk factors for MDR pathogens etc. Consult an infectious disease specialist or pulmonologist if the pneumonia is severe or the patient's background is complicated.

A. Community-acquired aspiration pneumonia:

Antibiotic regimen should cover typical CAP pathogens, gram-negative bacteria and anaerobes.
(a) For mild to moderate disease (Information from references 6-10)
Most patients need hospitalization. Initial empiric antibiotic regimen may be:
Co-amoxiclav (alone) 1.2 g IV 8-hourly

In some mild cases, if the patient is suitable for oral therapy, Co-amoxiclav 625 mg 8-horuly or 875 mg 12-hourly PO may be considered from the outset.
Alternative: Oral Amoxicillin Plus Metronidazole

If anaerobic infection is suspected but the infection is not severe (eg, putrid sputum, alcoholism, or severe periodontal disease), consider to add metronidazole 500 mg IV 8-hourly with Co-amoxiclav 1.2g IV 8 hourly.

Alternative to IV co-amoxiclav ±metronidazole:
Levofloxacin (500mg/ day IV) or Ceftriaxone (1-2g/day)
Plus
Clindamycin or metronidazole IV

Clindamycin monotherapy is the preferred empiric antibiotic therapy in nonsevere community-acquired aspiration pneumonia by many physicians (especially in the USA) although this drug does not cover aerobic gram-negative bacteria.[4]
Dose of Clindamycin: 600 mg 8-hourly IV initially until significant improvement, then 300 mg 6-hourly PO when oral medication is possible.

If unresponsive to any of the above initial regimens, consider escalation of the antibiotic therapy.

(b) For severe disease (Information from references 1,10)

Piperacillin- Tazobactam (4.5 g IV 6-8 hourly) or Carbapenem
±
Vancomycin or linezolid

Alternative regimen (for severe penicillin allergy) may be: Levofloxacin (500mg BD IV) **Plus** metronidazole (500 mg IV 8-hourly) ± either Vancomycin or linezolid

If patients with community-acquired severe aspiration pneumonia have risk factors for MDR pathogens (eg, Pseudomonas aeruginosa and or MRSA), appropriate empiric antibiotic coverage for them should be considered as mentioned in the treatment of severe CAP.
For details please see the treatment of severe CAP in the chapter 'community acquired pneumonia'.

According to IDSA, pneumonia in hospitalized CAP patients with any one of the following: (1) requirement intensive care, (2) necrotizing or cavitary lesion, or (3) empyema should be considered severe community acquired pneumonia where empiric MRSA coverage should be provided.[11]

Addition of coverage for atypical bacteria in community-acquired aspiration pneumonia:

In doubtful cases of community acquired aspiration pneumonia, addition of atypical bacteria coverage (eg, azithromycin or clarithromycin) to the empiric antibiotic regimen may be rational, particularly in severe pneumonia unless the regimen contain any drug which can provide the atypical coverage (eg, fluoroquinolone).

Notes:

- Penicillin or metronidazole alone is usually inadequate for the treatment of aspiration pneumonia. Although metronidazole is highly effective against almost all anaerobes, it does not cover aerobic and microaerophilic streptococci, so not suitable for monotherapy in aspiration pneumonia. It can be combined with a β-lactam or other antibiotics when necessary.
- Empiric anaerobic coverage: although recent studies show that anaerobes are infrequently involved in aspiration pneumonia, inclusion of some anaerobic coverage in all empiric antibiotic regimens for aspiration pneumonia is still a common practice. However, specific anaerobic coverage (eg, with metronidazole or clindamycin) may be considered only when anaerobic pneumonia is suspected.
- Anaerobic coverage of piperacillin-tazobactam, imipenem and meropenem: each of these drugs are active against virtually all anaerobic bacteria including those involved in anaerobic pulmonary infection.[5,12] So when any of these drugs is included in the empiric antibiotic regimen, additional anaerobic coverage (eg, as with metronidazole or clindamycin) is usually unnecessary.[12]
- Clindamycin has excellent activity against gram-positive cocci, and both gram-positive and gram-negative anaerobes. Its anaerobic coverage may be broader than that of most cephalosporins, but it is not effective against aerobic gram-negative bacteria.[13]

B. Nosocomial aspiration pneumonia:

- Empiric antibiotic regimen should cover gram-negative bacteria including Pseudomonas; S. aureus; Pneumococcus; and anaerobes. Therefore***, empiric antibiotic regimens for nosocomial aspiration pneumonia are mostly similar to those for nosocomial pneumonia without aspiration, except the regimen for nosocomial aspiration pneumonia should also have adequate anaerobic coverage.***
- Some drugs, such as Cefepime or Levofloxacin, although can be used in HAP/VAP, they do not have adequate anaerobic coverage which is generally considered for nosocomial aspiration pneumonia, so they should not be used without additional anaerobic coverage (eg, additional metronidazole) in nosocomial aspiration pneumonia.
- ***Empiric regimens:***
    a) *For patients with nonsevere nosocomial aspiration pneumonia without any risk factors for MDR pathogens:*[4]
    Piperacillin-tazobactam or carbapenem (eg, meropenem)

    b) *For patients with severe nosocomial aspiration pneumonia or nonsevere nosocomial aspiration pneumonia with high risk for both MRSA and Pseudomonas aeruginosa:*
    Piperacillin-tazobactam/ Meropenem
    Plus
    An aminoglycoside (Gentamicin/ tobramycin/ amikacin) or Levofloxacin
    Plus
    An anti -MRSA drug (Vancomycin/ Linezolid)

However, when a nonsevere nosocomial aspiration pneumonia patient has high risk for either MRSA or Pseudomonas (not for both the pathogens), he or she can receive the coverage for that particular pathogen only.*(For details please see 'Treatment of hospital-acquired pneumonia/ ventilator-associated pneumonia' in the chapter 'Nosocomial pneumonia.')*

Empiric antibiotic therapy should be reviewed in unresponsive patients or after obtaining microbiological test results.

Route of antibiotic administration in aspiration pneumonia:

Most patients with aspiration pneumonia need intravenous antibiotic initially, and then the antibiotic can be switched to oral form when the patient is clinically improved (eg, afebrile, no hemodynamic derangement and no hypoxia) and fit for oral medication.

Duration of antibiotic treatment

- There is no definitive recommendation for the duration of antibiotic treatment in bacterial aspiration pneumonia. However, a 7-or 8- day course may be adequate for nonsevere uncomplicated cases (eg, no necrotizing pneumonia, lung abscess, empyema, or bronchopleural fistula).
- Patients with complications, such as abscess or empyema, may need drainage along with a longer duration of antimicrobial therapy.[4]

Aspiration pneumonitis/ chemical pneumonitis

- Aspiration pneumonitis or chemical pneumonitis is the effect of chemical injury caused by aspirated materials.
- Many experts agree that aspiration of gastric content > 0.3 ml/Kg body weight (20 to 25 ml in adults) with a pH of <2.5 is required for the development of aspiration pneumonitis.[2]

Pathophysiology: Immediate chemical injury caused by gastric acid and other materials of the aspirate followed by inflammatory reactions;

Clinical features:

Aspiration pneumonitis typically develops in patients with depressed level of consciousness (eg, stroke, sedative overdose, general anesthesia) and the episode of aspiration may be witnessed.
Clinical presentation varies:

- Patients may present with abrupt onset (within minutes to hours after an observed or suspected episode of aspiration) of breathlessness, cough, wheeze, low-grade fever, cyanosis, hypoxemia, pulmonary edema, hypotension etc.
- In many patients, only cough or wheeze develops;[2]
- Some patients are asymptomatic or only have arterial desaturation with radiologic evidence of aspiration.[2,4]

As these symptoms of aspiration pneumonitis overlap with those of bacterial aspiration pneumonia, in many cases, differentiation between the two entities may be difficult, particularly when the symptoms of aspiration pneumonitis develop slowly.

Clinical course of aspiration pneumonitis[14]

Clinical course of aspiration pneumonitis also varies. In one retrospective study of 50 patients with observed aspiration of gastric content, the onset of clinical signs were prompt after aspiration in all patients and the subsequent course had following three patterns:

1. About 60% of patients improved clinically and radiologically rapidly, with resolution of the pulmonary infiltrates within a few days.
2. About 15% of patients deteriorated rapidly, progressing to hypoxia, hypotension, severe acute respiratory distress syndrome and death shortly.
3. The remaining about 25% of patients develops secondary bacterial infection after an initial improvement and have high mortality rate (>60%).

Treatment of aspiration pneumonitis/ chemical pneumonitis

- The mainstays of treatment of uncomplicated chemical pneumonitis are supportive and symptomatic such as:
  - Airway clearing
  - Bronchodilator for bronchospasm
  - Oxygen therapy
  - Ventilatory support
- Patients condition should be monitored closely to detect secondary bacterial infection and chest X-ray should be repeated.
- Antibiotic and corticosteroid use are controversial in chemical pneumonitis.[4]

Empiric antibiotic therapy in chemical pneumonitis:

(a) When aspiration of gastric content is witnessed or strongly suspected, prophylactic antibiotic use is generally not recommended although antibiotics are frequently prescribed.[2,4] However, empiric broad-spectrum antibiotic therapy should be considered for these patients if:

1. the pneumonitis is not resolved within 48 hours (when secondary bacterial infection should be suspected)[2,9] or
2. there is any risk factor for bacterial colonization of the stomach such as gastroparesis, small bowel obstruction, or patients on any acid suppressant.[2]

(b) When the event of aspiration is neither witnessed nor strongly suspected and it remains unclear whether the pneumonitis syndrome is due to chemical injury or bacterial infection, it is rational to start antibiotic therapy empirically after obtaining lower-respiratory specimens for microbiological tests. The antibiotic therapy can be stopped if the patient improves clinically and radiologically rapidly (within 48 to 72 hours) and microbiological test results are negative. But if the patient does not improve or microbiological test results are positive, appropriate antibiotic therapy should be continued.[4]

Steroid in chemical pneumonitis:

Use of steroid in this condition is controversial.[4,5,9] Although infiltrate on the chest radiograph may improve more quickly with steroid treatment, it has no overall mortality benefit and may increase the risk of pneumonia with gram-negative bacteria; therefore, corticosteroids are not recommended in chemical pneumonitis.[9]

Prevention of aspiration syndromes:[2,4,5]

Following measures can reduce the incidence of aspiration syndromes:

- Elevation of the head end of the bed can minimize gastroesophageal reflux and subsequent aspiration.
- Patients should be placed on their sides if there is vomiting.
- Among patients who are at high risk of aspiration, good oral and dental care can reduce the incidence of aspiration pneumonia by reducing the oral bacterial load.
- In patients with dysphagia, a comprehensive swallowing test by a speech therapist can identify those who are at higher risk of aspiration. Evaluation of cough and gag reflexes is not reliable in this regard. For patients at higher risk of aspiration, dietary, behavioral and medical interventions, such as soft diet; and feeding strategies like keeping chin tucked and small bite size may reduce the risk of aspiration.
- Swallowing reflex may be altered temporarily in patients with endotracheal intubation even when the intubation lasted for a short period of time such as 24 hours. However, this difficulty usually resolves within 48 hours after extubation. So oral feeding can be withheld for at least 6 hours after extubation, and then gradual institution of oral feeding can be considered, starting with pureed food followed by soft food for at least 48 hours.[2]

Percutaneous endoscopic gastrostomy, orogastric, or nasogastric tubes cannot protect from aspiration.[4] However, in patients with dysphagia, gastrostomy tubes are often preferred for long-term nutritional support to avoid discomfort, poor cosmesis and other problems associated with nasogastric tubes. But gastrostomy tubes should not be considered for patients who are likely to regain their ability to swallow within a few weeks.[2]

Lung abscess

Lung abscess can be defined as the localized collection of pus within the lung due to microbial infection.

Necrotizing pneumonia is the condition in which multiple small abscesses are formed in contiguous areas of the lung. Although similar pathologic process is involved in both lung abscess and necrotizing pneumonia, necrotizing pneumonia usually occurs due to infection with more virulent pathogens.

Mechanisms of lung abscess formation

In most cases, lung abscess is developed as a complication of aspiration pneumonia.[15]
Other mechanisms of lung abscess formation include:

- **Lung abscess formation as a complication of other types of pneumonias** (eg, CAP or HAP), particularly when caused by S. aureus or Klebsiella pneumoniae.
- **Infection of a collapsed lobe or segment** which often occurs as a complication of bronchial obstruction by a neoplasm or foreign body.
- **Cavitation of pulmonary infarcts associated with infection**: on CT, cavity detected in up to 32% of patients with pulmonary infarction and on plain radiograph, in up to 7%. In most cases of pulmonary infarction due to venous thromboembolism, initially aseptic necrotic cavity is formed, where superinfection develops later in about 50% of cases.[16]
- **Hematogenous spread through septic emboli or bacteremia:** Septic emboli, which usually contain staphylococci, commonly originate from bacterial endocarditis of tricuspid valve in IV drug abusers. On the other hand, bacteremia generally results from abdo-

minal sepsis, cannula site infections etc. Multiple lung abscesses may develop in these cases.

- **Infection of a preexisting bulla or lung cyst**
- **Spread from subphrenic abscess**
- **Pulmonary tuberculosis**
- **Fungal infections** eg, Histoplasmosis, Blastomycosis, Coccidioidomycosis etc

Notes:

- In some cases, lung abscess may be formed directly without going through the preceding stage of pneumonic consolidation,[17]
- Although by definition not considered as lung abscess, cavitary lesions in the lung may develop in many noninfectious conditions such as necrotizing tumors and Wegener's granulomatosis.

Common sites of lung abscess:

It depends on the cause. When it occurs as a complication of aspiration pneumonia, the affected parts are same as in aspiration pneumonia:

1. Apical and basal segments of the lower lobe and or
2. Posterior segment of the upper lobe

Tuberculosis commonly affects upper lobes.

Microbiology

The likely pathogens depend on the circumstance where the lung abscess has developed as well as host factors such as presence or absence of risk factor for aspiration and immune status.

A. Lung abscess developed in community setting:

When related to aspiration (most cases of lung abscess fall in this category)
Polymicrobial infection is common. Commonly isolated organisms are:[16-19]

- **Anaerobes** (Peptostreptococci, Fusobacterium, Prevotella , Bacteroides species etc; multiple species of anaerobes may be present in an abscess)
- **Streptococcus species** (particularly Streptococcus mitis, Streptococcus milleri, Streptococcus pneumoniae especially type 3)
- **Gemella species** (some of these gram-positive cocci are commensals of the oral cavity of normal individuals)
- **Klebsiella pneumoniae**

When unrelated to aspiration[16]

- Although in community-acquired pneumonia lung cavities are not common, many of the patients with aspiration unrelated lung abscess are otherwise healthy and lung abscess is developed as a complication of CAP. **Streptococcus pneumoniae, Haemophilus influenzae, Klebsiella pneumoniae, S. aureus (including CA-MRSA), endemic fungi etc. are commonly implicated.** Of these:
    - In Streptococcus pneumoniae or Haemophilus influenzae induced CAP, lung abscess is an occasional complication, whereas in K. pneumoniae pneumonia it is a common complication.

- S. aureus (including CA-MRSA) is an emerging cause of community acquired lung abscess. Community-acquired S. aureus pneumonia is often severe and cavitation on plain chest radiographs is also common in this pneumonia.

- In TB endemic areas, Mycobacterium tuberculosis is also common cause of cavitary lesion in the lung.

Immunocompromised hosts
Likely pathogens depend on the type of immunodeficiency such as:
- Neutropenia: Gram-negative bacteria (particularly K. pneumoniae), S. aureus, fungi etc.
- Impaired cell-mediated immunity: Mycobacteria species, Nocardia species, Aspergillus, Rodococcus equi etc.

B. Lung abscess developed in nosocomial setting:
Likely pathogens include
- Gram-negative bacilli including *P. aeruginosa and K. pneumoniae*
- Staphylococcus aureus including MRSA
- Anaerobes, particularly oropharyngeal

Clinical presentation:
In adults, lung abscess predominantly occurs in male; in some series about 80% were male.[17-19] Clinical presentation of lung abscess varies depending on the pathogens implicated.

A. When anaerobes are involved (true anaerobic or anaerobes as a part of mixed infection):
- *Patient characteristics:* Typically these patients have risk factors for aspiration; periodontal diseases are also common (in >60% cases);[18,19]
- *Symptoms:* Gradual onset (often over days or weeks) of cough, sputum, fever and weight loss. Sputum may be of copious amount, and is characteristically purulent and foul smelling. Some patients develop hemoptysis and pleuritic chest pain.
- In general, most patients seek medical attention within the first two weeks of onset of symptoms; however, 25% to 30% patients appear late with chronic abscess, four to eight weeks after the of onset of symptoms.[19]
- Clubbing may develop rapidly (within 10-14 days)
- On physical examination of the chest, crackles are commonly found; pleural rub and signs of consolidation may be found. However, the characteristic amphoric or cavernous breath sounds of a pulmonary cavity are only rarely detected.
- Usually the abscess is solitary; in two series, in about 95% cases of suspected or confirmed anaerobic lung abscess, single cavity was detected on CXR.[17,19]

B. When anaerobes are not involved:
- These patients' presentation is commonly more acute with symptoms and signs more like community acquired or hospital acquired pneumonia.
- In some cases, lung abscess may be formed rapidly without the preceding stage of pneumonic consolidation.

Actually, the differentiation between anaerobic- and non-anaerobic lung abscesses is not as easy as it was previously thought. A study in Taiwan[17] showed that like anaerobic lung abscesses,

Klebsiella pneumoniae lung abscesses may also be related to aspiration and alcoholism and may affect the same dependent segments of the lung. However, ***anaerobic lung abscesses more commonly have subacute or chronic clinical course, single abscess cavity, putrid sputum and an overall less aggressive disease.***

Lung abscesses due to fungi, Mycobacteria or Nocardia species tend to have an indolent clinical course with gradually progressive symptoms.[15]

Notes

1. In lung abscess caused by S. aureus or K. pneumoniae, multiple abscess cavities are relatively common.
2. In aspiration lung abscess, formation of a cavity in the lung or production of foul smelling sputum often takes at least 1-2 weeks after the event of aspiration.[20]
3. Foul smelling sputum:
   - Although foul smelling sputum is generally considered as characteristic of anaerobic lung abscesses, sometimes it is found in aerobic bacterial lung abscesses.
   - Putrid sputum is found in a variable percentage of patients with lung abscess. In one series of about 200 patients with anaerobe implicated aspiration lung abscess, 67% had foul smelling sputum.[19] But in another study of community acquired lung abscess where 28 patient had confirmed lung abscess with anaerobes (pure anaerobic or anaerobes as a part of mixed infection), only 25% had putrid sputum, and in about 7% cases, putrid sputum was present in confirmed aerobic bacterial lung abscesses.[17]
4. Cough may be unproductive in Klebsiella pneumoniae lung abscess; in one series, about one-third of such patients had dry cough.[17]
5. Many cases of *K. pneumoniae* lung abscess do not have the stage of consolidation before abscess formation.[17]

Investigations:

- CBC with CRP and ESR
- Sputum for Gram stain, Acid Fast Bacilli, Fungi, malignant cell and culture;
- Blood culture (aerobic and anaerobic; infrequently positive)
- Other routine tests
- Tuberculin skin test (if TB is suspected)
- Imaging
  - CXR (typical finding: cavity with an air-fluid level; pleural effusion may be present)
  - CT scans of the chest: CT is better than CXR in this regard. CT is more sensitive than CXR and can detect small cavities and obstructing endobronchial lesions; also, it can distinguish lung abscesses from air-fluid levels in the pleural cavity.[19]

How can anaerobic infection in lung abscess be confirmed?

Anaerobic culture of expectorated sputum or any upper respiratory specimen is not useful, because oral anaerobes, which are commonly implicated in lung abscess, are normal flora of the oral cavity and usually contaminate the upper respiratory samples. Some invasive procedures can be used to collect respiratory samples avoiding the contamination with upper airway flora. Special facilities and expertise are needed to perform these procedures. But empiric antibiotic therapy is often effective. So these procedures are not performed routinely and lung abscesses rarely have a confirmed microbial diagnosis.[17]

The specimens that can be considered uncontaminated (by oral anaerobes) include:[17,18]

1. Transthoracic needle aspiration [CT or Percutaneous ultrasound guided (PUTA)]
2. Surgical specimens (during open-lung biopsy)
3. Empyema fluid
4. Blood culture sample (the isolated organism can be regarded as the etiologic agent for lung abscess when lung infection is the only possible source for that blood culture isolate)

Bronchoscopic protected specimen brush (PSB) samples and bronchoalveolar lavage (BAL) fluids are ideally not uncontaminated specimens.[18]

If the same pathogen is isolated in simultaneous blood culture and respiratory specimen cultures, that pathogen can be considered as an etiologic agent.

There are no clear guidelines on the use of invasive procedures to collect pulmonary specimens for the diagnosis of lung abscess. However, most experts suggest their use only when the lung abscess is not responding to early antibiotic therapy.[17]

Complications of lung abscess

- Empyema (found in 5-20% of lung abscess patients in different series)[17-19]
- Bronchiectasis
- Fibrosis (Lung/ pleura)
- Bronchopleural fistula
- Septicemia
- Respiratory failure
- Metastatic brain abscess (rare)
- Amyloidosis (extremely rare; can occur in untreated chronic lung abscess)

Treatment of lung abscess

Empiric antibiotic therapy

- No recommendation on the antibiotic therapy of lung abscess is available from major societies and local practice varies significantly.
- Usually initial empiric antibiotic regimens depend on the circumstance where the lung abscess has developed as well as the clinical context and radiological findings which suggest possible causative pathogens.
- Empiric antibiotic therapy should be broad-spectrum covering mixed infection containing anaerobes, and aerobic gram-positive and gram-negative bacteria.
- In many cases, empiric antibiotic regimens are mostly similar to those for aspiration pneumonia described earlier.
- Empiric Antibiotic treatment should be reviewed after obtaining microbiological test results.

A. Community-acquired lung abscess

<u>Following antibiotics can be used for empiric therapy</u>: (Information from references 17,18,21)

- Co-amoxyclav
- Cefuroxime or Ceftriaxone Plus either Clindamycin or metronidazole
- Levofloxacin Plus either Clindamycin or metronidazole

- Piperacillin- Tazobactam
- Carbapenem (eg, meropenem)

If unresponsive to the initial empiric antibiotic regimen, the antibiotic therapy should be escalated and further investigation should be considered to find the cause. For difficult cases, a pulmonologist (and an infectious disease specialist) should be consulted.

Empiric antibiotic regimens for some common clinical contexts:
(a) For mild to moderate disease
The following initial antibiotic regimens appear reasonable:

- *Co-amoxiclav 1.2g IV 8 hourly*[17]
  Consider to add metronidazole with Co-amoxiclav if anaerobic infection is suspected (fetid sputum, single abscess cavity, severe periodontal disease, alcoholism etc.)
- Alternative to Co-amoxiclav ± metronidazole
  1) Cefuroxime or Ceftriaxone **Plus** either Clindamycin or metronidazole[17] or
  2) Levofloxacin **Plus** either Clindamycin or metronidazole

(b) ***For severe disease***
When lung abscess has developed as a complication of CAP: (eg, Patient's clinical presentation is acute, like CAP, but radiography is suggestive of lung abscess or necrotizing pneumonia). *The empiric antibiotic regimen may be like severe CAP with abscess formation.*
IDSA recommends empiric MRSA coverage for hospitalized CAP patients with abscess formation[11] and the empiric regimen may be:

Piperacillin- Tazobactam (4.5 g IV 6-8 hourly) or carbapenem (eg, meropenem)
Plus
Macrolide (eg, clarithromycin)
Plus
MRSA coverage (IV Vancomycin or linezolid)

If these patients with severe disease have additional increased risk for Pseudomonas infection, double anti-pseudomonal coverage should be considered and the regimen may be:

Piperacillin- Tazobactam + Vancomycin or linezolid + respiratory quinolone (if aminoglycoside is used instead of respiratory quinolone, additional macrolide is needed for atypical bacteria coverage).

Rarely, Legionella causes lung abscess.

(For details please see the treatment of severe CAP in the chapter 'Community acquired pneumonia).

B. Nosocomial lung abscess:

Empiric antibiotic treatment for this category of patients is not mentioned clearly in the literature. However, gram-negative bacteria (including Pseudomonas), S. aureus (including MRSA) as well as anaerobes are the likely pathogens. Therefore, *it seems rational to use the same empiric antibiotic regimens that are used in nosocomial aspiration pneumonia.*

(For details please see the treatment of nosocomial aspiration pneumonia described earlier)

Postural drainage and chest physiotherapy

Chest physiotherapy and postural drainage are controversial. They may cause spillage of the infected debris into other bronchi, and thus may spread infection to the unaffected part of the lung or may cause acute bronchial obstruction.

Other therapeutic measures that may need to consider:

- Adequate drainage if empyema is present;
- Bronchoscopic or percutaneous CT guided drainage of the abscess may be needed in some cases;
- Surgery (Lobectomy or pneumonectomy) may be needed in some cases (infrequently used now-a-days);

  Common indications for surgery:
  - Failure of adequate medical management
  - Neoplasm causing bronchial obstruction
  - Massive or recurrent hemoptysis

Response to treatment

Overall clinical improvement, with improvement of fever, is usually noticed within 3 or 4 days of initiation of antibiotic therapy; fever generally subsides within in 7-10 days. If fever persists beyond this period, the cause of therapeutic failure should be sought and further investigation (CT, bronchoscopy etc) may be needed.

***Causes of failure to improve with medical management include*:**

(1) Presence of bronchial obstruction
(2) Empyema without drainage
(3) Infection with relatively resistant bacteria (eg, P. aeruginosa), mycobacteria or fungi;
(4) Inappropriate antibiotic
(5) Incorrect diagnosis such as non-infectious causes of cavitary lesions like cavitating tumor, pulmonary infarction etc.

*The response to antibiotic therapy may be delayed if the abscess cavity is very large (>6cm in diameter), or when the infection occurs in a preexisting cyst, bulla or sequestrated part of the lung.

Duration of antibiotic treatment

- Antibiotics should be administered until the complete resolution of clinical and radiological abnormalities which usually takes 4-6 weeks.[18,20]
- Prolonged antibiotic therapy (3-6 months or longer) is usually needed for lung abscess due to Actinomyces and Nocardia.
- Antibiotics can be changed to oral form when the patient is afebrile and improved clinically.

Prognosis of lung abscess:

Overall prognosis is now good; in two recent series, the mortality rate was 1-4%.[18,19]

Summary of the empiric antibiotic therapy for aspiration pneumonia and lung abscess

Empiric antibiotic therapy for aspiration pneumonia

A. Community-acquired aspiration pneumonia:

(a) *For mild to moderate disease*

Co-amoxiclav 1.2 g IV 8-hourly

If anaerobic infection is suspected (eg, putrid sputum, alcoholism, or severe periodontal disease), consider to add metronidazole 500 mg IV 8-hourly with Co-amoxiclav 1.2g IV 8 hourly.

Clindamycin monotherapy is the preferred empiric antibiotic therapy in nonsevere community-acquired aspiration pneumonia by many physicians (especially in the USA) although this drug does not cover aerobic gram-negative bacteria.

Dose of Clindamycin: 600 mg 8-hourly IV initially until significant clinical improvement, then 300 mg 6-hourly PO when oral medication is possible.

(b) *For severe disease*

Piperacillin- Tazobactam (4.5 g IV 6-8 hourly) or Carbapenem (eg, meropenem)

±

Vancomycin or linezolid

If patients with community-acquired severe aspiration pneumonia have risk factors for MDR pathogens (eg, Pseudomonas aeruginosa and or MRSA), appropriate empiric antibiotic coverage for them should be considered as mentioned in the treatment of severe CAP.

Consider additional atypical bacteria coverage (eg, by adding clarithromycin) for doubtful cases of community-acquired aspiration pneumonia.

B. Nosocomial aspiration pneumonia:

(a) *For patients with nonsevere nosocomial aspiration pneumonia without any risk factors for MDR pathogens:*

Piperacillin-tazobactam or carbapenem (eg, meropenem)

(b) *For patients with severe nosocomial aspiration pneumonia or nonsevere nosocomial aspiration pneumonia with high risk for both MRSA and Pseudomonas aeruginosa:*

Piperacillin-tazobactam/ Meropenem

Plus

An aminoglycoside (Gentamicin/ tobramycin/ amikacin) or Levofloxacin

Plus

An anti -MRSA drug (Vancomycin/ Linezolid)

However, when a nonsevere nosocomial aspiration pneumonia patient has high risk for either MRSA or Pseudomonas (not for both the pathogens), he or she can receive the coverage for that particular pathogen only.

Empiric antibiotic therapy for lung abscess

A. Community-acquired lung abscess (regimens for some common clinical contexts)

(a) *For mild to moderate disease*
Co-amoxiclav 1.2g IV 8 hourly
Consider to add metronidazole with Co-amoxiclav if anaerobic infection is suspected (fetid sputum, single abscess cavity, severe periodontal disease, alcoholism etc.)
Alternative to Co-amoxiclav ± metronidazole
(1) Cefuroxime or Ceftriaxone Plus either Clindamycin or metronidazole[17] or
(2) Levofloxacin Plus either Clindamycin or metronidazole

(b) *For severe disease*
When lung abscess has developed as a complication of CAP:
Piperacillin- Tazobactam (4.5 g IV 6-8 hourly) or carbapenem
Plus
A macrolide (eg, clarithromycin)
Plus
MRSA coverage (IV Vancomycin or linezolid)

If these patients with severe disease have additional increased risk for Pseudomonas infection, double anti-pseudomonal should be considered.

B. Nosocomial lung abscess:
It seems rational to use the same empiric antibiotic regimens that are used in nosocomial aspiration pneumonia.

References

1. Marik PE. Pulmonary aspiration syndromes. **Curr Opin Pulm Med. 2011;** May;17(3):148-54

2. Paul E. Marik. Aspiration pneumonitis and aspiration pneumonia. **N Engl J Med 2001**; March 1, Vol. 344, No. 9

3. Jason C Kwong et al. New aspirations: the debate on aspiration pneumonia treatment guidelines. **MJA 2011**; 3 October 195 (7)

4. Ehab Daoud et al. Are antibiotics indicated for the treatment of aspiration pneumonia? **Cleve Clin J Med. 2010**; 77(9):573-6

5. Simon O'Connor et al. Aspiration pneumonia and pneumonitis. **Australian Prescriber 2003**; Vol. 26 No. 1

6. Relevant chapters of **Kumar &Clark's Clinical Medicine,** 8th edition; Parveen Kumar and Michael Clark (Editors). Edinburgh, Elsevier, **2012**

7. Relevant chapters of **Davidson's Principles and Practice of Medicine**, 21 edition, Nicki R. Colledge et al (editors). India, Elsevier, **2010**

8. Relevant chapters of **Current Medical Diagnosis and Treatment**; Maxine A. Papadakis et al (Editors). New York, McGraw-Hill, **2013**

9. Acute aspiration. **BMJ best practice 2014;** at: http://bestpractice.bmj.com/best-practice/monograph/528/treatment/step-by-step.htm

10. 'Clinical guideline for hospital management of community acquired pneumonia' on the website of **Royal Cornwall Hospitals (NHS trust, UK);** at: www.rcht.nhs.uk/GET/d10159534

11. Catherine Liu et al. Clinical Practice Guidelines by the Infectious Diseases Society of America for the Treatment of Methicillin-Resistant Staphylococcus Aureus Infections in Adults and Children. **Clin Infect Dis. 2011**; 52(3):285-92

12. 'Double Anaerobic Coverage: What is the role in clinical practice?' on the website of the **Nebraska Medical Center (USA)**; at: http://www.nebraskamed.com/app_files/pdf/careers/education-programs/asp/doubleanaerobiccoverage.pdf

13. Marek Smieja. Current indications for the use of clindamycin: A critical review. **Can J Infect Dis 1998;** 9(1): 22-28

14. Bynum LJ et al. Pulmonary aspiration of gastric contents. **Am Rev Respir Dis. 1976;** 114(6):1129-36.

15. Nader Kamangar. Lung abscess. **Emedicine** (2016). at: http://emedicine.medscape.com/article/299425-overview#showall

16. L. Beth Gadkowski et al. Cavitary Pulmonary Disease. **Clinical Microbiology Reviews, Apr. 2008**, p. 305–333

17. Jiun-Ling Wang et al. Changing Bacteriology of Adult Community-Acquired Lung Abscess in Taiwan: *Klebsiella pneumoniae* versus Anaerob**es. Clinical Infectious Diseases 2005;** 40:915–22

18. Noboru Takayanagi et al. Etiology and Outcome of Community-Acquired Lung Abscess. **Respiration 2010**; 80:98–105

19. JOSÉ DA SILVA MOREIRA et al. Lung abscess: analysis of 252 consecutive cases diagnosed between 1968 and 2004. **J Bras Pneumol. 2006;** 32(2):136-43

20. M. Allewelt et al. Ampicillin + sulbactam vs. clindamycin ± cephalosporin for the treatment of aspiration pneumonia and primary lung abscess. **Clin Microbiol Infect 2004**; 10: 163–170

21. Relevant chapters of **Harrison's Principles of Internal Medicine**; 18 th edition; Dan L Longo et al (Editors). New York, McGraw-Hill 2012

Chapter 7
Urinary Tract Infection (UTI)

Urinary Tract Infection (UTI)

UTI is a common bacterial infection and accounts for 1-2% of consultation in primary care.[1] It is predominantly a female disease except in infancy and after the age of 50. 50%-80% of women experience UTI in their lifetime. After the age of 50, urinary tract obstruction from prostatic hypertrophy increases the risk of UTI in male and the incidence of UTI among male and female becomes similar.[2]

There is a wide variation in practice with regard to the diagnosis and treatment of UTI.

The term UTI includes:

- Asymptomatic bacteriuria (ABU)
- Urethritis
- Prostatitis
- Cystitis
- Pyelonephritis

Risk factors for UTI

1) Female sex (because of short urethra and absence of bactericidal prostatic secretion)
2) Pregnancy
3) Incomplete bladder emptying
   - Urinary tract obstruction at any site (by BPH*, calculus, tumor etc)
   - Neurological disorders (e.g. diabetic neuropathy, multiple sclerosis, spinal cord lesions)
   - Gynecological problems (e.g. uterine prolapse, cervical tumor)
   - Vesicoureteric reflux
4) Impaired natural defenses
   - Diabetes mellitus**; other immunosuppressive diseases or drugs
   - Atrophic urethritis or vaginitis in post-menopausal females
5) Impaired renal function
6) Foreign body in the urinary tract (eg, Urinary catheter, ureteric stent)
7) Being sexually active - UTI is more common among sexually active women; in female, minor urethral trauma during sexual intercourse facilitates infection.
8) Certain types of birth control measures (e.g. Diaphragm and spermicides)
9) History of previous UTI

*BPH: Benign Prostatic Hypertrophy
**Diabetic women (but not men) have two- to threefold increased risk of asymptomatic bacteriuria (ABU) and UTI compared to non-diabetic women.[2]

Classification of UTI

A clear classification of UTI is important for clinical decision making, but there is no widely used such a classification available in the literature.

(1) Depending on the site of infection

- *Upper and Lower UTI:*

- Upper UTI: Infection of the kidney and ureter;
- Lower UTI: Cystitis and urethritis are usually considered as lower UTI. However, in clinical practice, the term 'lower UTI' is frequently used synonymously with 'cystitis.'

(2) Depending on recurrence

- *Relapsing UTI and reinfection*
  - Relapsing UTI: It is the recurrence of UTI with the same organism within two weeks of the end of treatment for the preceding episode.[3] Relapsing UTI indicates that the antibiotic has failed to eradicate the infection.[3] If relapse occurs despite appropriate treatment, the patient should be evaluated for complicating factors for UTI.
  - Reinfection: When a new episode of symptoms of UTI starts at least two weeks after the previous episode, then it is considered as reinfection. Usually it is an infection with a new organism.[4] Reinfection is not always associated with complicating factors; instead, it may be repeated attack of uncomplicated UTI. The recurrence rate is about 20%-30% among women who have experienced one episode of UTI.[2]

Differentiation between relapsing UTI and reinfection ideally needs pre-and post treatment urine culture results. Clinically, if the symptoms of UTI recur within two weeks after the clinical recovery of the preceding episode then it can be considered as relapsing UTI.

(3) Depending on the presence or absence of complicating factors:

- *Complicated and uncomplicated UTI*
  - Generally, acute lower UTI in premenopausal nonpregnant otherwise healthy adult women without any known structural and functional abnormalities of the urinary system is considered as **uncomplicated UTI**, while all other cases are considered as **complicated UTI**.[5-7]
  - Actually the classification of UTI into uncomplicated or complicated is done in two stages: during clinical assessment and during interpretation of lab test results. When clinically the infection appears complicated, some additional lab tests (eg, renal tract imaging) are often performed, which may confirm or rule out the clinical diagnosis of complicated UTI. Treatment of complicated UTI is often different. So the clinical suspicion is very important to avoid the hazards of delayed or missed diagnosis of complicated UTI.

When should UTI be considered complicated?

UTI associated with one or more of the following complicating factors should be considered as complicated UTI:[5,8]

a) Structural and functional abnormalities of the urinary tract
b) Pregnancy
c) Diabetes mellitus
d) Immunosuppressed state
e) Renal impairment
f) Urinary calculi
g) History of recent instrumentation of the urinary tract
h) Foreign body (eg, catheter or ureteric stent) in the urinary tract

i) Presence of any risk factor(s) for health care associated infections such hospitalized for a prolonged period, resident of a nursing home etc. These individuals are at risk of infection with drug resistant bacteria.

Additionally, the following categories of UTIs in adults are generally considered as complicated and should be investigated looking for complicating factors:[5,7,9]

- UTI in men
- UTI in postmenopausal women
- Acute pyelonephritis
- Recurrent UTI

However, some experts do not consider the following forms of UTIs always as complicated UTI; so they do not suggest further tests (eg, urinary tract imaging) in these patients to rule out complicating factors.

1. UTI in Postmenopausal women: Some experts do not consider cystitis in otherwise healthy postmenopausal women as complicated UTI.[10,11] So they do not order further tests in these patients to rule out complicating factors (eg, urinary system ultrasound) unless the attack is severe or recurrence occurs.

2. Acute pyelonephritis: Some experts do not consider acute pyelonephritis in otherwise healthy premenopausal nonpregnant women as complicated UTI.[9,10] So they do not suggest further testing (eg, urinary tract imaging) to rule out complicating factors unless the infection is severe, response to antibiotic is not prompt, or recurrence occurs.

3. UTI in patients with well-controlled diabetes without long term urological complications (such as autonomic neuropathy affecting bladder emptying or diabetic nephropathy);[10]

4. Recurrent UTI: Recurrent cystitis (reinfection) is common in otherwise healthy nonpregnant premenopausal women. Therefore, in clinical practice, some physicians do not suggest further investigations looking for complicating factors (eg, urinary tract imaging) in this group of patients unless the recurrences are frequent (≥3/ year or ≥2/ six month) or unusually severe.[12]

Microbiology:

A. *Uncomplicated UTI*:
Causative organisms are similar for upper and lower UTI;[2] they are usually enteric gram negative bacilli as follows-

- *E. coli* (75-95% cases)[6,13]
- *Staphylococcus saprophyticus/ epidermidis* (5-20%) (more common in younger women)[2,6]
- *Proteus mirabilis, Enterococcus fecalis, Klebsiella aerogenes* and other bacteria (5-10%)[2]

B. *Complicated UTI (including hospital acquired):*[2,12]

- *E. coli* still predominates
- Gram-negative bacilli (Klebsiella, Proteus, *Pseudomonas aeruginosa* etc) are more frequent.

- Gram-positive organisms (Enterococci, *S. aureus* etc.) and yeasts are also important.

Pathogenesis:

Normally bacteria may be found only in the lower end of the urethra. Rest of the urinary tract is free of organisms.[12] Urinary tract infection is usually ascending infection from the urethra to kidney following contamination with enteric bacteria. Hematogenous spread occurs in <2% of cases, and usually very virulent organisms such as Salmonella or *Staph. Aureus* are involved in such cases.[2]

Clinical features of UTI

A. Clinical features of acute lower UTI (cystitis)[12,14,15]

- Acute onset of urinary frequency, urgency and dysuria;
- Suprapubic pain during and after micturition
- Strangury (painful urge to pass more urine after micturition due to spasm of the inflamed bladder)
- Turbid urine
- Foul smelling urine
- Hematuria

These symptoms are due to inflammation of bladder and urethra. Symptoms of only urethritis include urethral discharge, dysuria and urethral pruritus. In clinical practice, the term 'cystitis' and 'lower UTI' are often used interchangeably.[1]

Notes:

1) In women with one symptom of UTI (dysuria, frequency, or hematuria) in the absence of any other apparent explanation for the symptom, the probability of UTI is about 50%.[8,16] Specific combinations of symptoms, such as dysuria and frequency in the absence of vaginal discharge or irritation, increase the probability of UTI to > 90%.[8,16]

2) In women who have symptoms of cystitis as well as vaginal discharge or irritation, vaginal examination and urine culture should be performed. In such cases, it is rational to delay the antimicrobial therapy (if possible) until the test results are available.[9]

3) ***Systemic symptoms, such as fever and rigors, are usually absent in UTI unless upper urinary tract or prostate is involved.***[6,12,15]

B. Clinical features of acute pyelonephritis

- Fever which may be associated with chills and rigors;
- Flank pain and costovertebral angle tenderness;
- Nausea and vomiting are also common[15]
- Symptoms of lower urinary tract infection, such as dysuria, frequency and urgency of micturition, are present only in about one-third of the patients.[12]
- In the elderly, confusion may be the only symptom;[14]

Typical presentation: fever with flank pain and costovertebral angle tenderness;

Suspect acute pyelonephritis in the following conditions:

1) When fever is associated with loin pain and or costovertebral angle tenderness;
2) UTI with fever in female, even in the absence of loin pain or costovertebral angle tenderness;
3) UTI with costovertebral angle tenderness, even in the absence of fever;
4) New-onset confusion in the elderly (as it is a presentation of infection in older people);

Notes

1) In female, fever is the main differentiating feature between acute cystitis and acute pyelonephritis.[2]
2) In male, UTI with fever may be due to acute pyelonephritis or acute prostatitis.[2,15]

C. Clinical features of acute prostatitis

- Fever
- Urinary frequency, urgency and dysuria;
- Perineal, sacral or suprapubic pain;
- Sometimes obstructive voiding symptoms such as poor stream, interrupted urine flow and even retention of urine develop.
- Prostate is highly tender on digital rectal examination (***During rectal examination prostate should be palpated gently; vigorous manipulation may precipitate septicemia***).

Differential diagnosis:

Differential diagnoses of lower UTI

Symptoms similar to those of lower UTI may be produced in many other conditions which include:

1) Urethritis due to sexually transmitted diseases, particularly due to chlamydia[12]
2) Urethritis due to Reiter's syndrome[12]
3) Vaginitis including atrophic vaginitis in postmenopausal females (Vaginitis is more likely than UTI if dysuria is associated with vaginal discharge and irritation)[16]
4) Genital herpes (may cause urethritis and or cystitis)[16]
5) Irritant urethritis, cystitis, or vaginitis (due to contraceptive gel, toiletries etc)
6) Urethral injury related to sexual intercourse
7) Bladder calculi[14] (a chronic condition)
8) Interstitial cystitis (a chronic condition)
9) Bladder cancer (a chronic condition)

Differential diagnoses of acute pyelonephritis

1) Acute appendicitis
2) Pelvic inflammatory disease[14]
3) Diverticulitis
4) Ruptured ovarian cyst
5) Ectopic pregnancy
6) Cholecystitis

7) Perinephric abscess (Characterized by: high fever, toxic appearance, marked loin pain and tenderness often associated with bulging in the loin; but there is no urinary symptoms, pyuria, or bacteriuria)[12]

Urethral syndrome (also known as abacterial cystitis)

The term 'urethral syndrome' has been used by some authors to describe a clinical state of lower urinary tract symptoms (urinary frequency, urgency, dysuria, and suprapubic discomfort) with negative urine culture. However, it has no clear definition and it overlaps with other defined entities such as urethritis due to chlamydia; vaginitis; atrophic vaginitis or urethritis in post-menopausal women; urethritis or vaginitis due to environmental irritants (contraceptive gel, soap etc); and interstitial cystitis. As a result, use of the term 'urethral syndrome' remains controversial. For this reason, 'urethral syndrome' has not been mentioned on the list of differential diagnoses of lower UTI in this chapter.

Interstitial cystitis

Interstitial cystitis (also called painful bladder syndrome) is now considered as a fairly common condition. This chronic condition is characterized by:[17]

1) Pain, pressure, or discomfort in the suprapubic region or surrounding area related to the urinary bladder.
   Plus
2) One or more lower urinary tract symptoms (frequency, urgency etc) for at least six weeks, in the absence of UTI and other detectable causes for the symptoms.

Etiology:

- The exact cause of the disorder is unknown.[15]
- Many patients with interstitial cystitis have other chronic pain disorder such as irritable bowel syndrome and fibromyalgia.
- Several autoimmune disorders such as systemic lupus erythematosus, rheumatoid arthritis and Sjogren's syndrome are more frequent in patients with interstitial cystitis.[18,19]
- Many researchers think interstitial cystitis may be a bladder manifestation of a systemic disorder rather than a particular organ disorder.[19]

Age of onset: It is more common among women, and is typically diagnosed in middle aged individuals although in many cases the disease possibly starts much earlier.[17,18]

Symptoms:

- ***Pain or discomfort in the suprapubic region or surrounding area is considered as an essential diagnostic criterion;*** urinary frequency is a common symptom followed by urgency.[18]
- In interstitial cystitis, daytime urinary frequency is typically >10,[20] while the frequency including nocturia may be up to 60 times/ day.[19] Previously nocturia was regarded as an essential symptom for the diagnosis of interstitial cystitis, but now it is considered that it may develop later in the course of the disease.[18]
- Initially, symptoms may be mild and intermittent.[18]

Diagnosis of interstitial cystitis:

- Interstitial cystitis has no characteristic symptoms or signs. Its presentation is similar to that of many other urological and gynecological disorders, especially urinary infections and bladder carcinoma.[17] As a result, it is a diagnosis of exclusion[19] and the diagnosis is often difficult and delayed.
- Urinalysis and urine culture are always performed to exclude UTI. Urine cytology and cystoscopy are often required.
- The patient should be referred to a nephrologist or urologist when the condition is suspected.

Investigations of UTI

A. For apparently uncomplicated lower UTI

- **In uncomplicated lower UTI** with a clear history (dysuria and frequency in the absence of vaginal discharge or irritation; or any features of acute pyelonephritis) in an otherwise healthy nonpregnant woman of child-bearing age, antibiotic therapy can be given without any investigations[2,8] although urine dipstick test (leukocyte esterase and nitrite test) is often performed.

  A positive dipstick test reinforces the diagnosis; but when the history is strongly suggestive of UTI, negative results of the both dipstick tests do not reliably exclude the infection.[9] In such cases, empiric antibiotic is often effective, so should be prescribed.[5]

- **In all other cases,** *urinalysis* (including dipstick test and urine microscopy) and *urine culture* should be performed.

Notes:

1) ***In cystitis, urine microscopy shows pyuria in almost all cases*** and hematuria in about 30% cases.[2]

2) Bacterial count in urine culture should be interpreted in the light of clinical probability. In symptomatic lower UTI, a colony count $>10^2$ colony forming units (cfu)/ mL in women, and $>10^3$ cfu/ mL in men on midstream (voided) urine culture should be considered as significant bacteriuria.[2] For asymptomatic cases, the $>10^5$ cfu/ml is usually considered as significant bacteriuria (asymptomatic bacteriuria). However, normally bladder urine is sterile, and identification of any bacteria in the suprapubic aspirate is significant.[12]

3) In adult women with uncomplicated symptomatic lower UTI, the sensitivity of urine culture (voided urine) is about 50% when the threshold for positive is considered $>10^5$ cfu/ml traditionally, while the sensitivity is increased to about 95% (with specificity 85%) when the threshold for positive is considered $>10^2$ cfu/ml.[2,21]

4) In practice, most clinical labs (in the USA) do not count the bacterial colonies below a threshold of 10^4 cfu/ml in voided urine samples and a report of 'no growth' is given in such cases. Therefore, a 'no growth' report in women with urinary symptoms should be interpreted cautiously,[9] as many of them actually have UTI with low colony count.

B. For patients with fever, suspected pyelonephritis, or complicated UTI:

- **Commonly considered tests:**
  Urinalysis; urine culture; CBC; CRP; blood glucose; urea, creatinine and electrolyte; blood culture; imaging of the urinary system; digital rectal examination in male and pelvic examination in female;[12]
- **Additional tests may need to perform:**
  - *Cystoscopy* in patients with persistent hematuria or when bladder pathology such as neoplasm is suspected[12]
  - *Urodynamic studies* to evaluate voiding dysfunction in some patients

Imaging study of the urinary system:

- Usually *ultrasonography or CT scan* is considered[1,12] with ultrasound being the most commonly performed first imaging.
- CT is better than Ultrasonography in this regard.[1]
- Sometimes, conventional IVU or CT urogram, or MRI is considered.
- Ultrasound may be more effective than IVU in detecting incomplete bladder emptying. In contrast, ultrasound is not as effective as IVU in detecting urinary calculi; however, addition of plain X-ray with ultrasound can solve this problem.[22]
- MRI can be used instead of CT in patients with iodinated contrast allergies.[1]

Notes:

1) In women with recurrent uncomplicated cystitis or pyelonephritis without any complicating factors, routine evaluation with ultrasonography or CT generally has a low diagnostic yield.[9]

2) In developed countries, most labs now use automatic analyzers for microscopic examination of urine. The automatic analyzers may be 4-5 times more sensitive than conventional manual microscopy;[23] so cell counts will be much higher.

3) Urgent renal tract ultrasound should be considered in a patient presenting with high fever, loin pain and costovertebral angle tenderness to rule out obstructed pyonephrosis.[1]

4) CT Urogram is the single most yielding imaging for the evaluation of the urinary tract for calculi and neoplasms.[24] However, cystoscopy is still required to detect bladder pathology in some conditions, such as in some cases of hematuria.

5) Patients with macroscopic hematuria or persistent microscopic hematuria after resolution of a UTI should be evaluated for bladder and upper urinary tract pathology by cystoscopy and CT urogram; also a urology consultation should be considered.[14]

Some essential information on urine testing

A. Urine dipstick tests in UTI:

For the diagnosis of UTI, urine dipstick tests for leukocyte esterase and nitrite are often performed.

a) Leukocyte esterase dipstick test can detect significant pyuria.

b) Nitrite dipstick test can detect significant bacteriuria.

- ***Leukocyte esterase test:*** The enzyme leukocyte esterase is released by polymorphonuclear leukocytes. Leukocyte esterase test can detect this enzyme when polymorphonuclear leukocytes (intact or lysed) are present in urine.

  Causes of false positive results:
  1) Conditions that cause sterile pyuria[25]
  2) Urine sample contaminated by vaginal secretions.[24]

- ***Nitrite test:*** Normally, nitrates are excreted by the kidneys, but nitrites are not found in urine. Some bacteria can reduce urinary nitrates to nitrites; dipstick for nitrite test can identify the urinary nitrite. Gram-negative enteric bacteria (including *E. coli*), which are the most common cause of UTI, reduce nitrate in urine to nitrite.

  Causes of false negative results of nitrite test:
  1) Gram positive uropathogens such as *Staphylococcus saprophyticus* and Enterococcus usually do not produce the enzyme nitrate reductase which reduce nitrate to nitrite; therefore, in infection with these bacteria, the dipstick test for nitrite will be false negative.[24]
  2) Enough nitrite may not accumulate in urine to give a positive result for the nitrite test when dietary nitrate consumption is low[25] or when a woman with acute cystitis drinks a lot and urinates frequently.[2]

  The cause of false positive result of nitrite test:
  - The reagent of nitrite dipstick is sensitive to air exposure; if they are exposed to air for a long time, the test result may be false positive. The strip containers should be closed quickly after removing a strip.[25]

Sensitivity and specificity of dipstick tests in culture confirmed UTI[25]

Test	*Sensitivity (%)*	*Specificity (%)*
Leukocyte esterase	72-97	41-86
Nitrites	19-48	92-100
Leukocyte esterase or nitrites	46-100	42-98

Interpretation of the dipstick test results

- The positive result for either leukocyte esterase or nitrite can be considered as dipstick test positive for UTI.[2]
- Nitrite test is less sensitive but more specific for UTI than leukocyte esterase test.[25] When dip stick test for both leukocyte esterase and nitrite are positive, it is highly suggestive of acute UTI (sensitivity 75% and specificity 82%)[1]
- Positive dipstick test result reinforces UTI diagnosis when symptoms are suggestive. In doubtful cases of UTI, such as patients with only one symptom of UTI, positive dipstick test increases the probability of UTI from 50% to up to 80%.[2]
- False negative results of these tests are common.[1,26] Negative results even of both the tests do not exclude UTI when symptoms are suggestive. Urinalysis and urine culture should be

performed in such cases.[26] However, if clinical suspicion of UTI is strong, empiric antibiotic can be started pending the culture results.[5]

- In asymptomatic elderly with positive dipstick test for UTI, urine culture is not indicated.[27]

B. Urinalysis

Normal range of some very important components:

- Specific gravity: 1.003-1.030
- pH: 4.5-8; often acidic, between 5.5-6.5
- Urine microscopy (Manual microscopy)
  - Epithelial cells: <15-20/HPF
  - WBC: <2-5/HPF; in male usually <2 and in female <5/HPF[25]
  - RBC: theoretically none; may be 0-2/ HPF; however, in a properly collected sample, if one or more RBCs are found in each high power field, it may be pathological.[28]
  - Casts: Hyaline casts 0-5 /Low power field
  - Bacteriuria (Gram-stain): Reference range depends on clinical scenario and the specimen type. 5 bacteria/ HPF represent approximately 10^5 cfu/ml.[25]

Causes of sterile pyuria:[29,30]

- Antibiotic use before collecting the urine sample;
- Sexually transmitted infections (chlamydia, *Neisseria gonorrhoeae*, mycoplasma, ureaplasma, herpes simplex infection etc)
- Genitourinary tuberculosis
- Fungal UTI
- Gynecological infection
- Interstitial nephritis or analgesic nephropathy
- Interstitial cystitis
- Urinary calculi
- Urinary tract neoplasms
- Nonbacterial prostatitis
- Appendicitis (when the appendix is in contact with a ureter or the bladder)
- Recent injury or irritation to the urinary tract (eg, catheterization, instrumentation etc)

C. Contaminated urine sample

Urine sample may be contaminated during collection by periurethral and perineal materials. Usually contaminated samples are detected on urine microscopy and culture.

(1) *Contamination detection on Urine microscopy*

Suspect a urine sample as contaminated if microscopy shows high numbers of epithelial cells (on conventional microscopy: >15-20/HPF; on automated microscopy: >55/μL). Culture of such a sample with high epithelial cell count may be false-positive, so a positive urine culture in the presence of high epithelial cell count should be interpreted cautiously.[23]

However, the presence of some squamous epithelial cells in midstream urine is common, and only about one-fifth of the samples with some squamous epithelial cells have bacterial contamination. Therefore, in women, the presence of some squamous epithelial cells in urine is not a good indicator of bacterial contamination.[31]

(2) *Contamination detection on Urine culture*

Generally, the growth of a single type of bacteria at high colony counts is considered as positive urine culture.

Suspect contamination:

a) If the growth is polymicrobial or
b) If the bacteria grow at a low colony count or
c) If the grown bacteria are not usual uropathogen

a) Polymicrobial growth:

- True polymicrobial UTI is rare.[31] Therefore, suspect bacterial contamination if the growth is polymicrobial, particularly if the organisms include *Lactobacilli, Corynebacteria* or other common nonpathogenic vaginal or periurethral bacteria or skin flora. However, true polymicrobial UTI can occur in the presence of ileal conduit, neurogenic bladder, vesicocolic fistula, urinary calculi, or long term indwelling catheter.[31]

- In polymicrobial growth, if one type of bacteria is dominating with significantly higher colony counts than the others, for example, 10^6 colony forming units (cfu)/mL versus 10^2 cfu/mL, then the predominant bacteria is likely the pathogen, and its identification and susceptibility test should be considered.

b) Low colony count:

- Contamination is likely when only small numbers of bacteria grow,[31] particularly the growth of multiple bacteria at low colony counts generally indicates contamination. However, the growth of a single type of usual uropathogen at a low colony count in a symptomatic patient may be true UTI, so should be interpreted cautiously.
- The growth of a single type of usual uropathogen at a low colony count is particularly significant in men, since contamination is not common in men.[31]
- The low colony counts are also significant when the samples are collected using a technique that minimizes contamination, such as a sample collected via a catheter.

c) Growth of bacteria which are not usual uropathogen

- *Typical uropathogens:*
  - E. coli
  - Staphylococcus saprophyticus
  - Enteric Gram negative bacteria other than E. coli
- When culture grows other organisms than these typical uropathogens, contamination is generally suspected. Vaginal and skin floras are common contaminants. However, sometimes, non-uropathogens can cause UTI, particularly in immunocompromised hosts and following instrumentation of the urinary tract.
- *Vaginal flora:*
  - Lactobacilli, Diphtheroids, *Staphylococcus epidermidis, Staphylococcus aureus,* Streptococcus species, *E coli,* Klebsiella, Peptostreptococcus species, Bacteroides species etc.[32]
- *Skin flora:*
  - *Staphylococcus epidermidis, Staphylococcus aureus,* Diphtheroids etc.

What can be done, when contamination is suspected?

Consider to repeat urine testing with possible precautionary measures to avoid contamination and take the therapeutic decisions carefully. Collection of urine sample using a urethral catheter can minimize and by suprapubic aspiration can eliminate the risk of contamination.

Notes:

- **Contamination is uncommon in men.**[31]

- **During assessment of a urine culture report three additional factors (other than the information about the growth) need to consider:**
    1) How the sample has been collected (midstream urine/ catheter urine/ suprapubic aspirate)
    2) Urinalysis results
    3) Patient's symptoms and signs

- **No growth means?**
    - 'No growth' report of a urine culture does not necessarily mean no organisms have grown there; often, in clinical microbiology lab, colony count <10^3 or 10^4 cfu/ml are not counted and reported as 'no growth.'

Treatment of UTI

A. Treatment of UTI without complicating factors

- Among otherwise healthy nonpregnant premenopausal women who present with **dysuria and frequency without vaginal discharge or irritation the probability of cystitis is > 90%.**[8,9,16] Lab tests, such as dipstick test or urine culture, are not necessary for these cases before initiating antibiotic treatment.[2]
- Empiric antibiotic regimens are very diverse and largely depend on local resistance pattern.
- In the USA, trimethoprim- sulphamethoxazole (TMP-SMX) and nitrofurantoin are considered as the first-line empiric antibiotic for uncomplicated cystitis in premenopausal women, while the second-line agents are fluoroquinolones (eg, ciprofloxacin) and β-lactams (eg, cephalosporins).[9] However, trimethoprim- sulphamethoxazole (TMP-SMX) should be avoided if local resistance is > 20% or used for UTI in the last three months.[13]
- In some parts of the developing world, uropathogens resistance to TMP-SMX and fluoroquinolone is probably high, while cephalosporins and nitrofurantoin have good efficacy. In such areas, nitrofurantoin or a cephalosporin may be used preferentially.
- Generally, it is considered that the rate of pathogen eradication is lower with beta-lactam therapy, so rate of relapse is higher.[2] However, when beta-lactam antibiotics (eg, cephalosporins) are given for longer than 5 days, cure rates are higher, 77 to 92%.[21]
- Duration of treatment usually depends on the site of infection, presence or absence of complicating factors and the drug used. In general, **shorter course of antibiotic is associated with increased rate of relapse.**[33]

Empiric antibiotic regimens for UTI without complicating factors (Information from references 2, 9, 12, 15, 34)

Clinical state	***Drug***	***Dose***	***Duration***
Acute lower UTI /cystitis (in premenopausal nonpregnant otherwise healthy women and otherwise healthy young men)	(a) TMP-SMX, **or**	One DS tablet bid PO	For women 3 days; for men 10-14 days
	(b) Nitrofurantoin, **or**	100 mg bid or 50 mg 6 hourly PO	At least 5-7 days
	(c) Ciprofloxacin, **or**	250-500 mg bid PO	For women 3 days; for men 10-14 days
	(d) Cefuroxime, **or**	250 mg bid PO	7-10 days; for men 10-14 days
	(e) Cephalexin	250-500 mg 6 hourly PO	7-10 days; for men 10-14 days
Acute pyelonephritis (in nonpregnant women)	Outpatient therapy Ciprofloxacin, **or** Cefpodoxime In-patient therapy (a) Ciprofloxacin 400 mg bid, **or** (b) Cefuroxime 750 mg 8 hourly, **or** (c) Ceftriaxone 1g every 12 or 24 hour, **or** (d) Gentamicin 5mg/Kg daily (in 3 divided doses),**or** (e) Amikacin 15mg/Kg daily (in 3 divided doses), **or** (f) Ampicillin 1g 6 hourly + Gentamicin1mg/Kg 8 hourly In severe cases: Piperacillin-tazobactum 4.5g tid, **or**	Oral therapy can be considered for mild to moderate cases in otherwise healthy nonpregnant women) 500-750 mg bid PO 200 mg bid PO IV IV IV IM/ IV IM / IV IV IV	Usually 14 days for both outpatient and inpatient therapy.

	Imipenem-cilastatin, **or** Meropenem *An Aminoglycoside can be combined with ceftriaxone or Piperacillin-tazobactum		
Acute bacterial prostatitis	Ciprofloxacin 500-750 mg bid, **or** TMP-SMX One DS tablet bid; *(Most antibiotics can penetrate acutely inflamed prostate)*	PO	21-28 days
	For systemically ill patients: *(broad spectrum beta lactams are preferred)* (a) Piperacillin-tazobactam ± Aminoglycoside; **or** (b) Ceftazidime/ ceftriaxone ± Aminoglycoside *(add aminoglycosides in severe cases or when history of recent antibiotic therapy is present)*	IV	
Chronic bacterial prostatitis	Ciprofloxacin 250-500 mg bid, **or** Ofloxacin 200-400 mg bid	PO	4-6 weeks; for recurrence -12 weeks

Maintain adequate hydration if necessary with IV fluids.

Symptomatic treatment of dysuria

- Drink plenty of fluid
- Hot sitz bath
- Phenazopyridine 200 mg three times daily after meal (maximum for two days). Phenazopyridine is widely used but can cause significant nausea and headache. Urine and soft contact lenses may turn to yellow or red. So contact lens should not be used during treatment with this drug.
- Potassium citrate (a urine alkalinizing agent) may be helpful.
- Antispasmodics may help to reduce bladder spasm but should be used cautiously.

Response to treatment:

- Usually the response is rapid.

- For cystitis in women, if the symptoms persist or recur within two weeks of treatment, perform urine culture and sensitivity test; investigations to look for complicating factors may also need to consider. Empiric antibiotic therapy with a broad spectrum antibiotic such as a fluoroquinolone (or another agent, depending on the local resistance pattern) should be considered while awaiting the test results.[2,9]
- In acute pyelonephritis, fever usually subsides within 72 hours. Failure to respond may be due to the presence of one or more complicating factors, antimicrobial resistance, or inadequate treatment.[12,15] If the response is not prompt, reculture urine and perform renal tract imaging (ultrasound or CT) if not already done.[12,15]
- In acute pyelonephritis, continue the intravenous antibiotic (if initiated) for 24-48 hours after the fever subsides, then it can be changed to oral form.[15,33]

Follow-up:

- Follow-up urinalysis and urine cultures are usually not considered for women with uncomplicated lower UTI whose symptoms have resolved with treatment.[21] However, of these patients who had hematuria, for them, follow-up urinalysis and urine culture to confirm that the infection and hematuria have resolved are probably justified.
- In acute pyelonephritis, follow-up urinalysis and urine cultures should be performed 1-2 weeks after completion of the treatment.[21]

**Acute uncomplicated cystitis usually does not progress to severe disease, even if left untreated, but quick relief of symptoms is important.*[9]

B. Treatment of complicated UTI

- The therapeutic decision must be individualized. The complicating factors should be addressed properly. Consultation with urology or nephrology team and sometimes with infectious disease specialists may need to consider.
- Although E. coli is the predominant organism, a wide range of organisms can cause a complicated UTI[3,34] and multidrug resistant infection is also common.[9]
- Antibiotic therapy should be directed by the culture and sensitivity results. So when clinically feasible, antimicrobial therapy should not be started before the culture and sensitivity results are available.[3]
- If the antibiotic therapy cannot be delayed, empiric broad spectrum antibiotic therapy, considering the local resistance pattern, should be started.[34]
- The resistance pattern seen in the previous urine culture results[2] and the history of recent antibiotic exposure (usually recently used antibiotics are avoided) should also be taken into account during selecting empiric antibiotic for the current episode of the infection.

Empiric antibiotic regimens for complicated UTI

The recommendations for empiric antimicrobial therapy in complicated UTI are unclear in the literature. The following empiric regimens can be considered:

(a) For cystitis, oral therapy is often adequate.[3] A fluoroquinolone (eg, Ciprofloxacin) or another broad spectrum antibiotic depending on local resistance pattern can be used.[9] Duration of treatment: 7 days or longer[9]

(b) Highly effective parenteral drugs for complicated cystitis or pyelonephritis include:[3]

1) Aminoglycosides
2) Ceftazidime
3) Carbapenems
4) Piperacillin- tazobactam

(c) For complicated pyelonephritis with risk factor for MRSA:[9]
Piperacillin–tazobactam or carbapenem,
Plus
Vancomycin

Recommendations from European Association of Urologists on empiric antibiotic therapy in complicated UTI (cystitis/ pyelonephritis) [34]

(a) *Initial empiric treatment for mild or moderate complicated UTI*
1) Ciprofloxacin (PO/ IV), **or**
2) Ceftriaxone, **or**
3) Aminoglycoside (eg, gentamicin or amikacin)

*The above mentioned drugs can be used when local resistance is not high.

(b) *For severe infection, or when initial empiric therapy fails:*
A broader-spectrum antibiotic coverage including pseudomonas coverage should be considered:
1) Piperacillin-tazobactam ± aminoglycoside, **or**
2) Ceftazidime± aminoglycoside, **or**
3) Carbapenem± aminoglycoside

*Some patients with complicated pyelonephritis may need additional interventions; for example, percutaneous nephrostomy in acute pyelonephritis occurring in a patient with ureteral obstruction.

*Duration of antibiotic treatment for complicated pyelonephritis may be 14 -21 days.[9]

C. Treatment of UTI in some special situations:

(1) Treatment of UTI in postmenopausal women:

- This is a controversial issue. Generally, UTI (acute cystitis or pyelonephritis) in postmenopausal women is considered as complicated. However, some experts think postmenopausal women should be divided into two groups in this regard: (a) otherwise healthy postmenopausal women and (b) elderly frail with significant comorbidities.[11]

(a) UTI in otherwise healthy postmenopausal women
Acute cystitis in otherwise healthy postmenopausal women:

- This category of patients can be treated with the same drugs used in uncomplicated UTI in premenopausal women.[13]
- Longer duration of treatment, such as minimum of 7 days for cystitis, may be justified.
- Short-term antibiotic therapy is not well established for them.[11] Shorter courses have higher failure rates.[6]

- Although otherwise healthy postmenopausal women have higher rate of recurrent UTI, the risk of serious outcome is not higher compared to premenopausal women.[34,35]

Acute pyelonephritis in otherwise healthy postmenopausal women:
This group of patients can be treated with similar antibiotic therapy used for uncomplicated pyelonephritis in premenopausal nonpregnant women.[11]

(b) UTI in elderly frail women with significant comorbidities:
UTI due to more resistant Gram-negative organisms are common. So cystitis or pyelonephritis in these patients should be treated as complicated UTI.[35]

Which drug is more appropriate for cystitis in elderly women?
This is another controversial issue. In the USA, a multicenter study among elderly women (>65 years; both outpatient and institutionalized) with acute cystitis revealed, in general, eradication rate of bacteriuria was higher when treated with ciprofloxacin (250 mg bid for 10 days) than TMP-SMX (160/800 mg bid for 10 days), with 96% and 80% respectively.[6,36]

(2) UTI in Diabetic patients:

Generally, UTI in a diabetic patient is considered as complicated UTI. However, some experts have different opinions:
A. For acute cystitis in diabetic:
Some experts consider cystitis in otherwise healthy nonpregnant women with well-controlled diabetes as uncomplicated UTI, provided that the patient has no long term urologic complications of diabetes such as difficulty in bladder emptying due to autonomic neuropathy and diabetic nephropathy.[13,34]

They suggest these patients can be treated with the same drugs used for uncomplicated cystitis in premenopausal women. However, A shorter course of antibiotic therapy may not be suitable for them, as even well-controlled diabetes increases the risk of recurrent UTI (although it does not increase the risk of severe outcome).[34] Hence a minimum 7 days' antibiotic treatment can be considered.

B. For acute pyelonephritis in diabetic:
Serious complications of UTI, such emphysematous bladder or kidney, renal abscess, and renal papillary necrosis, are more frequent in diabetic.[37] Therefore, it may be prudent to treat all cases of acute pyelonephritis in diabetic as complicated UTI.

Suggestions in recent German guidelines are somewhat different:[11]

(a) Acute otherwise uncomplicated **cystitis** in women with well-controlled diabetes, without any long term complications of diabetes, can be treated as for uncomplicated cystitis in nondiabetics. Short term antibiotic treatment is justified in these cases.

(b) Acute otherwise uncomplicated **pyelonephritis** in women with well-controlled diabetes, without any long term complications of diabetes, can be treated as for uncomplicated pyelonephritis in nondiabetics. Duration of treatment depends on severity and response to treatment.

(3) UTI in pregnancy:

- Prevalence of UTI in pregnant women is approximately 1–4 %.[33]
- Pathogenesis:
  - Both hormonal and mechanical factors contribute to the development of UTI in pregnancy.
  - Progesterone is a smooth muscle relaxant causing dilatation of the ureter and relaxation of the detrusor muscle of the bladder.
  - Dilated ureter facilitates vesicoureteric reflux.
  - Relaxation of the detrusor muscles of the bladder and mechanical compression of the bladder by the gravid uterus may impede complete bladder emptying; thus facilitate bacterial growth in the bladder.
  - Glycosuria develops in up to 70% of pregnant women, which may also facilitate microbial growth in the urinary tract.[38]

- Microbiology: same as for nonpregnant women[38]

- Treatment of lower UTI (cystitis) in pregnancy:
  - Cephalosporins and nitrofurantoin are widely used.
  - Recently investigators have expressed their concerns about the safety of nitrofurantoin in pregnancy, particularly after 36 weeks because of the risk of hemolytic anemia in the newborn.[33]
  - Resistance of E. coli to ampicillin and amoxicillin is high (20-40%).[38,39]

- Treatment of pyelonephritis in pregnancy:
  - The patient should be hospitalized and antibiotic therapy should be guided by culture and sensitivity results.
  - For empiric antibiotic therapy: parenteral beta lactam drugs such as intravenous 2nd or 3rd generation cephalosporins can be used.

- Duration of antibiotic therapy:
  - For cystitis usually 7- 10 days.[33,38]
  - Shorter course, like 3-day's, is associated with increased rate of relapse in both pregnant and non-pregnant women. As recurrent infection in pregnant women may have serious outcomes, shorter course of antibiotics should be avoided.[33,38]

- Follow-up (test-of-cure) urine culture should be performed 1-2 weeks after finishing the antibiotic treatment, which is usually negative.[39]

(4) UTI (cystitis or pyelonephritis) in men[11]

- UTIs in men are usually complicated and investigations looking for the complicating factors (including urinary tract imaging) must be performed in all cases.[3,11]
- UTIs in men are usually treated as complicated UTI, except cystitis in otherwise healthy young men (<40 years).[10]
- Acute cystitis in otherwise healthy young men[10,11]
  - All cases must be investigated for the possible complicating factors. If no complicating factors are found, acute cystitis in these otherwise healthy young men can be

treated with the same drugs used in uncomplicated cystitis in premenopausal women. However, ***nitrofurantoin, pivmecillinam, and fosfomycin are usually not used in male UTI.***

- Duration of antibiotic therapy is usually longer for male UTI.

***Prostate penetrating abilities of different antibiotics**

- For acute prostatitis: Most antibiotics can penetrate the acutely inflamed prostate.
- For chronic prostatitis:[10]
  - Fluoroquinolones, and to a lesser degree trimethoprim, can achieve the highest concentrations in the prostatic tissue.
  - Nitrofurantoin has insufficient penetrating power.
  - For other drugs, no data are available.

***For suspected acute or chronic prostatitis**, consider urology consultation.

Asymptomatic bacteriuria (ABU)

- **Definitions:**[12,40,41]
  For midstream voided urine: isolation of $\geq 10^5$ cfu/ml of one species of bacteria in an asymptomatic individual.
  For urine sample collected through a urinary catheter: a colony count of $\geq 10^2$ cfu/ml of one species of bacteria in asymptomatic persons.

- **Significance of asymptomatic bacteriuria:**
  - Asymptomatic bacteriuria is a common condition, but not always harmful in adults.[40]
  - It is clearly harmful in pregnant women and patients who undergo traumatic urologic procedures; therefore, these two categories of individuals should be screened for asymptomatic bacteriuria and should be treated if found.[2,40] For all other adult individuals, asymptomatic bacteriuria is generally not considered harmful; therefore, screening for and treatment of asymptomatic bacteriuria in these people is usually discouraged.[2,40]
  - Individuals with asymptomatic bacteriuria are at an increased risk of symptomatic UTI, but treatment of asymptomatic bacteriuria cannot reduce the incidence of symptomatic infection or risk of complications, except in the two specific groups of people mentioned above.[40]
  - Pyuria accompanying asymptomatic bacteriuria is also not an indication for antibiotic treatment.[40]

- According to the IDSA guidelines for asymptomatic bacteriuria (2004),[40] treatment of asymptomatic bacteriuria does not improve outcomes in older people; or in patients with diabetes mellitus, spinal cord injuries or an indwelling catheter. Therefore, screening for and treatment of asymptomatic bacteriuria in these individuals are not recommended.

- **Treatment of asymptomatic bacteriuria** (detected during screening in pregnancy or before a traumatic urologic procedure) should be guided by urine culture and sensitivity results.[2]

Asymptomatic bacteriuria in pregnancy:

- The prevalence of asymptomatic bacteriuria in pregnant women is 2-10%.[33,40]
- **Why important:**
  - Women with asymptomatic bacteriuria have a high risk of developing acute pyelonephritis during pregnancy.
  - Asymptomatic bacteriuria also increases the risk of low–birth weight infants and preterm delivery.
  - Antibiotic therapy can reduce the risk of subsequent pyelonephritis from 20%–35% to 1%–4%.[40] It also reduces the frequency of low–birth weight infants and premature delivery.
- **What should be done for asymptomatic bacteriuria in pregnancy:**
  - All pregnant women should be screened for asymptomatic bacteriuria in the first trimester[41] and should be treated if the results are positive.
  - Cephalosporins or nitrofurantoin can be used.[1,41] However, recently investigators have expressed their concerns about the safety of nitrofurantoin in pregnancy, particularly after 36 weeks.[33]
  - Duration of treatment is usually 3-7 days.[40]
  - A follow-up urine culture should be performed one to two weeks after completion of therapy to ensure eradication of the bacteriuria.[33] Thereafter screening for recurrent bacteriuria should be performed periodically.

Candiduria

- Candiduria is a common laboratory finding.[42]
- Candida in urine may be present in:[43-45]
  - Upper or lower UTI caused by the fungus;
  - Colonization of the urinary catheter or bladder by the organism;
  - Contamination of the sample (commonly candida from the perineal area)
- Fungal UTI is almost always caused by candida species.[43]
- Yeast in urine almost always of candida species, so yeast in urine generally means candiduria.[42]
- Candiduria is mostly a nosocomial problem and rare among healthy individuals with normal urinary tract in the community.[46]
- Candida UTI constitutes 10-15% of nosocomial urinary tract infections.[46] Candiduria develops in about 80% of patients with a Foley's catheter for prolonged periods.[46] However, candidemia is uncommon (just over 1% to up to 10%) among patients with candiduria and usually occurs in patients with multiple underlying disorders.[43]
- Concomitant bacteriuria is identified at the time of funguria in about 25% cases.[43]

Risk factors (or predisposing factors) for candiduria:[42,43,44,46]

- Indwelling urinary drainage devices
- Recent use of antibiotics

- Structural and functional abnormalities of the urinary tract
- Diabetes mellitus
- Immunosuppressed state (due to drug or disease)
- Organ transplantation
- Instrumentation of the urinary tract
- Prolonged hospital stay
- Intensive care unit admission
- Surgery in the preceding months
- Old age
- Female sex

*No risk factors are found in about 10% of cases.[42,43]

Notes:

1) Use of indwelling urethral catheters or other form of urinary drainage devices for prolonged periods is associated with more than 80% cases of candiduria.[42]

2) History of nonfungal infections (often UTI or pneumonia) within one month of the detection of the funguria is present in about 85% of cases, and history of recent antibiotic use is present in about 90% cases of funguria.[43]

Pathogenesis:

Lower urinary tract candidiasis is usually an ascending infection whereas renal parenchymal infection is commonly due to candidemia.[44,46] However, ascending infection of the kidneys can occur in the presence of urinary tract obstruction, concomitant bacteriuria or severe immunosuppression.[44]

Clinical features:

Most patients with candiduria are asymptomatic; however, absence of symptoms does not exclude a treatable infection. A catheterized patient cannot perceive dysuria or frequency and many debilitated patients cannot vocalize symptoms.[42]

In symptomatic candiduria, clinical features of fungal UTI are indistinguishable from those of bacterial UTI.[45] Sepsis and septic shock (which are often associated with pyonephrosis), and renal abscess may develop;[46] fungus ball may also form.[46]

Notes:

1) Many experts think candiduria in neutropenic patients is a marker of disseminated candidiasis and should be treated accordingly.[42]

2) Candiduria with fever may be the only initial manifestation of invasive candidiasis in patients with high-risk of disseminated candidiasis such as neutropenic individuals, transplant recipients, or who have undergone invasive urologic procedure recently.[46]

3) Concomitant pyuria with candiduria generally supports the diagnosis of urinary candida infection. But it may be due to concomitant bacteriuria or mechanical injury to the bladder and urethra from a urinary catheter.[42,46]

4) In most cases, candiduria does not cause candidemia unless urinary tract obstruction is present.[46]

What should be done when candida species are detected in urine?

Contamination of the urine sample with the fungus is common. Therefore, the first step is to determine whether it is true candiduria or just a contaminated sample by repeating the urinalysis and urine culture.[45]

<u>To avoid contamination of the repeat sample, consider the followings:</u>[45]

1) Collection of a midstream clean-catch urine sample (often satisfactory);
2) If the patient is unable to collect a midstream clean-catch sample, collect specimen through a urethral catheter or suprapubic aspiration.
3) For patients with an indwelling catheter, replace the catheter with new one before collecting the repeat sample.

If no fungus is found in the repeat sample, further diagnostic workup is not necessary.[45]

Follow the algorithm and description below for detailed management.

Please see the next page for candiduria management algorithm.

Simplified algorithm for the management of candiduria (Mainly based on information from references 44-47)

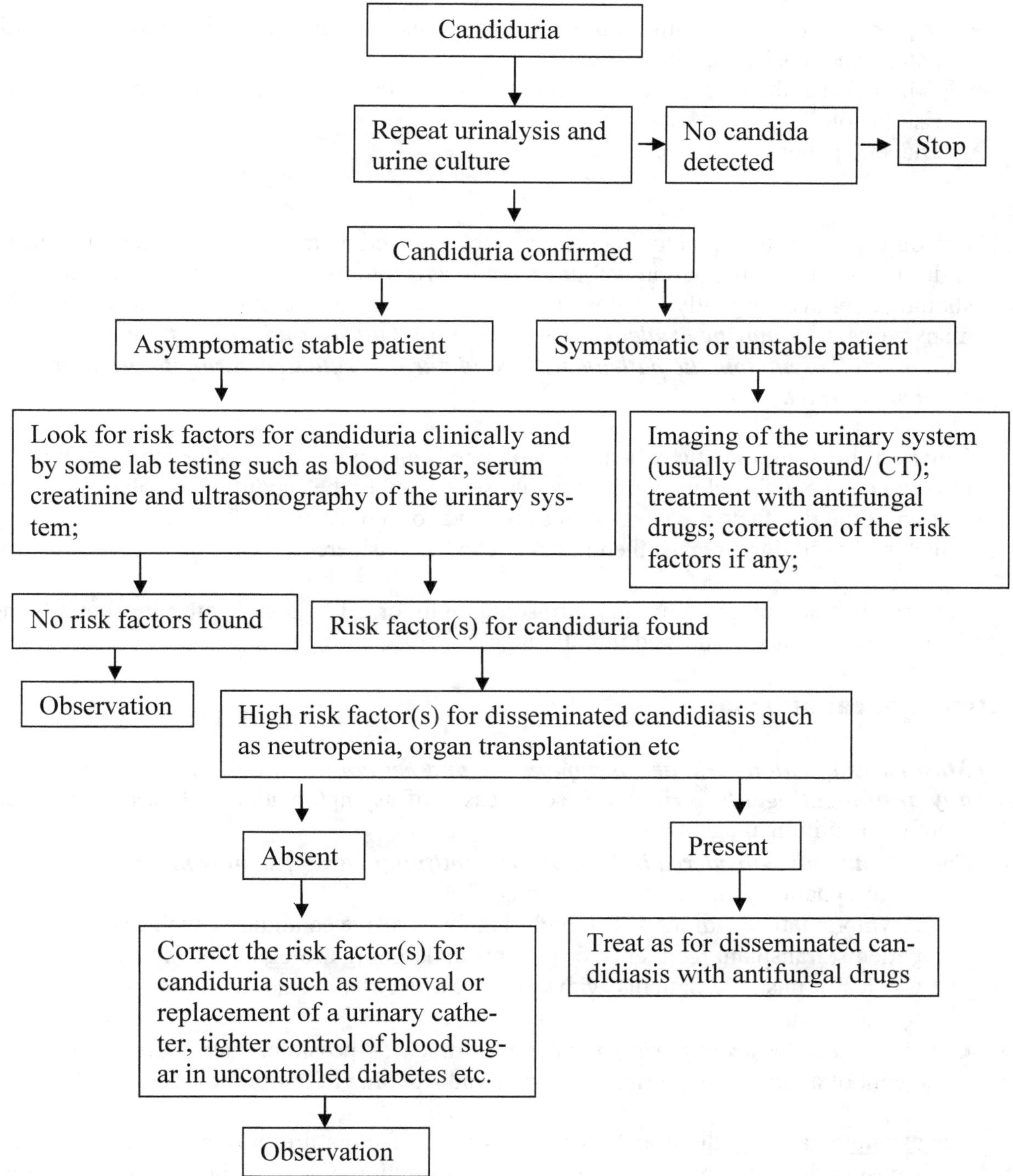

Indications for renal tract imaging in candiduria:

- For symptomatic cases: Imaging of the urinary system to rule out abscess, fungus ball, or urologic abnormalities is indicated in all symptomatic cases.[45]

- For asymptomatic patients: There is some controversy about when imaging should be performed in asymptomatic cases. Some physicians suggest that it should be performed in the following conditions:
  - Who need treatment with antifungal drugs[47] (eg, patients with high risk of disseminated candidiasis; unstable patients)
  - Who has risk factor(s) for candiduria, but the candiduria persists after correction of the risk factor[44]
  - Diabetic patients[44]

Notes:

1) Urologic abnormalities, including urinary tract obstruction, are risk factors for candiduria and if urinary tract obstruction is found even in asymptomatic patients with candiduria, it should be relieved urgently.[44] Clinically, urinary obstruction cannot be diagnosed in many cases, so ***it may be prudent to perform at least ultrasound study of the urinary system in all asymptomatic patients with candiduria to rule structural abnormalities of the urinary tract.***

   However, in asymptomatic patients, when there is an obvious risk factor for candiduria, imaging can be deferred in some cases to assess whether the candiduria resolves with correction of the risk factor, such as such as removal or replacement of an indwelling urinary catheter. If candiduria persist then imaging can be considered.

2) For urinary tract imaging, usually ultrasonography or CT is done, with ultrasound being the most commonly performed initial imaging.

Treatment of candiduria:

- ***Most cases of candiduria are asymptomatic and benign in nature, and resolve without any antifungal agents.***[44] However, some cases of asymptomatic candiduria need treatment with antifungal agents.
- ***Some commonly considered indications for antifungal drug use in candiduria:***
  - Symptomatic cystitis or pyelonephritis[44,47]
  - Asymptomatic candiduria with high risk for invasive candidiasis such as neutropenic patients, transplant recipients; or patients undergoing urologic procedures.[46,47]
  - Clinically unstable patients with candiduria even when no symptoms of cystitis or pyelonephritis.[44]
- ***Correction of the predisposing factor(s)*** as much as possible, such as removal or replacement of an indwelling urinary catheter and stopping of antibiotic, is essential.

  For asymptomatic candiduria: When predisposing factors are present, correction of the predisposing factors may be sufficient for the resolution of the candiduria in many cases. For example:
  - Indwelling urinary catheter associated asymptomatic candiduria may be eliminated after replacement or removal of the catheter in 20 – 40% of cases;[44,46]
  - Asymptomatic candiduria in an elderly patient with uncontrolled diabetes may resolve completely with tighter glycemic control;[44]
  - Antibiotic associated candiduria often disappears shortly after stopping the antibiotics;[44]

- Candiduria in a patient with benign prostatic hyperplasia and mild obstruction can resolve with a peripheral α-adrenergic blocker. [44]

Close follow–up is needed for these asymptomatic candiduria patients with predisposing factors.

- **Antifungal drug selection for candiduria**
  - There are controversies about what anti-fungal agents are appropriate for a particular case of candiduria.[46]
  - All antifungal drugs cannot achieve good concentration in urine, so not suitable for the treatment of urinary tract candidiasis.
  - ***Fluconazole*** can achieve high concentration in urine in its active form and is relatively less toxic; therefore, this antifungal agent is usually considered as the drug of choice for the empiric therapy of candida infection of the urinary tract.[44,47] Oral form of the drug is usually adequate for cystitis and most cases of pyelonephritis.[44]
    Dose of Fluconazole:[44]
    For cystitis, 200 – 400 mg/day for14 days;
    For pyelonephritis, 400mg/day for 14 days
    Other azoles and echinocandins are generally not considered useful, as they cannot achieve good concentration in urine.[44,47]
    If isolated candida is resistant to fluconazole, oral flucytosine (more toxic than fluconazole and develops resistance when used alone) and or parenteral amphotericin B can be given.[44,47]
  - ***Bladder irrigation with amphotericin B***, which can clear candiduria, can be considered in fluconazole resistant candida cystitis and in patients with fungus ball. However, the therapy is uncomfortable for non-catheterized patients and relapse rate is high; hence this option is not commonly used.[44,47]
  - ***Urinary fungus ball:*** Systemic anti-fungal drug therapy along with aggressive surgical debridement and sometimes local irrigation with amphotericin B is usually performed.[44,47]

Note:

- Some patients with asymptomatic candiduria with risk factor(s) for candiduria will need treatment with anti-fungal agents (as mentioned above), but the differentiation between the patients who need and who do not need treatment with antifungal drugs is difficult in some cases. No diagnostic tests or clinical criteria are available to distinguish between the two groups reliably.[46] As a result, empiric use of antifungal agents is likely to continue inappropriately in many cases.[44]
- Consultation with nephrology team and sometimes with infectious disease specialists may be needed for difficult cases.

Catheter-associated urinary tract infection (CA-UTI)

- In the USA, urinary catheters are used in 15-25% of hospitalized patients.[48]
- There are controversies regarding definition and treatment of CA-UTI.
- Simply, symptomatic significant bacteriuria in a catheterized patient can be considered as CA-UTI.

- UTIs are the fourth most common form of healthcare-associated infections in the USA and accounts for >12% of healthcare associated infections.[49] Virtually all healthcare-associated UTIs are related to instrumentation[49] with about 75% being associated with a urinary catheter use.[48]
- All forms of urinary catheters- indwelling urethral, suprapubic, or condom catheters- impose some risk for UTI. However, condom catheters may be less hazardous.

Definitions:

Catheter-associated urinary tract infection (CA-UTI)

CA-UTI can be defined as significant bacteriuria ($\geq 10^3$ cfu /ml) with otherwise unexplained symptoms and signs of UTI in a patient with a urinary catheter or who was catheterized within the last 48 hours.[50]

Catheter associated asymptomatic bacteriuria (CA-ASB)

The term catheter associated asymptomatic bacteriuria (CA-ASB) refers to significant bacteriuria ($\geq 10^5$ cfu/ml) in a catheterized patient without any symptoms and signs attributable to UTI.[50,51]

Catheter-associated bacteriuria (CA-bacteriuria)

It is a nonspecific term used to describe bacteriuria in a catheterized patient. It can be used when no distinction has been made between catheter associated asymptomatic bacteriuria (CA-ASB) and catheter-associated UTI (CA-UTI).[50]

Epidemiology:

Following insertion of an indwelling urinary catheter, the daily incidence of bacteriuria is 3-8%.[50] and within a few weeks, almost all patients develop bacteriuria.[51] However, in most cases, the bacteriuria is asymptomatic (i.e. CA-ASB) and only a small percentage of CA-ASB patients develop symptomatic urinary infection (i.e. CA-UTI) from time to time.[51]

Microbiology:[50,51]

- ***E. coli is the most frequently isolated organism*** although it is isolated in less than one-third of cases.[50]
- ***Isolated other organisms include:***
    - Other Enterobacteriaceae, e.g., *Klebsiella*, *Proteus*, *Serratia*, and *Enterobacter* species; Nonfermenters e.g., Pseudomonas aeruginosa;
    - Gram-positive cocci e.g., coagulase-negative *Staphylococci* and *Enterococci*;
    - Fungus- mostly Candida species

Notes:

1) In CA-UTI, polymicrobial infection is common with long-term catheterization, while monomicrobial infection is common with short-term catheterization.[50]
2) Proteus mirabilis is commonly found in CA-UTI with long-term catheterization.[51]
3) Antimicrobial-resistant organisms are frequently isolated in CA-UTI.[51]

Pathogenesis:[50,51]

- The infection is usually ascending. In catheter-associated bacteriuria, about two-thirds of the uropathogens enter into the bladder along the external surface of the catheter.[50]

- Biofilm formation plays the most important role in the pathogenesis of catheter-associated bacteriuria.[51]
- Biofilm is a layer of living bacteria with mucopolysaccharide produced by them; Tamm-Horsfall protein and urinary salts are also incorporated into the biofilm.[50,51]
- Biofilm is formed on both the inner and outer surfaces of the catheter. It provides a protected environment for the bacteria. Bacteria multiply in the biofilm and shed from it.[50,51]

Clinical features of CA-UTI:

- Patients with CA-UTI usually do not have typical clinical features of UTI, as catheterized patients cannot perceive dysuria, urinary frequency or urgency. However, the classic features may develop after removal of the catheter.
- Symptoms and signs of CA-UTI are usually nonspecific and include new-onset or worsening of fever, rigors, confusion, malaise, or lethargy without any other identified cause.[50]
- ***Most patients present with new onset or worsening of fever without localizing features.***[50,51]
- Localizing features such as flank pain, renal angle tenderness, acute hematuria, or suprapubic pubic pain or discomfort help to identify urinary origin of the fever, but these features are not commonly present.[51]
- Foul smelling and or turbid urine in a catheterized patient is often considered as evidence of CA-UTI, but actually clinical significance of these features is controversial. Odorous or turbid urine can occur without bacteriuria;[50] hence, probably it is not justified to order urine culture or initiate antimicrobial therapy in a catheterized patient just for the presence of foul smelling or turbid urine.

Notes:

1) As fever, new-onset confusion, malaise, lethargy etc. are non-specific symptoms of infection, so probable other causes for those symptoms should also be sought carefully before considering them due to UTI in a catheterized patient.
2) ***Fever with bacteriuria in a catheterized patient does not necessarily mean CA-UTI.***
3) In patients with spinal cord lesion, increased spasticity, autonomic dysreflexia, or sense of unease are also suggestive of CA-UTI.[50]

Key investigations when CA-UTI is suspected:

- Urinalysis
- Urine culture and sensitivity
- Blood culture if systemic features of infection (eg, fever, rigors etc.) are present;
- Imaging of the urinary tract (Ultrasound/CT) in some cases;

Urine sample collection[50,51]

1) Patients with short term catheterization (<2 weeks): usually the sample is collected from the catheter port or puncturing the catheter tube with a needle and syringe (if no port is present).
2) Patients with long term catheterization (>2 weeks): replace the old catheter with new one and collect specimen from the new catheter.

*If an indwelling catheter is in place for more than two weeks mature biofilm is usually formed. Urine sample collected through these catheters are generally contaminated by the organisms in the biofilm; therefore, the number of species and the quantity of organisms isolated from these samples may not reflect those in bladder urine.[51]

Pyuria in catheterized patients:

- Pyuria is almost universal among patients with long term indwelling catheterization.
- In catheterized bacteriuric patients, pyuria is usually seen in both asymptomatic (CA-ASB) and symptomatic groups (CA-UTI). However, it can develop in the absence of bacteriuria because of catheter induced inflammation of the bladder.[51]
- Pyuria (of any degree) is not helpful to differentiate between asymptomatic bacteriuria (CA-ASB) and symptomatic UTI (CA-UTI) in catheterized patients.[50]
    - In catheterized bacteriuric patients, the presence of any degree of pyuria alone is neither suggestive of a symptomatic infection (i.e. CA-UTI) nor an indication for antimicrobial therapy.[51]
    - Antimicrobial treatment is not indicated in pyuria accompanying CA-ASB.[50]
- ***A diagnosis other than CA-UTI should be considered if pyuria is absent in a symptomatic patient.***[50]

Diagnosis of CA-UTI:

CA-UTI = Symptoms and signs attributable to UTI in a catheterized patient + significant bacteriuria (i.e., $\geq 10^3$cfu/ml).[50]

The symptoms and signs should not have other explanations.

Significant bacteriuria (According to IDSA guideline 2009)[50]
(1) *To define CA-UTI:*: $\geq 10^3$ cfu /ml

However, in most cases of CA-UTI colony counts are $\geq 10^5$ cfu/ml.

(2) *To define CA-ASB*: $\geq 10^5$ cfu/ml

Notes:

1) In the absence of localizing genitourinary features, identification of the same organism on both the urine and a simultaneous blood culture is suggestive of CA-UTI if no other source of the bacteremia is present.[51]
2) Bacteriuria and pyuria almost always develop in patients with a urinary catheter in place for more than a few weeks; hence only their presence does not necessarily mean CA-UTI.

Treatment

A. Treatment of CA-UTI:

- Remove or replace the urinary catheter.
- Antimicrobial resistance is high in CA-UTI. Therefore, antimicrobial therapy should be directed by culture and sensitivity results.
- Wherever possible, empiric antimicrobial treatment should be delayed until the urine culture and sensitivity results are available.[52] However, in severe cases, or in patients with systemic features of infection or features of pyelonephritis empiric antimicrobial treatment should be started without delay as for complicated UTI.

B. ***Treatment of Catheter-associated asymptomatic bacteriuria (CA-ASB):***

- Treatment is generally not indicated in CA-ASB, unless:[50]
  1) The patient is pregnant, or
  2) The patient undergoes a potentially traumatic urologic procedure.
- Screening for and treatment of CA-ASB is not recommended in other cases (except the above mentioned two groups), as it does not reduce subsequent episodes of symptomatic UTI (CA-UTI); instead, antibiotic resistant strains of the bacteria could emerge.[50]
- In patients with neurogenic bladder managed with intermittent catheterization, screening for and treatment of CA-ASB are not beneficial.[50]
- In general, asymptomatic patients with short- or long-term indwelling urethral catheters do not need to undergo periodic urine testing to check whether there is an infection; and if incidentally bacteriuria (of any degree) is detected in them, it does not need any treatment.
- Because of nonspecificity of symptoms and signs, differentiating CA-UTI from CA-ASB is difficult in many cases; as a result, inappropriate use of antimicrobials in catheter-associated bacteriuria is frequent.

Duration of antibiotic treatment

- The duration of antibiotic therapy is usually 7-14 days.[2]
- When the response is prompt a shorter course of 7 days may be adequate, while for delayed response 10-14 days' treatment should be considered.[50]

Prevention of CA-UTI:

- Of the catheter-associated UTIs up to 69% can be avoided with strictly following infection-prevention guidelines.[53]
- Avoid unnecessary catheterization and remove the catheter as early as possible.[50,51]
- Use condom catheter instead of an indwelling catheter whenever possible.[50,51]
- When feasible, intermittent catheterization is better than an indwelling catheter use, such as in some form of neurogenic bladder (eg, atonic bladder).[54]
- CDC (USA) does not recommend changing chronic indwelling catheters or drainage bags at routine fixed intervals. Instead, it suggests changing catheters and drainage bags depending on clinical indications, such as obstruction or other malfunction in the drainage system, or before initiating antimicrobial therapy for CA-UTI.[54]

Treatment and prevention of recurrent UTI without complicating factors in women

Recurrence of uncomplicated cystitis is common in women.

Main risk factors for recurrent cystitis in otherwise healthy women are:

1) Frequent sexual intercourse
2) Use of spermicides or diaphragm (destroys lactobacilli in vagina)
3) Estrogen deficiency (in post menopausal women)

However, in many cases recurrence occurs without any apparent risk factors.

Empiric treatment of recurrent cystitis without complicating factors in women:

- For initial (first) recurrence: The same first-line drugs (eg, cotrimoxazole or nitrofurantoin) used in the first attack of an uncomplicated cystitis can be used.[16,] however, if the recurrence is within six months of the first attack, a first-line drug other than that was used in the previous attack may be better, because of higher possibility of resistance to the recently used drug.[9]
- For subsequent attacks: A fluoroquinolone or another broad spectrum antibiotic depending on local resistance pattern may be appropriate.

Test-of-cure urine culture

In recurrent UTI, a test-of-cure urine culture may be performed about one to two weeks after completion of the antibiotic treatment to confirm clearance of the bacteriuria.[16]

Prevention of recurrent cystitis without complicating factors in women:

The following preventive measures can be considered: (Information from references 2,9,16)

A. *Antibiotic prophylaxis*
   1) Continuous prophylactic antibiotic
   2) Post coital prophylaxis
   3) Patient initiated therapy

B. *Behavioral modification*

C. *Others*

A. *Antibiotic prophylaxis*

Antibiotic prophylaxis can reduce the risk of recurrence by 95%.[9]

Who should receive antibiotic prophylaxis for recurrent UTI?

- It should be limited to women with three or more recurrences per year, or two or more recurrences per six months where nonantibiotic measures were not effective.[9]
- Patient's preference should also be considered about the preventive strategies.[2]

(1) Continuous prophylaxis:

- Before starting prophylactic antibiotic, urine culture should be negative which confirms that the current episode of the UTI has resolved completely.[9]
- Antibiotic selection is largely influenced by local resistance pattern.
- *Drugs for continuous prophylaxis:*[9,12,16]
  Single daily dose of anyone of the following drugs should be taken at bedtime which helps to achieve a good concentration of the drug in the bladder for a prolonged period.
  a) TMP-SMX 40/200, **or**
  b) Nitrofurantoin 50 – 100 mg, **or**
  c) Trimethoprim 100 mg, **or**
  d) Cephalexin 125-250 mg;
- *Duration:* Usually continuous prophylaxis is initially given for six months, then the antibiotic is discontinued and the patient is observed.[9,16] If recurrent UTIs develop again, prophylaxis is reinstituted and can be continued for longer period (may be 2-5 years).[16]

(2) Post-coital prophylaxis:

For post-coital prophylaxis, single dose of anyone of the following drugs should be taken as soon as possible following intercourse (within 2 hours of the sexual intercourse)[9,16]

a) TMP-SMX 40/200- 80/400 mg, **or**
b) Nitrofurantoin 50 – 100 mg, **or**
c) Trimethoprim 100 mg, **or**
d) Cephalexin 250 mg;

(3) <u>Patient initiated therapy</u> (not strictly a prophylactic measure)
Patients are instructed to commence antibiotic at the start of the first symptom of UTI (with one of the same drugs used in uncomplicated UTI); duration is usually 3 days; if no improvement within 48 hours, the patient should be evaluated by a clinician.[16] These patients can be supplied with urine culture materials with instructions to start urine culture before initiating the antibiotic therapy. The urine culture can be refrigerated until delivered to the caring physician's office as soon as possible.[2]

B. *Behavioral modification:*

1) Reduction in the frequency of coitus (often not feasible)[9]
2) Avoidance of the use of spermicide and diaphragm[9]
3) Drinking plenty of fluid (at least two liters/day)[12]
4) Regular complete bladder emptying
5) Bladder emptying before and after coitus
6) Cleaning of the valva and perineum before and after sexual intercourse;
7) Cleaning front-to-back after urination or defecation;
8) Taking showers rather than bath

However, there is controversy about the efficacy of these behavioral modifications except the first two strategies.

C. *Others*

1) Cranberry juice: Drinking cranberry juice may be useful.
2) Topical estrogen: In post menopausal women, use of estrogen vaginal cream (0.5 mg) at every night for two weeks, then twice a week for 8 months can reduce the incidence of recurrent UTIs.[16]

Treatment and prevention of complicated recurrent UTI

- Complicating factors should be addressed properly. Urology, nephrology, or infectious disease specialist consultation may be required.
- <u>Antimicrobial therapy is not well defined for this category of patients.</u>[16]
    - It should be guided by urine culture and sensitivity results. So when clinically feasible, antimicrobial therapy should not be started before the culture results are available.
    - If antibiotic therapy cannot be delayed, empiric antibiotic should be of broad spectrum.
    - Antibiotic regimens and duration of treatment used for complicated UTI (described earlier under '*treatment of complicated UTI*') can be considered.

- ***Antibiotic prophylaxis is not recommended for complicated recurrent UTI.***[16] When the complicating factor cannot be removed, suppressive dose of antibiotics may be useful.[12,16]

Summary of the management of UTI

Upper and Lower UTI:

Upper UTI: Infection of the kidney and ureter

Lower UTI: Cystitis and urethritis are usually considered as lower UTI. However, in clinical practice, the term 'lower UTI' is frequently used synonymously with 'cystitis.'

Complicated and uncomplicated UTI

Generally, acute lower UTI in premenopausal nonpregnant otherwise healthy adult women without any known structural and functional abnormalities of the urinary system is considered as uncomplicated UTI, while all other cases are considered as complicated UTI.

Microbiology: UTIs are mainly caused by E. coli and other enteric gram-negative bacilli.

Typical clinical features:

- Lower UTI (Cystitis):
  - Acute onset of urinary frequency, urgency and dysuria;
    Systemic symptoms, such as fever and rigors, are usually absent unless upper urinary tract or prostate is involved.

- Acute pyelonephritis:
  - Fever associated with chills and rigors
  - Flank pain and costovertebral angle tenderness;
  - Accompanying symptoms of lower UTI such as dysuria, frequency and urgency are present in about one-third of cases.

  * In female, fever is the main differentiating feature between acute cystitis and acute pyelonephritis; UTI with fever in them is generally suggestive of acute pyelonephritis.

- Acute prostatitis:
  - Fever
  - Urinary frequency, urgency and dysuria;
  - Perineal, sacral or suprapubic pain;
  - Prostate is highly tender on digital rectal examination;

  *In male, UTI with fever may be due to acute pyelonephritis or acute prostatitis.

Investigations:

- Apparently uncomplicated lower UTI in women

- *No investigations are generally needed* for otherwise healthy premenopausal nonpregnant women with clear history of uncomplicated lower UTI (such as frequency and dysuria without any vaginal symptoms).
- *Urinalysis, and urine culture and sensitivity* are necessary for all other cases;

- For patients with fever, suspected pyelonephritis, or complicated UTI:
  - *Commonly considered tests:*
    Urinalysis; urine culture; CBC; CRP; blood glucose; urea, creatinine and electrolyte; blood culture; imaging of the urinary system (often ultrasound); digital rectal examination in male and pelvic examination in female;

Treatment of UTI

Empiric antibiotic therapy for UTI without complicating factors

A. *For acute cystitis*

- Otherwise healthy nonpregnant premenopausal women who present with dysuria and frequency without vaginal discharge or irritation, the probability of cystitis in them is > 90%; no lab tests are necessary for these cases before initiating antibiotic treatment.
  What antibiotic can be given to them?
  - One of the first-line antibiotics can be given.
  - Empiric antibiotic regimens are very diverse and largely depend on local resistance pattern.
  - In the USA, trimethoprim- sulphamethoxazole (TMP-SMX) and nitrofurantoin are considered as the first-line empiric antibiotic for uncomplicated cystitis in premenopausal women, while the second-line agents are fluoroquinolones (eg, ciprofloxacin) and β-lactams (eg, cephalosporins).
  - In some parts of the developing world, uropathogens resistance to TMP-SMX and fluoroquinolone is probably high, while cephalosporins and nitrofurantoin have good efficacy. In such areas, nitrofurantoin or a cephalosporin may be used preferentially as the first-line agents.

B. *For acute pyelonephritis*

- Out-patient therapy: oral Ciprofloxacin or Cefpodoxime;
- In-patient therapy:
  - *In most cases:* Intravenous Ciprofloxacin or 2nd or 3rd generation Cephalosporins or an Aminoglycoside;
  - *In severe cases:* Piperacillin-tazobactum;
    An Aminoglycoside can be combined with Piperacillin-tazobactum or an IV 3rd generation Cephalosporin;

Empiric antibiotic therapy for recurrent uncomplicated cystitis in women:

- For initial (first) recurrence: The same first-line drugs (eg, cotrimoxazole or nitrofurantoin) used in the first attack of an uncomplicated cystitis can be used.[16,] however, if the recurrence is within six months of the first attack, a first-line drug other than that was used in the previous attack may be better because of higher possibility of resistance to the recently used drug.
- For subsequent attacks: A fluoroquinolone or another broad spectrum antibiotic depending on local resistance pattern may be appropriate.

Empiric antibiotic therapy for complicated UTI

- When clinically feasible, antimicrobial therapy should not be started before the culture and sensitivity results are available.
- If antibiotic therapy cannot be delayed, a broad spectrum empiric antibiotic regimen considering local resistance pattern should be considered, which may be:
  - *For mild or moderate complicated UTI (cystitis/ pyelonephritis)*
    Ciprofloxacin (PO/ IV), **or**
    Ceftriaxone, **or**
    An aminoglycoside (eg, gentamicin or amikacin)

    *For cystitis, oral therapy is often adequate.

  - *For severe infection (cystitis/ pyelonephritis), or when initial therapy fails:*
    A broader-spectrum antibiotic coverage including *Pseudomonas* coverage should be considered:
    Piperacillin-tazobactam ± aminoglycoside, **or**
    Ceftazidime± aminoglycoside, **or**
    Carbapenem± aminoglycoside

  Complicating factor(s) should be addressed properly. Referral to a nephrology or urology team may be need.

Treatment of UTI in some special situations:

(1) Treatment of UTI in postmenopausal women:

Generally, UTI (acute cystitis or pyelonephritis) in postmenopausal women is considered as complicated. However, some experts think postmenopausal women should be divided into two groups in this regard: (a) otherwise healthy postmenopausal women and (b) elderly frail with significant comorbidities.

a) *UTI (acute cystitis/ pyelonephritis) in otherwise healthy postmenopausal women*
   - This category of patients can be treated with the same drugs used in uncomplicated UTI (acute cystitis/ pyelonephritis) in premenopausal women.

b) *UTI (acute cystitis/ pyelonephritis) in elderly frail women with significant comorbidities:*
   - UTI due to more resistant Gram-negative organisms are common. So cystitis or pyelonephritis in these patients should be treated as for complicated UTI.

(2) UTI in Diabetic patients:

Generally, UTI in a diabetic patient is considered as complicated. However, some experts have different opinions about otherwise healthy nonpregnant women with well-controlled diabetes without long term urologic complications of diabetes, such as difficulty in bladder emptying due to autonomic neuropathy and diabetic nephropathy:

- Acute cystitis in these patients can be treated with the same drugs used for uncomplicated cystitis in premenopausal women. However, it may be prudent to treat all cases of acute pyelonephritis in diabetic as complicated UTI.

(3) UTI (cystitis or pyelonephritis) in men

- UTIs in men are generally considered as complicated UTI.

- All cases of UTI in adult men must be investigated for complicating factors. If no complicating factors are found, acute cystitis in otherwise healthy young men (<40 years) can be treated with the same drugs used for uncomplicated cystitis in premenopausal women. However, Nitrofurantoin, pivmecillinam, and fosfomycin are usually not used in male UTI. All other cases of UTI in men should be treated as complicated UTI.

Asymptomatic bacteriuria:

- Asymptomatic bacteriuria is a common condition, but not always harmful in adults.
- It is clearly harmful in pregnant women and patients who undergo traumatic urologic procedures; therefore, these two categories of individuals should be screened for asymptomatic bacteriuria and should be treated if found.
- For all other adult individuals, asymptomatic bacteriuria is generally not considered harmful; therefore, screening for and treatment of asymptomatic bacteriuria in these people are usually discouraged.

***In asymptomatic candiduria or catheter-associated asymptomatic bacteriuria (CA-ASB)** antimicrobial therapy is not always indicated (for details please see 'Candiduria; CA-UTI' in the text)

References:

1. Relevant chapters of **Kumar &Clark's Clinical Medicine,** 8th edition; Parveen Kumar and Michael Clark (Editors). Edinburgh, Elsevier, **2012**.

2. Relevant chapters of **Harrison's Principles of Internal Medicine**; 18 th edition; Dan L Longo et al (Editors). New York, McGraw-Hill 2012

3. LE Nicolle. Complicated urinary tract infection in adults. **Can J Infect Dis Med Microbiol 2005**;16(6):349-360.

4. Shawn Dason et al. Guidelines for the diagnosis and management of recurrent urinary tract infection in women. **Can Urol Assoc J 2011**; 5(5):316-22

5. Laboratory investigations of UTI. **The Best Practice Advocacy Centre New Zealand (bpac^nz); 2006;** New Zealand. At: http://www.bpac.org.nz/Supplement/2006/July/uti.aspx

6. Susan A. Mehnert-Kay. Diagnosis and Management of Uncomplicated Urinary Tract Infections. **Am Fam Physician 2005;** 72:451-6,458.

7. Three-day courses of antibiotics for uncomplicated urinary tract infection. **NICE guidelines, UK; 2015**; at: nice.org.uk/guidance/ktt10

8. Stephen Bent et al. Does this woman have an acute uncomplicated urinary tract infection? **JAMA 2002**; 287(20): 2701-10

9. Thomas M. Hooton. Uncomplicated Urinary Tract Infection. **N Engl J Med 2012**;366:1028-37.

10. S.E. Geerlings et al. **SWAB Guidelines** for Antimicrobial Therapy of Complicated Urinary Tract Infections in Adults **2013**. At: http://www.swab.nl/swab/cms3.nsf/uploads/41949F6BD9ED10EDC1257B7F00212560/$FILE/revised%20uti%20guideline%20FINAL%20010413.pdf

11. Florian M E Wagenlehner et al. Epidemiology, diagnostics, therapy and management of uncomplicated bacterial community acquired urinary tract infections in adults. **Chemother J 2011**. 20:158-68

12. Relevant chapters of **Davidson's Principles and Practice of Medicine**, 21 edition, Nicki R. Colledge et al (editors). India, Elsevier, **2010**

13. Kalpana Gupta et al. International Clinical Practice Guidelines for the Treatment of Acute Uncomplicated Cystitis and Pyelonephritis in Women: A 2010 Update by the Infectious Diseases Society of America and the European Society for Microbiology and Infectious Diseases. **Clinical Infectious Diseases 2011**; 52(5):e103–e120

14. Assessment and management of lower urinary tract infection in adults. **Australian prescriber 2014**; February, Volume 37: Number 1

15. Relevant chapters of **Current Medical Diagnosis and Treatment**; Maxine A. Papadakis et al (Editors). New York, McGraw-Hill, **2013**

16. Charles M. Kodner et al. Recurrent Urinary Tract Infections in Women: Diagnosis and Management. **Am Fam Physician 2010**; 82(6):638-643.

17. Niall F. Davis et al. Interstitial cystitis/painful bladder syndrome: the influence of modern diagnostic criteria on epidemiology and on Internet search activity by the public. **Transl Androl Urol 2015**; 4(5):506-511

18. Dimitrios-Anestis Moutzouris et al. Interstitial Cystitis: An Unsolved Enigma. **Clin J Am Soc Nephrol 2009;** 4: 1844–1857

19. Interstitial Cystitis/Painful Bladder Syndrome. On the website of '**The national institute of diabetes and digestive and kidney diseases (NIDDK)**', USA. At: https://www.niddk.nih.gov/health-information/health-topics/urologic-disease/interstitial-cystitis-painful-bladder-syndrome/Pages/facts.aspx#what

20. 'Interstitial Cystitis/Bladder Pain Syndrome' on the website of **American Urological association.** At: https://www.auanet.org/education/guidelines/ic-bladder-pain-syndrome.cfm

21. Guidelines for 'Urinary Tract Infection', May 2011. **University of Michigan Health System (UMHS).** At: http://www.med.umich.edu/1info/FHP/practiceguides/uti/uti.pdf

22. 'UTI' in **GP Notebook, UK**. At: http://www.gpnotebook.co.uk/simplepage.cfm?ID=1214971922&linkID=34803&cook=yes

23. Guide to interpretation: Urine microscopy**.** On the website of **Nottingham University Hospitals, UK.** At: http://www.nuh.nhs.uk/healthcare-professionals/microbiology/guide-to-interpretation/

24. Interpreting urine dipstick tests in adults: a reference guide for primary care**. The Best Practice Advocacy Centre New Zealand (bpac^{nz}) 2013;** At: http://www.bpac.org.nz/BT/2013/June/urine-tests.aspx

25. Jeff A. Simerville et al. Urinalysis: A Comprehensive Review. **Am Fam Physician 2005**; 71:1153-62

26. Simati B et al. FPIN's clinical inquiries: Dipstick urinalysis for the diagnosis of acute UTI. **Am Fam Physician. 2013** May 15;87(10):Online.

27. 'Diagnosis of UTI: Quick reference guide for primary care' by **British Infection Association**. At: https://www.gov.uk/government/uploads/system/uploads/attachment_data/file/323398/UTI_guidelines_with_RCGP_logo.pdf

28. Urinalysis. **UTAH University (USA) Tutorial**. At: http://library.med.utah.edu/WebPath/TUTORIAL/URINE/URINE.html

29. Gilbert J. Wise et al. Sterile Pyuria. **N Engl J Med 2015;** 372:1048-54

30. Sanchia Goonewardene et al. Sterile pyuria: a forgotten entity. **Ther Adv Urol 2015**. 7(5): 295–298

31. Martina Franz and Walter H. Horl. Common errors in diagnosis and management of urinary tract infection. I: Pathophysiology and diagnostic techniques. **Nephrol Dial Transplant 1999**; 14: 2746-53

32. Bryan Larsen et al. Understanding the Bacterial Flora of the Female Genital Tract. **Clinical Infectious Diseases 2001**; 32:e69–77

33. Managing urinary tract infections in pregnancy. **The Best Practice Advocacy Centre New Zealand (bpac^{nz}) 2011;** BPJ 35; at: http://www.bpac.org.nz/BPJ/2011/april/pregnant-uti.aspx

34. Guidelines on urological infections by **European Association of Urology 2015**. At: http://uroweb.org/wp-content/uploads/19-Urological-infections_LR2.pdf

35. Raul Raz. Urinary Tract Infection in Postmenopausal Women. **Korean J Urol 2011**;52:801-808

36. Gomolin IH et al. Efficacy and safety of ciprofloxacin oral suspension versus trimethoprim-sulfamethoxazole oral suspension for treatment of older women with acute urinary tract infection. **J Am Geriatr Soc. 2001;** 49(12):1606-13.

37. Shengsheng Yu et al. Disease burden of urinary tract infections among type 2 diabetes mellitus patients in the U.S. **Journal of Diabetes and Its Complications 2014**; 28: 621–626

38. John E. Delzell, JR. et al. Urinary Tract infections during pregnancy. **Am Fam Physician 2000**; 61(3):713-720

39. Urinary tract infections in pregnancy. **Emedicine.** At: http://emedicine.medscape.com/article/452604-overview

40. Lindsay E. Nicolle et al. Infectious Diseases Society of America Guidelines for the Diagnosis and Treatment of Asymptomatic Bacteriuria in Adults. **Clinical Infectious Diseases 2005;** 40:643–54

41. Richard Colgan et al. Asymptomatic bacteriuria in adults. **Am Fam Physician 2006;** 74:985-90

42. Carol A. Kauffman. Candiduria. **Clinical Infectious Diseases 2005**; 41:S371–6

43. Carol A. Kauffman et al. Prospective multicenter surveillance study of funguria in hospitalized patients. **Clinical Infectious Diseases 2000**; 30:14–8

44. John F. Fisher et al. Candida urinary tract infections—treatment. **Clinical Infectious Diseases 2011**;52(S6):S457–S466

45. Carol A. Kauffman et al. Candida urinary tract infections—diagnosis. **Clinical Infectious Diseases 2011**;52(S6):S452–S456

46. Bukhary ZA. Candiduria: A Review of Clinical Significance and Management. **Saudi J Kidney Dis Transpl 2008**;19 (3):350-60

47. Peter G. Pappas et al. Clinical Practice Guidelines for the Management of Candidiasis: 2009 Update by the Infectious Diseases Society of America. **Clinical Infectious Diseases 2009**; 48:503–35

48. Catheter-associated Urinary Tract Infections (CAUTI). **CDC (USA);** October 2015. At: https://www.cdc.gov/HAI/ca_uti/uti.html

49. Urinary Tract Infection (Catheter-Associated Urinary Tract Infection [CAUTI] and Non-Catheter-Associated Urinary Tract Infection [UTI]) and Other Urinary System Infection [USI]) Events. **CDC (USA); January 2016**. At: http://www.cdc.gov/nhsn/pdfs/pscmanual/7psccauticurrent.pdf

50. Thomas M. Hooton et al. Diagnosis, Prevention, and Treatment of Catheter-Associated Urinary Tract Infection in Adults: 2009 International Clinical Practice Guidelines from the Infectious Diseases Society of America. **Clinical Infectious Diseases 2010;** 50:625–663

51. Lindsay E Nicolle. Catheter associated urinary tract infections. **Antimicrob Resist Infect Control. 2014**; 3: 23.

52. Nicolle LE. Catheter-related urinary tract infection. **Drugs aging. 2005**; 22(8):627-39.

53. Sanjay Saint et al. A Program to Prevent Catheter-Associated Urinary Tract Infection in Acute Care. **N Engl J Med 2016**; 374:2111-2119

54. Carolyn V et al. Guideline for Prevention of Catheter-Associated Urinary Tract Infections **2009**. **CDC, USA**; at: http://www.cdc.gov/hicpac/pdf/CAUTI/CAUTIguideline2009final.pdf

Chapter 8

Skin and soft tissue infections

Skin and soft tissue infections (SSTIs):

Folliculitis (inflammation of the hair follicle): Most cases of folliculitis are superficial infection of the hair follicle often caused by *Staphylococcus aureus*;

Boil (or furuncle):

Boils (also called furuncle) are deep infection of the hair follicles usually caused by *Staphylococcus aureus*.

Carbuncle:

A carbuncle is a cluster of boils connected to each other subcutaneously. Usually it occurs on the back of the neck, particularly in individuals with diabetes. Generally, carbuncles are larger and deeper than furuncles.[1]

Impetigo:

- It is a highly contagious, superficial, purulent infection of the skin caused by staphylococcus or streptococcus. It is more common among children.
- There are two types of impetigo: non-bullous (about 70% of cases) and bullous.[2,3]
- Non-bullous impetigo, in which single or multiple vesicles or pustules are formed, may be caused by either staphylococcus or streptococcus or a combination of the two. In contrast, bullous impetigo, where one or more pus filled blisters appears on the skin, is mainly caused by staphylococcus.[2] In both the types of impetigo, usually characteristic honey-colored crust is formed upon rupture of the lesions, and removal of the crust leaves a denuded red area.
- Gram stain and culture of the pus or discharge from the lesions can be used to identify the causative pathogen.
- *Staphylococcus aureus* isolates from impetigo are usually methicillin susceptible.[1] However, MRSA is increasingly found in skin and soft tissue infections.[1,4]
- Treatment: Topical mupirocin or retapamulin (ointment) twice daily for 5 days may be attempted when the number of lesions are limited.[1,5] However, in most cases, oral antibiotics are used.[5] A first generation cephalosporin (eg, cephalexin, 250-500 mg 4 times daily, or cephradine); dicloxacillin (250-500 mg QID)/ flucloxacillin (500mg QID); or co-amoxyclav (625mg TID) for 7-10 days is usually effective.[1,4,6] If community-acquired MRSA (CA-MRSA) infection is suspected or confirmed oral clindamycin (monotherapy), 300mg QID, can be given.[1]
- For recurrent or resistant impetigo, test nasal swab (Gram stain and culture) of the patient, and also consider checking close contacts. Intranasal mupirocin ointment 2-3 times daily for 5-7 days or rifampicin 500 mg daily for 5 days may clear the nasal colonies of *Staphylococcus aureus*.[1,4,5] Daily decontamination of the personal items such as towels, bed-sheets and cloths is also important.[1] Check CBC (for neutrophil disorders) and blood sugar of the patient if not already checked.
- Glomerulonephritis may develop after skin infection with certain types of streptococcus.

Erysipelas

It is a superficial infection of the skin and subcutaneous tissue usually caused by streptococcus. The lesion is characterised by highly painful, intensely erythematous, well demarcated plaque on the face or extremities. Blisters may appear on it on the second or third day. Erysipelas may be difficult to distinguish from cellulitis. In European countries, the term erysipelas is often used synonymously with cellulitis.[1,7] Treatment of erysipelas is mostly similar to that of typical (nonpurulent) cellulitis (described below).

Cellulitis

- Cellulitis is an acute spreading infection of the skin and subcutaneous tissue. Most commonly it occurs on the lower leg.[4,5]
- The lesion is characterized by a painful, erythematous, warm plaque with spreading edge with or without vesicles or blisters on it. The lesion expands quickly, over hours, and patients usually present within 6-36 hours of onset.[5] Systemic features such as fever, chills, malaise and hypotension may develop.

Microbiology

Most common pathogens:

- Cellulitis occurs most commonly due to streptococcus particularly group A β-hemolytic streptococcus, or *Staphylococcus aureus*;[5,7] however, staphylococcus is less frequently involved than streptococcus. Staphylococcal cellulitis is often associated with skin infection such as boil or abscess, or penetrating injury including IV drug use.[3]
- The number of cellulitis cases due to MRSA is increasing. In the USA, community-acquired MRSA (CA-MRSA) is involved in 15 to 74% of all skin and soft tissue infections (SSTIs), depending on the different regions of the country.[8] CA-MRSA has been identified in >80% of all community-acquired *S. aureus* infections in some locations in the USA.[9] However, MRSA is an unusual cause of nonpurulent cellulitis.[1]

Less common organisms:

1) Gram-negative bacteria, including pseudomonas, induced cellulitis commonly occurs in immunocompromised individuals or diabetic patients, and in hospital settings. As multidrug resistance is a concern in these groups of patients, so culture and sensitivity tests are very important.[4,10]

2) Animal (dog or cat) bite related cellulitis: The infection is often polymicrobial. Various anaerobes and aerobes including of *Pasteurella species* are involved commonly.[3,10]

3) Human bite related cellulitis: The microbiology of these wounds is complex. The pathogens include aerobic bacteria such as Streptococci, Staph aureus and *Eikenella corrodens* along with different mouth anaerobes such as Fusobacterium and Peptostreptococcus.[1,7]

4) Contaminated water exposure related cellulitis:
   - *Freshwater*: *Aeromonas hydrophila, Plesiomonas shigelloides* etc. *Aeromonas hydrophila* can cause aggressive cellulitis.[10,11]
   - *Salt water:* A special concern is *Vibrio vulnificus and other* species of Vibrio.[11] *Vibrio vulnificus* can cause severe cellulitis, especially in immunocompromised individuals and patients with liver disease, following consumption of raw or under-

cooked sea-food or salt water exposure. Therefore, these individuals should avoid raw or undercooked seafood and salt water exposure. [12]

****Vibrio vulnificus infection should be suspected in*** patients with sepsis and severe skin lesions (severe cellulitis associated with bullae, ecchymoses etc), particularly when associated with gastrointestinal upset (eg, diarrhea, nausea and vomiting). This is a very rapidly progressive infection and may be fatal within 24 hours of onset of symptoms if not properly treated. Most cases of Vibrio vulnificus cellulitis and septicemia occurs in individuals with some sort of immunocompromised state when they consume raw or undercooked seafood. Therefore, ask patients with cellulitis about seafood consumption and seawater exposure.[12]

****Mycobacterium marinum***, sometimes found in aquarium water and swimming pool, can cause cellulitis or granulomatous skin lesions. In contaminated water exposure related cellulitis, suspect cellulitis with this organism when cellulitis remains unresponsive to appropriate antibiotics for the other possible pathogens, and consider wound biopsy for mycobacterial stains and culture.[3] Cotrimoxazole, tetracycline, or combined therapy with rifampicin and ethambutol may be effective.[10]

5) *Erysipelothrix rhusiopathiae*, a Gram-positive aerobic bacillus, can cause cellulitis in bone renders, meatpackers and fishmongers. This organism is sensitive to most β-lactam antibiotics, cephalosporins and clindamycin but is resistant to vancomycin.[10]

6) Anaerobes may be involved in cellulitis among immunosuppressed and diabetic patients.[4]

7) Fungi[5]

Conditions predispose to cellulitis:

1. Tinea infection in the interdigital area: In otherwise healthy individuals, skin damage due to tinea infection in the interdigital area is the most common portal of entry for leg cellulitis.[5]
2. Diabetes mellitus especially with neuropathy or callus skin[5]
3. Some focal infections such as infected traumatic wound; boil and folliculitis especially when manipulated[7,10]
4. Leg edema and lymphedema (may cause recurrent cellulitis)[1]
5. Skin ulcer[5]
6. Injection site[5]
7. Obesity[7]
8. Venous insufficiency[7]
9. Past history of erysipelas or cellulitis (increases the risk of recurrent infection at the same site)[1]

Bacteria usually enter into the deeper tissues through a break in the skin.[10] In some cases, the disrupted skin surface is obvious, but often it is small and clinically undetectable. [1]

Differential diagnosis[5,7]

1. Deep venous thrombosis (DVT) (usually present with swelling and pain *without significant erythema*)
2. Necrotizing fascitis (has been discussed later)
3. Sclerosing panniculitis (predominantly affects obese women with venous insufficiency; characterized by sudden onset of very tender erythematous plaque on the medial aspect of the leg without any systemic upset)
4. Acute severe contact dermatitis (characterized by the presence of erythema, edema with or without vesiculation like cellulitis but itching is present instead of pain)
5. Gout (erythema limited to joint area)

Investigations (Information from references 1,3,7,10)

For mild nonpurulent cellulitis without systemic features or comorbidities, only some routine investigations are generally sufficient; etiologic diagnosis is usually not considered in these cases.

In the other cases, the following investigations are considered:

- CBC with differential (leukocytosis, neutrophilia and left shift may be seen)
- CRP
- Blood sugar
- Urea, creatinine and electrolytes
- Creatine phosphokinase
- Tests for the definitive etiologic diagnosis:
  Blood culture; or cultures of cutaneous aspirates, biopsies or swabs are not recommended routinely.
  - If there is an open wound, discharge, or an obvious portal of microbial entry, swabs should be taken from the lesion for Gram-stain and culture. When there is purulent discharge, bulla, or abscess, Gram-stain and culture of the specimen collected from these lesions may be very yielding; for instance, the specimen collected from an abscess may be positive in about 90% cases.
  - Gram-stain and culture of the specimen collected from the inflamed area by needle aspiration is positive only in ≤5% to 40% of cases and punch biopsy is positive in 20-30% of cases. Therefore, these procedures should be considered only in some special circumstances such as severe disease, immunocompromised state, animal bite related infection, or contaminated water exposure related infection; also, they should be considered when the patient is unresponsive to the initial empiric antibiotic treatment.
  - Blood culture and sensitivity are generally low yielding, positive in ≤5% of cases, so should not be ordered routinely. However, blood cultures should be obtained in patients with significant systemic manifestations (eg, high fever and or hypotension); or unstable co-morbidities that may interfere with therapeutic response; or when an unusual organism is likely to be involved such as in immunodeficient state or animal bite related infection.
  - Streptococcal serology [(antistreptolysin-O titer (ASOT) and anti-DNase B)] may be useful for retrospective diagnosis only in selected refractory cases when there is

some doubt about the diagnosis.

In fact, in severe disease such as extensive limb threatening cellulitis or cellulitis with marked systemic upset, all possible measures should be considered to establish the microbial diagnosis.

Indications for hospitalization:[1,3,5]

1) Severe systemic manifestations such as fever, hypotension or altered mental status;
2) If there is suspicion of a deeper or necrotizing infection;
3) Severe immunocompromised state
4) Inadequate response to outpatient treatment
5) Noncompliant patient
6) Severe local symptoms and signs
7) If one or more of the following abnormal lab findings are present:
   - Raised serum creatinine level
   - Low serum bicarbonate level
   - Raised creatine phosphokinase level (generally 2–3 times the upper limit of normal)
   - Marked left shift in CBC with differential
   - CRP >13mg/L

For hospitalized patients, aggressive efforts should be made for a microbial diagnosis and surgical consultation is often considered.

Treatment of cellulitis

General measures:

Immobilization and elevation of the affected part may help reduce edema; use of bed cradles, cool and wet dressings can reduce local discomfort.

Empiric antibiotic therapy in cellulitis

For the purpose of empiric antibiotic therapy, cellulitis can be categorized as follows:

A. cellulitis **without** purulent discharge, ulcer, or associated abscess (Nonpurulent cellulitis)
B. Cellulitis **with** purulent discharge, ulcer, or associated abscess (Purulent Cellulitis)

Each of the two broader categories (Nonpurulent and purulent) can be graded again into:[1,7]

1. Mild: Limited area involvement with no systemic features of infection or uncontrolled comorbidities* that can affect patient outcome.
2. Moderate: Local lesion is not extensive; some systemic features of infection are present but not marked, or systemically well but one or more co-morbidity is present.
3. Severe: Presence of anyone of the followings--
   - Marked systemic toxicity such as (a) systemic signs of infection: temperature >38°C (100.4°F), tachycardia (heart rate >90/minute), tachypnea (respiration rate >24/minute),

hypotension etc. or (b) abnormal WBC count (>12 000 or <4000 cells/μL), or (c) evidence of organ dysfunction

- Failure of oral antibiotic therapy
- Immunocompromised state
- Extensive local lesion or clinical evidences of deeper infection such as bullae, skin sloughing etc.

*Comorbidities include peripheral arterial disease, chronic venous insufficiency, morbid obesity etc. which may complicate or delay resolution of the infection.

Indications for empiric MRSA coverage in cellulitis[1,3,13,14,15]

1) Cellulitis with purulent drainage, ulcer or abscess;
2) Cellulitis associated with penetrating injury including those from IV drug use;
3) Presence of MRSA infection elsewhere or MRSA colonization of the nose;
4) Where β-lactam antibiotic therapy has failed;
5) Severe cellulitis
6) History of recent hospitalization (within three months);
7) History of recent antibiotic use;

There is no consensus on optimal antibiotic treatment in skin and soft tissue infections, resulting in substantial variation in practice. ***As cellulitis is most commonly caused by group A β-hemolytic streptococcus or Staphylococcus aureus, in all cases empiric antibiotics should cover these organisms adequately.***[5,7]

Empiric antibiotic regimens

A. Cellulitis without purulent discharge, ulcer, or associated abscess (nonpurulent cellulitis)

In these cases, the most likely organism is streptococcus and the possibility of MRSA or any unusual pathogen involvement is low.

(1) ***For mild infection, consider any of the followings (can be given on outpatient basis):***[1,3,11]

a) Amoxicillin-clavulanate 625 mg 8 hourly (or 875 mg 12 hourly) PO, **or**
b) Cephalexin 500 mg 6 hourly PO, **or**
c) Flucloxacillin/Dicloxacillin 500mg 6 hourly PO, **or**
d) Clindamycin 300-450 mg TID or QID PO (can be used in patients with penicillin allergy)

*Dicloxacillin is a newer agent than flucloxacillin with probably less adverse effects than flucloxacillin, and can be used as a substitute for flucloxacillin.

When MRSA coverage indicated:

a) Clindamycin 300-450 mg TID or QID PO, **or**
b) Doxycycline 100 mg BID PO **Plus** a β-lactam (eg, cephalexin 500 mg 6 hourly or amoxicillin 500 mg 8 hourly), **or**
c) Trimethoprim-sulfamethoxazole 1-2 DS tabs BID PO **Plus** a β-lactam (eg, cephalexin or amoxicillin)

(2) ***For moderate infection (these patients should be hospitalized)***[1,11]

a) Cefazolin 1 g IV 8 hourly, **or**
b) Ceftriaxone IV 1-2 gm daily, **or**
c) Nafcillin (penicillinase resistant penicillin) 1-2 g IV 4 hourly, **or**
d) Clindamycin 600 mg IV 8 hourly;

When MRSA coverage indicated:
Recommended antimicrobial coverage should include both Streptococcus and MRSA.
The antibiotic regimen may be monotherapy with:

Vancomycin 15 mg/kg (usual maximum 1g) IV 12 hourly;
Or
Linezolid 600 mg BID IV

If the patient is unresponsive to monotherapy with vancomycin or linezolid, a broader coverage may be given by combining a β-lactam antibiotic (eg, cefazolin or ceftriaxone) with vancomycin or linezolid.[13]

Is there any exception to the above mentioned therapeutic approach to moderate nonpurulent cellulitis?

- Yes. Some experts think in moderate nonpurulent cellulitis with systemic toxicity, CA-MRSA coverage may be considered even when otherwise not indicated.[13]
- Some physicians prefer to give a broader coverage often with combination of cefazolin plus clindamycin in all patients with moderate nonpurulent cellulitis when there is no indication for MRSA coverage mentioned above. Clindamycin is effective against both *Streptococcus* and *Staph aureus* including CA-MRSA. However, in moderate nonpurulent cellulitis, when there is any indication for MRSA coverage (mentioned above), probably it would be more justified to use a stronger anti-MRSA drug (eg, vancomycin or linezolid) than clindamycin.

(3) ***For severe infection***[1]

Piperacillin-tazobactam 3.375g -- 4.5 g 6–8 hourly IV
Plus
Vancomycin 15 mg/kg (usual maximum 1 gm) IV 12 hourly;

Switching to oral antibiotics can be considered when the patient is improving (afebrile and skin findings are resolving).[1,16] In uncomplicated cellulitis, usually patients can be switched safely to oral antibiotics within 3-5 days of therapy.[16] Use of parenteral antibiotics for longer than 3-4 days generally does not offer better outcomes.[7]

Suitable drugs for oral switching:
In most cases, an oral form of the parenteral drug, if available, will be the most appropriate oral agent. Co-amoxyclav, flucloxacillin/dicloxacillin, first or second generation cephalosporins, or clindamycin is suitable in many cases; clindamycin (300 mg tid or qid) or clarithromycin (500mg BID) is usually suitable in the penicillin allergic patients.[7]

Use of anti-inflammatory agents in the treatment of nonpurulent cellulitis[1]

Anti-inflammatory drugs, nonsteroidal anti-inflammatory agents (eg, Ibuprofen 400 mg QID for 5 days) or systemic corticosteroids (Prednisone 40 mg daily for one week), can cause significantly faster resolution of nonpurulent cellulitis when combined with antimicrobial therapy. Before prescribing systemic corticosteroids in cellulitis, it needs to be ensured that the patient is nondiabetic and there is no deeper tissue involvement such as necrotizing fasciitis.

B. Cellulitis with purulent discharge, ulcer or associated abscess (Purulent Cellulitis)

Staphylococcus aureus is the most common organism and the risk of MRSA is much higher than in nonpurulent cellulitis. In a study of patients with purulent SSTI presented to 11 emergency departments throughout the USA, *Staph aureus* was isolated from about 75% of cases, (about 60% were CA-MRSA and about 15% were MSSA), while β- hemolytic Streptococcus was identified only in about 3% of cases.[13] Empiric antibiotic regimen for this category of patients should cover both *Staph aureus* including MRSA and streptococci.[15] These patients also need appropriate surgical intervention.

(1) *For mild disease* (can be treated as outpatient basis)
Consider anyone of the following antibiotic regimens:

a) Clindamycin 300-450 mg TID or QID PO[3,15], **or**
b) Doxycycline 100 mg BID PO **Plus** a β-lactam (eg, cephalexin 500 mg 6 hourly or amoxicillin 500 mg 8 hourly)[15], **or**
c) Trimethoprim-sulfamethoxazole 1-2 DS tabs BID PO **Plus** a β-lactam (eg, cephalexin or amoxicillin)[15]

Activity of TMP/SMX and doxycycline against streptococci is unknown,[1] so they should be combined with a β-lactam (eg, Cephalexin or amoxicillin) to ensure adequate streptococcal coverage.

(2) *For moderate to severe disease:* (Hospitalization is required)

Vancomycin 15 mg/kg (usual maximum 1g) IV 12 hourly (also preferred for hospital acquired infection)[3,11,15]
Or
Linezolid 600 mg 12 hourly IV[11]

*Daptomycin, Ceftaroline, or Telavancin can also be used.[11]

In practice, among patients with cellulitis who need hospitalization, only about one-third of them receive specific treatment for gram-positive bacteria and the remaining two-thirds receive very-broad-spectrum antibiotic regimens.[1]

- If empiric broader coverage is considered for moderate purulent cellulitis, a β-lactam antibiotic (eg, cefazolin or ceftriaxone) may be combined with either vancomycin or linezolid.
- In severe purulent cellulitis, giving a broader coverage with vancomycin plus piperacillin-tazobactam until the microbial diagnosis is known or a medical microbiologist's opinion is available, is probably not an uncommon practice.

In severe cellulitis of any category:

(1) Rule out necrotizing fasciitis (described below in 'necrotizing fasciitis')
(2) Consult a surgeon urgently for possible surgical intervention.
(3) Consult an infectious disease specialist or a medical microbiologist.

Duration of treatment

In most cases of uncomplicated cellulitis antimicrobial therapy of 7-14 days is adequate; however, complicated cases (eg, associated abscess or infected ulcer) may need prolonged therapy depending on response.[7,16] The average duration of antimicrobial therapy for patients who need hospitalization is two weeks.[1]

Response to treatment

The progression of cellulitis may stop within 24 hours of initiation of antibiotic. However, it may appear to progress with increasing erythema in the first 24-48 hours of antibiotic therapy (even when the antibiotic is effective) possibly due to toxin release from the destructed bacteria.[1,7,11] Clear evidences of improvement are usually seen within 2-3 days.

Causes of failure of empiric antibiotics in Cellulitis

1. Infection with unusual organisms which can occur in immunodeficiency, injury sustained in water, human or animal bite related infection etc. (Treatment given below)
2. Infection with drug resistant organisms (may need switching to an antibiotic regimen with broader coverage).
3. Inappropriate drug or dose;
4. Involvement of the deeper tissues such as necrotizing fascitis;

*Cellulitis may recur at the same site; each attack may cause some lymphatic damage and repeated attacks may lead to lymphedema. Measures should be taken to prevent recurrent cellulitis considering the predisposing factors such as treatment of tinea pedis or venous eczema when present.

Anti-microbial coverage of some commonly used antibiotics in cellulitis:

Antibiotic	*Antimicrobial coverage*	*MRSA coverage*
Co-amoxyclav	Polymicrobial: Gram-positive (including *Streptococci* and *Staph aureus*), Gram-negative and some anaerobes	No MRSA coverage
Flucloxacillin	*Streptococci* and *Staph aureus*	No MRSA coverage
Cephalosporins	Polymicrobial: Gram-positive (including *Streptococci* and *Staph aureus*), Gram-negative and some anaerobes (do not cover *Bacteroides fragilis*) The first generation cephalosporins have the strongest Gram-positive coverage. Each newer generation of cephalosporins has significantly stronger gram-negative coverage than the preceding generation	No MRSA coverage

	but in most cases weaker activity against gram-positive organisms, except 4th generation cephalosporins; they (4th generation) are truly broad spectrum with almost similar activity against Gram positive as 1st generation along with stronger Gram-negative activity than 3rd generation.	
Clindamycin	Gram-positive bacteria (including *Streptococci* and *Staph aureus*) and many anaerobes. Its anaerobic coverage may be broader than that of most cephalosporins, but no significant Gram-negative coverage.	Covers CA-MRSA
TMP-SMX	Broad-spectrum; covers gram negative and gram-positive organisms including *Staph aureus* but streptococcus coverage is unknown.	Covers CA-MRSA
Doxycycline	Broad-spectrum; covers gram negative and gram-positive organisms including *Staph aureus* but streptococcus coverage is unknown like TMP-SMX.	Covers CA-MRSA
Vancomycin	A narrow-spectrum antibiotic effective against Gram-positive bacteria (including *Streptococci* and *Staph aureus)*	Covers both CA-MRSA and hospital acquired MRSA
Linezolid	Gram-positive bacteria (including *Streptococci* and *Staph aureus*); no Gram-negative coverage; (Linezolid can be used as an alternative to vancomycin, when vancomycin cannot be used)	Covers both CA-MRSA and hospital acquired MRSA
Piperacillin-tazobactam	Polymicrobial: Strong Gram positive, Gram negative including pseudomonas coverage and also covers almost all anaerobes like metronidazole	No MRSA coverage

Vancomycin versus Teicoplanin:[9,17]

- Vancomycin and teicoplanin both are glycopeptides effective against Gram-positive bacteria including MRSA.
- The two drugs have similar mechanisms of action and almost similar spectrum of activities.
- Their efficacies are similar, but teicoplanin has significantly lower rate of adverse effects. Total adverse effects, nephrotoxicity and red man syndrome are significantly less common with teicoplanin.
- Vancomycin is administered twice daily. In contrast, the half-life of teicoplanin is longer, which allows once daily administration after the loading dose.

- Probably teicoplanin is not approved for use in the USA, while it is more commonly used than vancomycin in some European countries.

Empiric antibiotic treatment of cellulitis in special circumstances

A. Animal bite (including dog and cat) related infection:

For empiric antibiotic therapy, polymicrobial coverage of various anaerobes and aerobes including *Pasteurella species* are commonly considered.

For nonsevere infection

1. Monotherapy with: Co-amoxiclav 625mg tid (or 875mg bid) PO [1,7]

2. Alternative oral regimens:[1,14]
   a) Cefuroxime 500 mg bid
      Plus
      Anaerobic coverage with either Metronidazole 500 mg tid or clindamycin 300 mg tid;

   Or

   b) Levofloxacin 750 mg OD PO/ or TMP-SMX 1 DS Tablet bid PO
      Plus
      Anaerobic coverage with either Metronidazole 500 mg tid or clindamycin 300 mg tid;

      [Moxifloxacin monotherapy (400mg OD) is also effective]

For severe infection

Piperacillin-tazobactam or carbapenem

B. Human bite related infection:

The bacteriological characteristic of human bite wound is complex. For empiric antibiotic therapy, polymicrobial coverage of both aerobic and anaerobic bacteria including *Eikenella corrodens* is considered.

For nonsevere infection

Monotherapy with: Co-amoxiclav, 625mg TID PO[1,7,16]

Alternatives for β-lactam allergic patients:[1]
Ciprofloxacin or levofloxacin
Plus
Anaerobic coverage with metronidazole (but not with clindamycin, as a potential pathogen *Eikenella corrodens* is resistant to this drug)

[Moxifloxacin monotherapy (400mg OD) is also effective]

For severe infection

Piperacillin-tazobactam or carbapenem

*Bite wound related patients should consult vaccination department for possible vaccine (tetanus and rabies) requirement.

C. Cellulitis of a wound sustained in aquatic environment:

Give coverage for common pathogens of cellulitis such as streptococci and staphylococcus aureus plus aquatic bacteria particularly of Vibrio species for salt water exposure related and *Aeromonas hydrophila* for fresh water exposure related infections.

For saltwater water associated infection:[3,12,15,18]
Ceftazidime 2g IV 8 hourly Plus Doxycycline 100mg BID PO / IV;

(Doxycycline to cover Vibrio species mainly although ceftazidime also covers Vibrio)

Alternative regimens
(a) Ceftriaxone 1 g daily Plus Doxycycline 100mg BID PO / IV
Or
(b) Ciprofloxacin 750 mg bid PO (or 400mg IV bid)

For freshwater associated infection:[3,7]
Ciprofloxacin 750mg bid PO
Plus
Flucloxacillin/ Dicloxacillin 500 mg 6 hourly

(Flucloxacillin/ Dicloxacillin for Streptococcus and Staphylococcus coverage)

Alternative regimen[3,10]
A third- or fourth-generation cephalosporin (ceftazidime or cefepime) monotherapy;

D. Cellulitis in immunocompromised host:

- Hospitalize the patient.
- Consult the team caring for the primary disorder (eg, Oncology or hematology) and an infectious disease specialist.

Empiric antimicrobial regimens depend on type of the immunodeficiency.

a) *Cellulitis during the initial episode of fever and neutropenia:*
Consider an empiric antibiotic regimen that covers gram-positive and gram-negative bacteria including MRSA and Pseudomonas. The empiric regimen may be:
Piperacillin-tazobactam or a carbapenem
Plus
Vancomycin

b) *Cellulitis during persistent or recurrent episodes of fever and neutropenia:*
Empiric antifungal coverage should be added to an appropriate antibiotic regimen.

For neutropenic patients consider adjunct therapy with:
1. Colony-stimulating factor
Granulocyte colony-stimulating factor [G-CSF] or

Granulocyte macrophage colony-stimulating factor [GM-CSF]

Or

2. Granulocyte transfusions

However, these adjunct therapies are not routinely recommended.

c) *Severe cellulitis in patients with impaired cell mediated immunity*

- In life-threatening situations, empiric antibiotics, antifungals, and/ or antivirals should be considered.
- Specific agents should be selected after immediate consultation with the team caring for the primary disease (eg, Oncology or Hematology) along with dermatology and infectious disease teams.

Necrotizing fasciitis

It is a rapidly progressive infection of the subcutaneous tissue and fascia. It spreads along the fascial plane and involves all tissues between skin and the underlying muscle.[1,3] Concomitant myonecrosis occurs in about 50% cases of streptococcal necrotizing fasciitis.[10]

Most cases are community acquired and involve limbs, especially lower limbs. Predisposing conditions are usually present which include diabetes mellitus, atherosclerosis, venous insufficiency, ulcer, injection drug use etc. In about 50% cases of streptococcal necrotizing fascitis, the infection occurs at the site of nonpenetrating injury (such as bruise or muscle strain) without any obvious portal of entry.[1]

*Fournier's gangrene is a form of necrotizing fasciitis involving the scrotum and perineal area.[3]

Microbiology

- The infection may be monomicrobial or polymicrobial.
- **Monomicrobial infection is commonly caused by** *Streptococcus pyogenes, Staphylococcus aureus, Vibrio vulnificus, Aeromonas hydrophila,* or anaerobic streptococci (Peptostreptococcus).[1]
- **Polymicrobial infection is usually caused by** numerous different anaerobic and aerobic bacteria, mostly coliforms and anaerobes from the gut or genitourinary flora. On average, five pathogens are isolated from each infection.[1]
- Necrotizing fasciitis may develop as a part of gas gangrene due to *Clostridium perfringens*.[10]

Clinical features

The initial presentation is like cellulitis.[5] However, unlike cellulitis, in many cases, severe pain may be the initial symptom with little cutaneous manifestation.[2]

When to suspect necrotizing fascitis in a cellulitis like presentation[1,2,5]

Features suspicious of necrotizing fasciitis include:

1. Severe and constant pain out of proportion to the physical findings;
2. Edema and induration extending beyond the erythema;
3. **Wooden hard consistency of the affected area which is a distinguishing feature;**

4. Unlike cellulitis, in fasciitis fascial planes and muscles cannot be separated during palpation.
5. Violaceous bullae (violaceous bullae are characteristics of deeper tissue infection; bullae with clear fluid may develop in both cellulitis and necrotizing fasciitis and are not characteristics of deep infection);
6. Skin necrosis and sloughing
7. Widespread petechiae and ecchymoses on the involved skin, especially when associated with systemic toxicity
8. Skin anesthesia (a late feature due to cutaneous nerve damage);
9. Crepitus (due to formation of gas in the soft tissue);
10. Very rapid progression
11. Marked systemic toxicity such as fever and hypotension;
12. Elevated levels of serum creatine phosphokinase (CPK)
13. Unresponsive to initial empiric antibiotic therapy;

Unfortunately, most of these features often appear late and the patient may look deceptively well. Therefore, in a cellulitis like presentation when the pain is severe, the induration is extending beyond the erythema, there is a tense swelling of the affected area, or the progression is very rapid, deeper tissue involvement should be suspected and a surgeon should be consulted urgently.

Diagnosis

- The disease may be difficult to recognize at the early stage.[3] Clinical assessment is the most important factor in diagnosis.[1]
- The appearance of the subcutaneous tissues or fascial planes during surgery is the most important feature for definitive diagnosis of the infection;[1,16] a small, exploratory incision made in the area of maximum involvement can be useful to confirm or rule out the diagnosis by direct visualization of the involved tissues.[1,16]
- Surgical team should be consulted immediately when necrotizing fascitis is suspected clinically rather than waiting for the investigation results.

Key investigations

Gram stain and culture

- Culture of specimens from the superficial wound may be misleading because deeper tissue may have different pathogens.
- Specimens (fluid) for Gram-stain and culture can be collected by direct needle aspiration of the lesion, or exudate from the exploratory incision (made for direct visualization of the involved tissue) can be used as specimen. Gram-stains of the exudate can provide a guide to the initial antimicrobial therapy.
- For the definitive microbial diagnosis, Gram-stain and culture of the deeper tissue collected during surgery should be performed. Blood culture when positive also establishes a definitive bacteriologic diagnosis.

Serum creatine phosphokinase (CPK)

Elevated creatinine phosphokinase may be an initial clue to the diagnosis of necrotizing fasciitis, but in many cases CPK remains within the normal limit. In monomicrobial necrotizing fasciitis, its levels are elevated in >55% of cases when the infection is caused by Gram-positive bacteria while the levels are often normal (in about 90% of cases) when the infection is caused by Gram-negative bacteria.[19]

Imaging:

- **MRI** is the most yielding imaging. Both CT and MRI may show edema along the fascial planes.[1] However, MRI can provide strong evidence of an inflammatory process involving the fascial planes.[3]
- **Ultrasonography** especially with color Doppler can also provide useful information in many cases.
- **Plain radiographs** to detect gas in the soft-tissue, which is sometimes formed in polymicrobial or clostridial necrotizing fasciitis, are of little or no value in the diagnosis of necrotizing fasciitis.[3] The absence of gas in the soft tissue does not exclude necrotizing fasciitis and the presence of gas does not confirm clostridial infection. In necrotizing fasciitis caused by group-A streptococcus or MRSA, gas is usually not formed in the lesion.[10] On the other hand, *E. coli, Peptostreptococcus*, and *Bacteroides* can also form gas in the tissue.[3]

Treatment

Necrotizing fascitis is a surgical emergency and surgery is the mainstay of treatment. Repeated wound debridement is usually needed. Therefore, when necrotizing fascitis is suspected, commencing an empiric antibiotic regimen and calling the surgical team are both urgent. General measures and adequate supportive care are also very important.

Empiric antibiotic therapy

Empiric antibiotics should be started immediately. The initial regimen should be broad, covering aerobic gram-positive bacteria (including MRSA), gram-negative organisms and anaerobes.[1,3]

The following regimen can be considered:[1]

Piperacillin-tazobactam or a carbapenem
+
Vancomycin or linezolid

Dose:
Piperacillin-tazobactam 3.375g -- 4.5 g 6–8 hourly IV
Vancomycin 15mg/kg (usual maximim1g) IV 12 hourly

***Another regimen may be*:** Ceftriaxone **Plus** metronidazole **Plus** either vancomycin or linezolid

Antibiotic coverage should be modified appropriately when definitive microbial etiology is known.

***The regimen for documented group-A streptococcal or clostridial necrotizing fasciitis**[1]

Penicillin 2–4 million units 4–6 hourly IV
Plus
Clindamycin 600–900 mg every 8 hourly IV

Clindamycin inhibits streptococcal toxin and cytokine production in addition to its antimicrobial role.[1]

Summary of the empiric antibiotic therapy in cellulitis and necrotizing fasciitis

For the purpose of empiric antibiotic therapy, cellulitis can be categorized as follows:
A. cellulitis **without** purulent discharge, ulcer, or associated abscess (Nonpurulent cellulitis)
B. Cellulitis **with** purulent discharge, ulcer, or associated abscess (Purulent cellulitis)

> Indications for MRSA coverage in cellulitis:
> (1) Cellulitis with purulent drainage, ulcer, or abscess; (2) Cellulitis associated with penetrating injury including those from IV drug use; (3) Presence of MRSA infection elsewhere or MRSA colonization of the nose; (4) Where β-lactam antibiotic therapy has failed; (5) Severe cellulitis; (6) History of recent hospitalization (within three months); (7) History of recent antibiotic use;

A. Cellulitis without purulent discharge, ulcer, or associated abscess (nonpurulent cellulitis)

(1) ***For mild infection, consider any of the followings (can be given on outpatient basis):***
When MRSA coverage not indicated:

a) Amoxicillin-clavulanate 625 mg TID (or 875 mg BID) PO, **or**
b) Cephalexin 500 mg 6 hourly PO, **or**
c) Flucloxacillin/Dicloxacillin 500mg QID PO, **or**
d) Clindamycin 300-450 mg TID or QID PO (can be used in patients with penicillin allergy)

When MRSA coverage indicated:

a) Clindamycin 300-450 mg TID or QID PO, **or**
b) Doxycycline 100 mg BID PO **Plus** a β-lactam (eg, cephalexin 500 mg QID or amoxicillin 500 mg TID), **or**
c) Trimethoprim-sulfamethoxazole 1-2 DS tabs BID PO **Plus** a β-lactam (eg, cephalexin or amoxicillin)

(2) ***For moderate infection (these patients should be hospitalized)***
When MRSA coverage not indicated

a) Cefazolin 1 g IV 8 hourly, **or**
b) Ceftriaxone IV 1-2 gm daily, **or**
c) Nafcillin (penicillinase resistant penicillin) 1-2 g IV 4 hourly, **or**
d) Clindamycin 600 mg IV 8 hourly;

When MRSA coverage indicated:

Vancomycin 15 mg/kg (usual maximum 1g) IV 12 hourly;
Or
Linezolid 600 mg BID IV

(3) ***For severe infection***

Piperacillin-tazobactam 3.375g -- 4.5 g 6–8 hourly IV

Plus
Vancomycin 15 mg/kg (usual maximum 1 gm) IV 12 hourly;
Consult a surgeon urgently and rule out necrotizing infection.

B. Cellulitis with purulent discharge, ulcer or associated abscess (Purulent cellulitis)

(Empiric MRSA coverage should be considered for all patients)

(1) ***For mild disease*** (can be treated as outpatient basis)
Consider any one of the following antibiotic regimens:

a) Clindamycin 300-450 mg TID or QID PO, **or**
b) Doxycycline 100 mg BID PO **Plus** a β-lactam (eg, cephalexin 500 mg QID or amoxicillin 500 mg TID), **or**
c) Trimethoprim-sulfamethoxazole 1-2 DS tabs BID PO **Plus** a β-lactam (eg, cephalexin or amoxicillin);

(2) ***For moderate to severe disease:*** (Hospitalization is required)
Vancomycin 15 mg/kg (usual maximum 1g) IV 12 hourly **Or** Linezolid 600 mg 12 hourly IV;

Notes:

- In practice, among patients with cellulitis who need hospitalization, only about one-third of them receive specific treatment for gram-positive bacteria and the remaining two-thirds receive very-broad-spectrum antibiotic regimens.
- In severe purulent cellulitis, some physicians prefer to give very broad coverage (like severe nonpurulent cellulitis) with piperacillin-tazobactam plus vancomycin.

Animal and human bite related infection (nonsevere cases)

Monotherapy with: Co-amoxiclav 625mg tid (or 875mg bid) PO;

In severe cellulitis of any category:

(1) Rule out necrotizing fasciitis.
(2) Consult a surgeon urgently for possible surgical intervention.
(3) Consult an infectious disease specialist or a medical microbiologist.

Necrotizing fasciitis

Piperacillin-tazobactam (3.375g -- 4.5 g 6–8 hourly IV) or a carbapenem
Plus
Vancomycin (15mg/kg (usual maximim1g) IV 12 hourly) or linezolid;
Another regimen may be**:** Ceftriaxone **Plus** metronidazole **Plus** either vancomycin or linezolid

References:

1. Dennis L. Stevens et al. Practice Guidelines for the Diagnosis and Management of Skin and Soft Tissue Infections: **2014 Update** by the Infectious Diseases Society of America.

(**IDSA Practice Guidelines for SSTIs**). **Clin Infect Dis. 2014** Jul 15;59(2):e10-52. At: http://cid.oxfordjournals.org/content/59/2/147.full.pdf+html

2. Relevant chapters of **Davidson's Principles and Practice of Medicine**, 21 edition, Nicki R. Colledge et al (editors). India, Elsevier, **2010**

3. Impetigo; cellulitis; necrotizing fasciitis. **Emedicine**. At: http://emedicine.medscape.com

4. Relevant chapters of **Kumar &Clark's Clinical Medicine,** 8th edition; Parveen Kumar and Michael Clark (Editors). Edinburgh, Elsevier, **2012**

5. Relevant chapters of **Current Medical Diagnosis and Treatment**; Maxine A. Papadakis et al (Editors). New York, McGraw-Hill, **2013**

6. Charles Cole et al. Diagnosis and Treatment of Impetigo. **Am Fam Physician 2007**; 75(6):859-864. At: http://www.aafp.org/afp/2007/0315/p859.html

7. 'Guidelines on the Management of Cellulitis in Adults' **(2005)** by Clinical Resource Efficiency Support Team (**CREST), Northern Ireland**. Available at: http://www.acutemed.co.uk/docs/Cellulitis%20guidelines,%20CREST,%2005.pdf

8. Thana Khawcharoenporn et al. Risk Factors for Community-associated Methicillin-resistant Staphylococcus Aureus Cellulitis – and the Value of Recognition. Hawaii Med J. 2010 Oct; 69(10): 232–236

9. Shuli Svetitsky et al. Comparative Efficacy and Safety of Vancomycin versus Teicoplanin: Systematic Review and Meta-Analysis. **Antimicrobial Agents and Chemotherapy, Oct. 2009**; P. 4069–4079

10. Relevant chapters of **Harrison's Principles of Internal Medicine**; 18 th edition; Dan L Longo et al (Editors). New York, McGraw-Hill 2012

11. 'Cellulitis' in **Johns Hopkins Antibiotic guide**. At: http://www.hopkinsguides.com/hopkins/view/Johns_Hopkins_ABX_Guide/540106/all/Cellulitis

12. Michael H. Bross et al. *Vibrio vulnificus* Infection: Diagnosis and Treatment. **Am Fam Physician 2007**;76:539-44, 546.

13. Catherine Liu et al. Clinical Practice Guidelines by the Infectious Diseases Society of America for the Treatment of Methicillin-Resistant Staphylococcus Aureus Infections in Adults and Children. **Clinical Infectious Diseases 2011**; 1–38

14. 'Cellulitis: Treatment guideline' in **Antimicrobial stewardship, Pennsylvania University**. At: http://www.uphs.upenn.edu/antibiotics/Skin_and_Soft_Tissue_Infections.html

15. 'Skin and Soft Tissue Infections' in the **antibiotic stewardship program** by **University of California Los Angeles**. At:

http://www.asp.mednet.ucla.edu/files/view/guidebook/Infectious_Syndromes-Skin_and_Soft_Tissue_Infections.pdf

16. Morton N. Swartz. Cellulitis. **N Engl J Med 2004**; 350:904-12.

17. Vancomycin and Teicoplanin. **British National Formulary** 64, September 2012; page: 368-69

18. Vibrio Cellulitis**. Family Practice Notebook.** At: http://www.fpnotebook.com/Derm/Bacteria/VbrCllts.htm

19. D. Yahav et al. Monomicrobial necrotizing fasciitis in a single center: the emergence of Gram-negative bacteria as a common pathogen. **International Journal of Infectious Diseases 2014**; 28: 13–16

Chapter 9
Diabetic foot infections

Diabetic foot infections

How important is diabetic foot infection?

- Foot infection in the diabetic is a potentially limb- and life-threatening condition.
- In the USA, 15% of diabetic patients are likely to develop foot ulcer during their lifetime.[1] Most diabetic foot infections begin in a foot ulcer. More than 60% of non-traumatic lower-limb amputations are performed in diabetics, mainly in patients with complicated foot infection.[1]
- The possibility of serious complications in diabetic foot infections is even higher in developing countries where access to adequate medical care is limited.

Microbiology of diabetic foot infection

- Most diabetic foot infections are polymicrobial although monomicrobial infection can also occur. Most frequently isolated pathogens are aerobic gram-positive cocci, predominantly *Staphylococcus* species.
- In acute mild infections without a history of recent antibiotic use, Gram-positive cocci, such as *Staph aureus* and beta-hemolytic streptococci, are the most common organisms.[1,2] In many cases, the infection is monomicrobial. These trends are similar to those found in non-diabetic patients with skin and soft-tissue infections.[1]
- Chronic, severe, or recently antibiotic treated infections are often polymicrobial with a variable combination of aerobic gram-positives, aerobic gram-negatives and anaerobes.[1,2] However, in these cases too, Gram-positive cocci predominates while Gram-negatives and anaerobes are frequently part of mixed infections[1]. Commonly involved Gram-negative bacteria include E coli, Klebsiella and proteus.[1] Anaerobes are typically found in ischemic or necrotic foul smelling wounds; commonly isolated anaerobes are *Bacteroides, Clostridium* and *Peptostreptococci*.[1,2]

Diabetic wound without infection:

- All wounds in diabetic patients are usually colonized with microorganisms, but only the presence of bacterial colonies is generally not an indication for antibiotic treatment.[2,3]
- Antibiotic is usually not recommended for an ulcer or wound without purulent discharge or any features of inflammation (i.e., redness, pain, tenderness, warmth or induration).[2,3] However, controversies exist regarding this. Some physicians believe that diabetic foot wounds without clinical signs of infection may have subclinical infection which may impair wound healing if not treated. Additionally, features of inflammation may not be present in an ischemic and neuropathic limb.[4]

Clinical evaluation of diabetic foot infection:

Optimal approach to the diagnosis and treatment of diabetic foot infection is unclear.

Clinical classification of diabetic foot infection:

A. Uninfected wound:

- A wound without any clinical features of inflammation (redness, pain, tenderness, warmth, or induration) or purulent discharge is generally considered as uninfected;
- Ideally, neither a culture nor antibiotic therapy is recommended for clinically uninfected wounds.

B. <u>Infected wound:</u>

Generally, a wound is considered as infected when at least 2 features of inflammation (redness, pain, tenderness, warmth, or induration) or purulent discharge is present.[4]

However, some patients with infected wounds may not have these classical features, especially those who have limb ischemia (causing reduced erythema, warmth, and induration) or peripheral neuropathy (leading to decreased pain or tenderness). In such a situation, the presence one or more of the following secondary features may be considered as evidence of infection and an indication for antibiotic therapy:[4]

1. Nonpurulent discharge
2. Discolored or friable granulation tissue
3. Foul smell
4. Undermined wound edge
5. Recent increase in wound pain or tenderness
6. Unresponsive to adequate wound care and other measures

Grading of infected wounds (Information from references 2-4)

1. <u>Mild</u>

<u>When all the following criteria are fulfilled:</u>

a. Localized superficial infection involving only skin and subcutaneous tissue;
b. Cellulitis or erythema around the wound (when present) $\leq$2 cm, and no local complications;
c. The patient is metabolically stable and no systemic features of infection (fever, hypotension, tachycardia etc)

2. <u>Moderate</u>

The patient must be metabolically stable and systemically well, and must have at least one of the following features:

a. Cellulitis or erythema > 2 cm around the wound
b. Involvement deeper structures beneath the subcutaneous tissue (eg, abscess, fasciitis, osteomyelitis, septic arthritis etc)
c. Lymphangitic streaking

3. <u>Severe</u>

Patients with:

- Systemic toxicity [eg, fever or hypothermia, hemodynamic instability, leukocytosis or leukopenia (WBC >12,000/μL or <4000/ μL) etc.] **or**
- Metabolic instability (eg severe hyperglycemia) **or**
- Potentially limb-threatening local infections (eg, extensive local infection)

Osteomyelitis complicating diabetic foot infection

- Osteomyelitis, a serious complication of diabetic foot infection, develops in 20-66% cases of diabetic foot infection.[5]
- <u>Suspect osteomyelitis</u> and consider orthopedic consultation if an infected foot ulcer is deep or large; over a bony prominence; or chronic.

- Probe-to-bone test (PTB test):
  - This test may be helpful to diagnose or rule out diabetic foot osteomyelitis. It should be performed in all diabetic foot infection with an open wound.
  - In this test, the wound is gently explored with a blunt sterile metal probe. PTB test is considered positive when the underlying bone is palpable with the tip of the probe (often as a hard or gritty object).
- In diabetic foot infection, visible or palpable bone (on PTB test) is suggestive of osteomyelitis.
- ***Osteomyelitis is unlikely when ESR is normal***; a very high ESR (>70mm per hour) is supportive of a clinical suspicion of osteomyelitis.[2]

Actually, for a complete clinical evaluation of a diabetic foot infection, the evaluation should be done at three stages: first the patient as a whole, next the affected limb and finally the wound. Most diabetic foot infections begin in an ulcer. Vascular and or neurological abnormalities can predispose and complicate such an ulcer. Therefore, during clinical evaluation, any evidence of vascular abnormalities and neuropathy should be sought with special attention.

Key investigations for diabetic foot infection:

1. Gram-stain and culture of the wound specimen

Culture is not indicated for clinically uninfected wounds and may not be necessary for a mild infection if there is no history of recent antibiotic use.[4] In other cases, appropriately collected wound specimens should be sent to the lab for Gram-stain and culture before commencing empiric antibiotic therapy if possible.

Appropriate way of wound specimen collection:
- Clean and debride the wound before specimen collection[2]
- Collect tissue specimen by scraping with a sterile scalpel or dermal curette, or biopsy from the base of a debrided wound.
- Aspiration of any purulent discharge if present with a sterile needle and syringe is an acceptable alternative.[2]
- Avoid swabs specimens, particularly from inadequately debrided wounds, as they are often contaminated with skin flora or colonizers, giving rise to false-positive results.[4]
- Quickly send the specimens to the lab in a sterile container or appropriate transport media for aerobic and anaerobic culture, and Gram stain.

2. Imaging

Plain X-ray:
- IDSA recommends all patients with a new diabetic foot infection should have a plain X-ray of their affected foot.[4]
- A plain radiograph may reveal evidence of bone or joint abnormalities (eg, features of osteomyelitis, deformity), soft tissue gas, calcified arterial wall, foreign bodies etc. However, the sensitivity (54%) and specificity (68%) of plain X-ray are relatively low for confirming or excluding osteomyelitis.[4]
- The radiological features of osteomyelitis may not appear on plain radiograph in the first 2-4 weeks of initial infection.[2,6] Serial plain radiographs may be helpful when the first

film is negative. If repeat radiographs taken a few weeks apart also do not show any bony abnormalities, osteomyelitis is probably excluded.

MRI

- MRI is more sensitive and more specific than plain X-ray for detecting both osteomyelitis and soft tissue pathology. For osteomyelitis, diagnostic sensitivity of MRI is 90-100%[6] and specificity is about 80%.[7]
- MRI should be considered if the diagnosis of suspected osteomyelitis remains uncertain after plain radiograph or when deeper tissue involvement (fasciitis, myonecrosis, deep abscess etc) is suspected.

Nuclear imaging:

- Nuclear imaging is inferior to MRI for the diagnosis of osteomyelitis, so may be considered as alternative to MRI when MRI is contraindicated or unavailable.
- Combination of technetium bones scan with gallium scan or radio-labeled leukocyte scan may improve the diagnostic yield for osteomyelitis.[2]

3. Assessment of vascular patency

- Peripheral arterial disease (PAD) is present in nearly one-half of all patients with diabetic foot ulcers; infection in these ischemic foot ulcers is more common and associated with poor outcomes.[8]
- Ankle-Brachial Index (ABI) measurement is a simple and reliable screening test for PAD. When ABI is suggestive of PAD then Duplex ultrasound (DUS), Magnetic Resonance Angiogram (MRA), or (rarely) arteriogram may be needed for detailed anatomic information before an intervention.

4. Bone biopsy for culture and histology:

- Combination of bone culture and histology is the most definitive way to diagnose diabetic foot osteomyelitis.
- Bone biopsy for culture and histology should be considered when osteomyelitis is suspected clinically but the diagnosis remains uncertain after imaging.[2]

Treatment of diabetic foot infections

- Treatment of diabetic foot infection includes adequate antibiotic therapy, appropriate wound care, correction of the metabolic derangements, surgical measures and psychological support.
- **The optimal antimicrobial therapy for diabetic foot infection has yet to be determined.**[9] However, antibiotics are generally not recommended for clinically uninfected diabetic wounds.
- Consultation with surgeons and infectious disease specialists are usually needed in moderate and severe infections. Ideally, all patients with diabetic foot infections should be cared by a multidisciplinary foot care team.

Empiric antibiotic therapy for diabetic foot infection

General principles:

- Most mild and many moderate infections (eg, acute, superficial and limited moderate infection) can be treated on outpatient basis with relatively narrow-spectrum oral antibiotics that usually cover only aerobic Gram-positive cocci (Staphylococci and Streptococci).[4,9,10]
- Patients with severe infections, and more extensive or chronic moderate infections, should be hospitalized; empiric parenteral broad-spectrum antibiotic therapy with a regimen that covers gram-positive cocci, common gram-negative and obligate anaerobic bacteria should be started promptly.[4,9,10]
- Necrotic, gangrenous, or foul-smelling wounds generally require antianaerobic antibiotic.[2] However, dry gangrenes are generally not infected and may be autoamputed.

Empiric antibiotic regimens: (Information from references 2-4; 9-15)

Empiric antibiotic regimens vary considerably among hospitals and health systems.

A. ***Mild infection***

Commonly considered antimicrobial coverage: Gram-positive cocci such Staph aureus and Streptococci;

Anyone of the following drugs can be used:

- Amoxicillin-clavulanate (625 mg 8 hourly PO/ 875 mg 12 hourly PO), **or**
- Cephalexin (500 mg 6 hourly PO), **or**
- Clindamycin (300-450 mg 8 hourly PO) (can be used in severe penicillin allergic patients)

Probably the most commonly used drug for patients not allergic to penicillin is co-amoxiclav and for patients allergic to penicillin is clindamycin.

Some experts from the UK suggest flucloxacillin 500mg -- 1g QID PO for acute mild diabetic foot infection without ulceration (eg, mild cellulitis).[13,14]

Some patients may need empiric antibiotic regimen with polymicrobial and or MRSA coverage. Coverage of co-amoxiclav is polymicrobial, but not the coverage of cephalexin or clindamycin; cephalexin has weaker anaerobic coverage and clindamycin does not cover gram-negative bacteria. Of the three drugs mentioned above, only clindamycin has some MRSA coverage.

MRSA coverage in diabetic foot infection

In diabetic foot infection the prevalence of MRSA is 5-30% and IDSA recommends MRSA coverage in the following conditions: [4]

- History of previous MRSA infection (probably the most important risk factor for MRSA infection) or colonization within the last one year;
- High prevalence of MRSA in the community;
- The infection is severe enough where delayed treatment for possible MRSA may cause an unacceptable outcome.

However, there are some other risk factors for MRSA infection and the list of risk factors includes:

1. History of previous MRSA infection or colonization within the last one year
2. High prevalence of MRSA in the community
3. Recent antibiotic use

4. Recent hospitalization
5. Chronic wound
6. Concomitant osteomyelitis
7. Nasal carriage of MRSA

Notes:

- MRSA infection may be identified when apparently no risk factors for this infection are present.[2] On the other hand, isolation of MRSA from a wound does not necessarily mean infection with this organism; instead, it may be only colonization.[4]
- Clinical resolution of MRSA positive diabetic foot infection sometimes occurs with antibiotics that do not cover MRSA.[4]

Drugs suitable for MRSA coverage in diabetic foot infection:

- In mild infection, oral Doxycycline, Trimethoprim-sulfamethoxazole or Clindamycin can be used.
- In moderate to severe infection, IV Vancomycin is probably the most commonly used drug. Some experts have suggested other drugs also, such as linezolid[4,14] or teicoplanin,[14,15] particularly for moderate infection.

Antibiotic regimens with MRSA coverage for mild diabetic foot infection may be:

- A β-lactam (Amoxicillin-clavulanate or Cephalexin) **Plus** either Doxycycline (100 mg BID PO) or Trimethoprim-sulfamethoxazole (1-2 DS tabs BID PO);
  Or
- Monotherapy with Clindamycin 300-450 mg TID or QID PO;

Polymicrobial diabetic foot infection

Risk factors for polymicrobial diabetic foot infection include: [2,4]

- Chronic wound
- Recent use of antibiotic (in the past month);
- Ischemia or gangrene of the foot

Empiric antibiotic regimen for suspected polymicrobial infection (coverage: Gram positive, Gram negative and anaerobe) may be:

- Amoxicillin-clavulanate monotherapy
  Or
- Combination therapy with clindamycin **plus** a fluoroquinolone such as levofloxacin (500mg OD PO) or ciprofloxacin (500mg BID PO); (This regimen covers MRSA also and suitable for severe penicillin allergic patients)

Empiric antibiotic regimen for suspected polymicrobial including MRSA infection (coverage: Gram positive including MRSA, Gram negative and anaerobe) may be:

- Amoxicillin-clavulanate **Plus** either Doxycycline or Trimethoprim-sulfamethoxazole **Or**
- Clindamycin **plus** a fluoroquinolone such as ciprofloxacin or levofloxacin (suitable for severe penicillin allergic patients)

B. *Moderate infection:*

- Polymicrobial antibiotic coverage is most commonly considered. However, many patients who present with acute, limited, superficial infection without other complicating factors, such as peripheral vascular disease, can be treated with less aggressive antimicrobial therapy covering mainly Gram-positive cocci.

- In the other cases, particularly for patients with deeper structure involvement, poor glycemic control or peripheral arterial disease, more aggressive antibiotic therapy with stronger polymicrobial coverage may be appropriate.

*Many patients with deep infections do not have fever, leukocytosis, or markedly elevated acute phase reactants, but the absence of these features does not necessarily rule out a potentially serious infection.[4]

Less aggressive antibiotic regimens:

1. Amoxicillin-clavulanate (625 mg TID/ 875 mg BID PO; or 1.2g TID IV, if IV therapy necessary)
   Or
2. Cefpodoxime (400 mg PO 12 Hourly) **plus** Metronidazole (500 mg PO 12 Hourly) **Or**
3. Ampicillin/sulbactam (1.5 – 3.0 grams IV 6 Hourly)
   Or
4. Ceftriaxone (1-2 Gram IV daily) **Plus** either Clindamycin (600 mg IV 8 hourly) or Metronidazole (500 mg 8 hourly PO/ IV);

For severe penicillin allergy:
Levofloxacin (500 mg IV or orally OD) **Plus** clindamycin (600 to 900 mg IV or orally TID);

If MRSA coverage deemed necessary:

(a) No penicillin allergy: Amoxicillin-clavulanate **Plus** either Vancomycin (preferred) or linezolid;
(b) Severe penicillin allergy (Oral therapy): Linezolid 600mg BID **Plus** Ciprofloxacin 500mg BID **Plus** Metronidazole 400mgTID;[14]

More aggressive antibiotic regimen with stronger polymicrobial coverage:
Piperacillin-tazobactam **plus** vancomycin

C. ***Severe infection***

Aggressive antibiotic therapy with polymicrobial coverage including MRSA and *Pseudomonas aeruginosa* may be appropriate.

Piperacillin/tazobactam (4.5 grams IV 8 Hourly) or Meropenem (500mg QID)
Plus
Vancomycin 15 mg/kg (usual maximum 1g) IV 12 Hourly[3,13,14]

(Higher initial dose of vancomycin may need to consider)

For severe penicillin allergy[3,13]
(Consult infectious disease specialists)

Levofloxacin (750 mg IV daily) or Ciprofloxacin (400 mg IV 12 hourly)
Plus

Metronidazole (500 mg IV 8 Hourly)
Plus
Vancomycin IV

*Diabetic foot osteomyelitis often needs prolonged antibiotic therapy along with surgical measures. Consult orthopedic specialist urgently.

Response to therapy:

- Clinical response to empiric antibiotic regimen is usually evaluated 24-72 hours after initiation of the therapy, sometimes earlier depending on the severity, disease progression and availability of culture results.[2]
- Intravenous antibiotics can be changed to oral form when the patient is clinically improved and stable.[3]

Duration of antibiotic therapy in diabetic infection:

- The duration should be based on severity of the infection, clinical response to the treatment and whether there is osteomyelitis.
- Generally, antibiotics can be discontinued when the clinical symptoms and signs of infection have disappeared. There is insufficient evidence to support that continuing antimicrobial therapy until complete wound healing may be helpful to accelerate wound closure or prevent recurrent infection.[4]
- Although a fixed duration of antibiotic therapy cannot be suggested for all patients of a particular category, in general the duration is as follows:[3,10,13]
    1. Mild infection: 1-2 weeks
    2. Moderate to severe infection: 2-4 weeks
    3. Osteomyelitis: very variable, depending mainly on the nature of the surgery performed;

Pseudomonas aeruginosa in diabetic foot infection:[4,12,16]

Pseudomonas aeruginosa is a ubiquitous environmental bacterium and a common inhabitant of soil and water. Isolation of *P. aeruginosa* from a wound does not necessarily mean they are pathogenic bacteria in that wound; instead, they may be nonpathogenic colonizer only. Healing of a *P. aeruginosa* positive wound may occur with antibiotics without coverage for this organism.[4,12]

How common is P. aeruginosa in diabetic foot infection?

In developed countries, *P. aeruginosa* has been isolated from <10% of complicated skin and soft tissue infections including diabetic foot infections.[4] However, the reported prevalence is much higher in developing countries with tropical climate (about 30% in some series[16]). Probably this trend is related to increased water exposure of the feet, increased sweating into shoes, and wearing open or no footwear.

When should I consider empiric P. aeruginosa coverage in diabetic foot infection?

There is some debate about this issue. IDSA guideline states in diabetic foot infection empiric antibiotic coverage for *Pseudomonas aeruginosa* is usually unnecessary unless the patient has risk factors for true infection with this bacteria.[4] But investigators from tropical countries, where

Pseudomonas aeruginosa positive diabetic foot infection is supposed to be common, have expressed their concern; they believe disregarding this bacteria (when isolated from diabetic foot infection) considering it as commensals or contaminants may result in many more sepsis or amputation.[17] This area needs more studies. However, **at least in the following situations empiric antipseudomonal therapy can be considered:**

- Severe infection[4,9]
- Deep infection
- Wound with green-blue colored discharge
- Where nonpseudomonal antibiotic therapy has failed[9]

*Empiric antipseudomonal coverage may be considered more frequently in regions with high prevalence of pseudomonal infections and warm climate, and for patients who soak their feet frequently.

What are the cheaper antipseudomonal antibiotics?

Antipseudomonal antibiotics are generally expensive. Aminoglycosides (Amikacin, gentamicin), which are effective against *P. aeruginosa,* are the exceptions; so they may be considered as alternatives to other more expensive antipseudomonal drugs where health system runs with limited resources. Gentamicin is probably the cheapest of all in this category. Levofloxacin and ciprofloxacin have some antipseudomonal activity[9]

What can be decided about the empiric antibiotic regimen after obtaining culture results?

The isolated bacteria may be true pathogens or contaminants. Clinical response to the empiric antibiotic regimen is very important. If the response is adequate, the regimen may be continued, or even can be narrowed; but when the response is inadequate, the therapy should be broadened to cover all isolated organisms.[4]

Other treatments

Surgical treatment[4,11]

- Most diabetic foot infections need some sort of surgical interventions and surgery is the mainstay of treatment for deep infections.
- Surgical procedures range from simple incision and drainage to extensive debridement and amputation. Revascularization may be needed for limb ischemia.
- Adequate surgical measures in time can substantially reduce the possibility of catastrophic outcome. Urgent surgical consultation is mandatory for patients with clinical evidence of a life- or limb-threatening infection, or if the involved limb is markedly ischemic.

Wound care

Ideally wound care should be done by wound a specialist. Regular dressing and pressure offloading are particularly important.

Correction of metabolic derangements

Good glycemic control and correction of fluid and electrolyte imbalances are critical.

Adjunct therapy

Selective adjunctive therapies may be considered in some nonresponding patients which include maggot debridement therapy, growth factor (including granulocyte colony stimulating factor) therapy, hyperbaric oxygen therapy and topical negative pressure therapy (eg, vacuum-assisted closure). [2,4]

Summary of the empiric antibiotic therapy for diabetic foot infections:

A. Mild infection

- Amoxicillin-clavulanate (625 mg 8 hourly PO/ 875 mg 12 Hourly PO), **or**
- Clindamycin (300-450 mg 8 hourly PO) (for penicillin allergic patients)

Some patients may need empiric antibiotic regimen with polymicrobial* and or MRSA** coverage. Coverage of co-amoxiclav is polymicrobial, but not the coverage of clindamycin; however, clindamycin has some MRSA coverage.

Antibiotic regimens with MRSA coverage for mild diabetic foot infection:

- Amoxicillin-clavulanate **Plus** either Doxycycline (100 mg BID PO) or Trimethoprim-sulfamethoxazole (1-2 DS tabs BID PO);
  (This regimen provides polymicrobial coverage also)
  Or
- Monotherapy with Clindamycin 300-450 mg TID or QID PO;

*Risk factors for polymicrobial diabetic foot infection include: Chronic wound**;** recent use of antibiotic (in the past month); ischemia or gangrene of the foot
**IDSA recommends MRSA coverage in the following conditions: (1) History of previous MRSA infection or colonization within the last one year, (2) High prevalence of MRSA in the community, or (3) The infection is severe enough where delayed treatment for possible MRSA may cause an unacceptable outcome.

B. Moderate infection

- Polymicrobial antibiotic coverage is most commonly considered. However, many patients who present with acute, limited and superficial infection without other complicating factors, such as peripheral vascular disease, can be treated with less aggressive antimicrobial therapy covering mainly Gram-positive cocci.
- In the other cases, particularly for patients with deeper structure involvement, poor glycemic control or peripheral arterial disease, more aggressive antibiotic therapy with stronger polymicrobial coverage may be appropriate.

Less aggressive antibiotic regimens
Amoxicillin-clavulanate (625 mg TID/ 875 mg BID PO; or 1.2g TID IV, if IV therapy necessary)
If MRSA coverage deemed necessary:
Amoxicillin-clavulanate **Plus** either Vancomycin (preferred) or linezolid;

More aggressive antibiotic regimen with stronger polymicrobial coverage:

Piperacillin-tazobactam **plus** vancomycin

C. Severe infection

Piperacillin/tazobactam (4.5 grams IV TID) or Meropenem (500mg QID)
Plus
Vancomycin 15 mg/kg (usual maximum 1g) IV 12 hourly;
(Higher initial dose of vancomycin may need to consider)

References

1. Mark A Kosinski et al. Current Medical Management of Diabetic Foot Infections. **Expert Rev Anti Infect Ther. 2010**; 8(11):1293-1305.

2. Mazen S. Bader. Diabetic Foot Infection. **Am Fam Physician. 2008;** 78(1):71-79.

3. 'Antimicrobial treatment of diabetic foot infection' in **antimicrobial stewardship of Pennsylvania University Health System, USA**; at: http://www.uphs.upenn.edu/antibiotics/Skin_and_Soft_Tissue_Infections.html

4. Benjamin A. Lipsky et al. 2012 Infectious Diseases Society of America Clinical Practice Guideline for the Diagnosis and Treatment of Diabetic Foot Infections. **Clinical Infectious Diseases 2012**; 54(12):132–173

5. Lawrence A. Lavery et al. Probe-to-Bone Test for Diagnosing Diabetic Foot Osteomyelitis: Reliable or relic? **Diabetes Care 2007**; 30:270–274

6. William J. Jeffcoate et al. Controversies in Diagnosing and Managing Osteomyelitis of the Foot in Diabetes. **Clinical Infectious Diseases 2004;** 39:S115–22

7. Kapoor A et al. Magnetic resonance imaging for diagnosing foot osteomyelitis: a meta-analysis. Arch Intern Med. 2007 **Jan 22;167(2):125-32**

8. L. Prompers et al. Prediction of outcome in individuals with diabetic foot ulcers: focus on the differences between individuals with and without peripheral arterial disease. The EURODIALE Study**. Diabetologia (2008)**; 51:747–755

9. Gregory T. Matsuura et al. Update on the Antimicrobial Management of Foot Infections in Patients With Diabetes. **Clinical Diabetes 2013**; Volume 31, Number 2

10. Fassil W. Gemechu et al. Diabetic Foot Infections. **Am Fam Physician. 2013**; 88(3):177-184.

11. Michael Stuart Bronze. 'Diabetic Foot Infections Treatment & Management' in **Emedicine**; at http://emedicine.medscape.com/article/237378-treatment#showall

12. Paul Auwaerter. 'Diabetic Foot Infection' in **Johns Hopkins Antibiotic (ABX) Guide.**

13. 'Guideline for the treatment of diabetic foot infection' on the website of **Nottingham University Hospitals, NHS trust (UK)**. At: https://www.nuh.nhs.uk/staff-area/ clinical-guidelines/; clinical guideline clinical support Pathology-microbioloy anti→ biotic prescribing policy for diabetic foot disease.

14. Antimicrobial guidelines for the empirical management of diabetic foot infections. **University hospitals of Leicester, NHS trust**, UK; at: http://www.leicestershirediabetes.org.uk/uploads/123/documents/UHL%20Antimicrobial%20Guidelines%20Diabetic%20Foot%20Infections.pdf

15. 'Diabetic Ulcers (Without osteomyelitis)' in the antibiotic guidelines of the **Gloucestershire Hospitals.** At: http://www.gloshospitals.nhs.uk/en/Trust-Staff/Antibiotic-Guidelines/SkinSoft-tissueBoneJoint/Diabetic-Ulcers-Without-osteomyelitis/

16. Muhammad Kazim Rahim Najjad et al. Pseudomonas as trespassers in diabetic foot infections: More questions and fewer answers. **JPMA 2014**; 64: S-112 (Suppl. 2)

17. S Murugan et al. Prevalence and antimicrobial susceptibility pattern of Metallo β-lactamase producing *Pseudomonas aeruginosa* in diabetic foot infection. **International Journal of Microbiological Research 2010**; 1(3): 123-128

Chapter 10

Sepsis/ Severe sepsis/ Septic shock

Sepsis/ Severe sepsis/ Septic shock

Terms used to describe septic states: [1,2]

Systemic Inflammatory Response Syndrome (SIRS)

When two or more of the following conditions are fulfilled in a patient with inflammation:

1. Fever (oral temperature >38^{0}C or 100.4^0 F) or hypothermia (<36^{0}C or 96.8^0 F)
2. Tachypnea (respiration rate >20/min)
3. Tachycardia (heart rate >90/min)
4. Leukocytosis (>12000/μL), leucopenia (<4000/ μL), or Bands >10%;

Inflammation in SIRS might have infectious or noninfectious etiology. Noninfectious etiology of SIRS includes pancreatitis; burns or trauma; pulmonary embolism; myocardial infarction; concealed bleeding etc.

Bacteremia

Presence of viable bacteria in blood (detected by blood culture)

Septicemia

Presence of microorganisms (bacteria, viruses, or fungi) or their toxins in blood; it is a broader term than bacteremia.

Sepsis

- When SIRS is due to probable or proven infection;
- Simply sepsis can be defined as infection with systemic manifestations. Bacteremia may or may not be present in sepsis; in many cases, bacterial toxins or inflammatory mediators are responsible for systemic manifestations in the absence of bacteremia.
- Severity of sepsis may vary from mild to severe.

Severe sepsis

When sepsis is associated with sepsis-induced organ dysfunction or tissue hypoperfusion; Evidence of tissue hypoperfusion may be hypotension, elevated lactate, or oliguria (urine output <0.5 ml/kg/hour).

Septic shock

When sepsis-induced hypotension persists despite adequate fluid resuscitation; here hypotension is considered as systolic blood pressure <90 mm of Hg, or 40 mm of Hg less than the patient's usual blood pressure.

Severe sepsis and septic shock are common problem worldwide, with a mortality of 25% (or often higher).[1]

Microbiology of severe sepsis and septic shock

- It depends on the primary site of infection.
- Any type of organisms- Gram-positives, Gram-negatives and anaerobes- may be involved. Fungi and viruses may also be found in some special circumstances.
- Blood culture is positive for bacteria or fungi in only 20-40% cases of severe sepsis.[2]

Clinical features of severe sepsis and septic shock

General features:

- Fever or hypothermia; however, temperature may be normal (in about one third of cases) especially in the elderly; neonate; or in patients with renal failure or alcoholism.
- Altered mental state (eg, confusion, disorientation), particularly in the elderly;
- Tachypnea (respiratory rate may be normal in some patients)
- Tachycardia (rarely, pulse rate may be normal)
- Hypotension (systolic BP <90mm Hg or systolic BP decrease >40mm Hg from the usual of that individual or mean arterial BP <70 mm Hg)
- Significant edema
- Increased capillary refill time

Features of organ dysfunction include:

- Oliguria - urine output < 0.5 mL/kg/hr for more than 2 hours despite adequate volume resuscitation, uremia (manifestations of acute kidney injury)
- Ileus
- Respiratory distress (Acute Respiratory Distress Syndrome)
- Jaundice, coagulopathy (Hepatic dysfunction)
- Heart failure, arrhythmia (Cardiomyopathy)
- Anemia, bleeding (Bone marrow suppression)

Other features depend on the site of primary infection.

Causes of hypotension in septic shock

1. Direct vasodilating effects of inflammatory mediators;
2. Myocardial depression and or arrhythmia (eg, atrial fibrillation);
3. Hypovolemia (due to less intake, gastrointestinal fluid loss etc)

Investigations of severe sepsis and septic shock

There is no specific diagnostic test for sepsis. Investigations can be divided into two groups:

- **Investigations to confirm the primary source of infection:** depend on the clinical suspicion about the primary source;
- **Common investigations** (considered irrespective of the primary source of infection): below is a list of commonly performed tests with some possible findings in sepsis:
  - **CBC with CRP:** Leukocytosis (WBC count > 12,000 /μL) or Leukopenia (WBC count < 4000 /μL); left shift; neutrophils may have toxic granulations, Dohle bodies or cytoplasmic vacuoles; thrombocytopenia (platelet count < 100,000 /μL); WBC count remains normal in some patients.
  - **Plasma glucose**
  - **Serum albumin, calcium, magnesium and phosphate;**
  - **Urinalysis:** proteinuria; pyuria, hematuria if UTI is present;
  - **Urea, creatinine and electrolyte:** Variable abnormality depending on severity; high urea and creatinine, low bicarbonate etc.

- **Liver Function Test (LFT):** hyperbilirubinemia; raised alkaline phosphatase due to cholestasis; raised ALT and AST;
- **Serum lactate:** elevated in lactic acidosis due to tissue hypoperfusion;
- **CXR:** evidence of volume overload, widespread infiltration due to ARDS, or underlying pneumonia
- **ECG:** Tachycardia, nonspecific ST-T changes, arrhythmia (eg, atrial fibrillation);
- **Coagulation profile:** PT, APTT, fibrinogen, D-dimers to look for evidence of DIC.
- **Arterial blood gas analysis:** hypoxemia
- **For microbial diagnosis:**
  1. Blood culture: at least two samples from two different sites should be taken.
  2. Microscopy and culture of specimen from the primary site of infection (sputum, urine, any wound etc);
  3. PCR of peripheral blood or sample from the primary site of infection (in some cases);

Treatment of severe sepsis or septic shock

Treatment should be started as soon as possible based on the clinical diagnosis, and should not be delayed for laboratory results. The patient should be cared in ICU.

Mainstays of treatment:
- Infection control: includes antimicrobial therapy and primary source control;
- Supportive care

Here the empiric antimicrobial therapy and supportive care have been described briefly, especially those measures that can be started in General Medicine ward when transferring the patient to ICU is underway.

Antimicrobial therapy:

Empiric antibiotic regimen depends on:
- The possible primary site of infection;
- Local prevalence of pathogens and their antibiotic sensitivity patterns;
- Patient's background such as immune status; organisms of previous infection or colonization; recent hospitalization; recent antibiotic use (within last three months) etc.

The initial empiric antimicrobial regimen should be broad enough to cover all the likely organisms because these patients have little ability to tolerate an error in the therapy. Recently used antibiotics (including the ineffective current ones) are usually avoided.[1] Consult an infectious disease specialist or medical microbiologist as soon as possible.

Antimicrobial therapy should be started within the first hour of suspicion of severe sepsis or septic shock before the lab test results are available. Promptness and appropriateness of treatment given in the initial hours are likely to influence the outcome.[1]

Community- acquired sepsis: The patient is coming from the community with no history of recent hospitalization or staying at long term care facilities; or onset of symptoms within 3 days of hospitalization.

Hospital-acquired sepsis: The patient has a history of recent hospitalization or staying at long term care facilities; or onset of symptoms at least 3 days after hospitalization.

The following empiric antibiotic regimens (IV) can be considered in severe sepsis or septic shock (the dose given here is for patients with normal renal function)**:** [Information from references 2—5]

Primary site of infection	***Community-acquired***	***Hospital-acquired***
Pneumonia	Ceftriaxone 1-2gm 12 hourly **Plus** azithromycin **Plus** vancomycin For β – lactam allergy: Levofloxacin 750 mg daily **Plus** Vancomycin	(a) Piperacillin-tazobactam 4.5g 8 hourly or Cefepime **Plus** (b) Amikacin **Plus** (c) Vancomycin; [a+b+c] For β – lactam allergy: Levofloxacin 750 mg daily **Plus** Amikacin **Plus** Vancomycin
Unknown source	Piperacillin-tazobactam 4.5g 8 hourly/ meropenem **Plus** Vancomycin	Piperacillin-tazobactam **Plus** Amikacin **Plus** Vancomycin For β – lactam allergy: Levofloxacin 750 mg daily **Plus** Amikacin **Plus** Metronidazole 500 mg 12 hourly **Plus** Vancomycin
Abdominal infection (Most cases are surgery related so usually managed in surgical ICU)	(1) Piperacillin-tazobactam (monotherapy) Or (2) Meropenem (monotherapy) For β – lactam allergy: Levofloxacin 750 mg daily **Plus** Tobramycin **Plus** Metronidazole 500 mg 12 hourly **Plus** Vancomycin	Piperacillin-tazobactam **Plus** Amikacin **Plus** Vancomycin +/- Caspofungin (when bowel perforation is suspected) Alternative drugs for the above regimen: (1) Cefepime **Plus** Metronidazole can be used instead of piperacillin-tazobactam while other drugs of the above regimen will be the same. For β – lactam allergy: Levofloxacin Plus metronidazole can be used instead of piperacillin-tazobactam keeping the other drugs of the above regimen same.

Urinary source	Piperacillin-tazobactam/ cefepime For β – lactam allergy: Levofloxacin Plus tobramycin	Piperacillin-tazobactam/ cefepime **Plus** Amikacin For β – lactam allergy: Levofloxacin Plus Amikacin
Skin and soft tissue	Piperacillin-tazobactam + Vancomycin ± Clindamycin (600-900mg TID) *Consider adding clindamycin if necrotizing fasciitis or group A Streptococcus infection is suspected. Clindamycin inhibits streptococcal toxin and cytokine production.	Same as for community acquired infection
Neutropenia with Absolute neutrophil count (ANC) ≤ 500 or ≤ 1000 but with a possibility of dropping to ≤ 500	**Prompt consultation with infectious disease specialists particularly important;** Piperacillin-tazobactam **Plus** Amikacin **Plus** Vancomycin **Plus** Caspofungin, first loading dose 70 mg then 50 mg daily; *Lower dose of Caspofungin should be given if there is hepatic impairment. *If there is recent piperacillin exposure, **meropenem 1g IV 8 hourly can be considered instead of piperacillin-tazobactam while other drugs of the regimen will remain the same.** For β – lactam allergy: Levofloxacin **Plus** Amikacin **Plus** Vancomycin **Plus** Caspofungin (+metronidazole if abdominal infection is suspected)	Same as for community acquired infection
Central line related	Piperacillin-tazobactam **Plus** Amikacin **Plus** Vancomycin	Same as for community acquired infection

Meningitis (Cover Listeria infection in community acquired meningitis if: age >50 years; brain-stem signs present; or patient pregnant, immunocompromised, diabetic, or alcoholic)	Ceftriaxone 2g 12 hourly **Plus** Vancomycin 15 mg/kg 8 Hourly ± Ampicillin 2g 4 hourly (Add ampicillin when Listeria coverage is necessary)	Post-surgical cases Meropenem 2g 8 hourly **Plus** Vancomycin 15 mg/kg 8 hourly

Note:

Antifungal coverage: During choosing empiric antimicrobial regimen clinicians should consider the possibility systemic candidiasis. Risk factors for candidemia include:[1]

- Immunosuppressed state (eg, neutropenia)
- Previous intense antibiotic therapy
- Candida colonies in multiple sites

De-escalation of antibiotic therapy:

- Empiric antimicrobial therapy should be reassessed daily for possible de-escalation.
- In most cases, when the causative organism and its sensitivity pattern are known the empiric regimen can be narrowed to more appropriate one; however, occasionally combined antimicrobial treatment may need to continue.[1] Seek advice from infectious disease specialists.

Duration of antimicrobial therapy:[1]

- Typically the duration is 7–10 days;
- Longer courses may be needed in patients with slow clinical response; undrainable source of infection; Staph. aureus bacteremia; some fungal or viral infections; or immunosuppressed state etc.

Identification and elimination of the potential primary source of infection

1. When appropriate, any identified source of infection should be removed or drained as soon as possible after successful initial resuscitation.
2. Consider removal (when possible) or replacement of all indwelling devices such as vascular catheter, urinary catheter and endotracheal tube. It should be done promptly when a particular device is a likely source of infection. For intravascular catheters, existing ones should be removed after inserting new ones at different sites.
3. To eliminate a source of infection, the procedures which are likely to be physiologically least deranging should be used; for example, percutaneous drainage instead of open surgical drainage when possible.
4. When the source of sepsis is not clear:
    - Look for potential sites of occult infection which include-
        - Abdomen or chest infection: Consider ultrasonography of the abdomen and plain x-ray of the chest; CT or MRI of the abdomen and chest. Chest CT may

reveal an unsuspected source of chest infection even when the plain x-ray is normal.

- <u>Cardiac infection:</u> Any new murmur, particularly in patients with a history of IV drug use;
- <u>Rectal and perianal infection:</u> look for cutaneous erythema and tenderness in the perineal area, particularly in immunocompromised patients;
- <u>Infected decubitus ulcer</u>
- <u>Paranasal sinusitis in a patient with nasal intubation;</u>

Supportive care

- Hemodynamic support
- Other supportive measures (oxygen, ventilatory support, metabolic support etc.)

Hemodynamic support

A. Fluid challenge or volume resuscitation
B. Vasopressor therapy
C. Steroid therapy

<u>When should hemodynamic resuscitation be started in sepsis?</u>
Hemodynamic resuscitation should be started if a patient with sepsis has (otherwise unexplained) any one of the following features of tissue hypoperfusion:

- Hypotension (generally systolic BP < 90 mmHg) or
- Blood lactate level ≥ 4 mmol/L.

<u>Why elevated blood lactate is considered as an independent marker of tissue hypoperfusion in sepsis?</u>
In some cases of septic shock, blood lactate is found elevated before the development of hypotension. Sepsis patients (not yet hypotensive) with lactate level ≥ 4 mmol/L are at high risk for septic shock.[6] Therefore, although lactate elevation in sepsis is not a specific evidence of hypoperfusion, lactate level ≥ 4 mmol/L is generally considered as an evidence of tissue hypoperfusion and an indication for starting hemodynamic resuscitation even in the absence of hypotension.

However, during the initial presentation of patients with severe sepsis, lactate elevation alone (without hypotension) is found in only about 5% of cases, whereas hypotension with or without lactate elevation is found in about 65% cases.[1] Therefore, in possible sepsis-induced hypoperfusion, hypotension is present (alone or associated with elevated lactate) in more than 90% cases.

In all patients at risk for septic shock, blood lactate should be checked.[6]

In severe sepsis, blood lactate levels have higher prognostic value than oxygen-derived variables.[6]

A. Fluid challenge or volume resuscitation

Fluid challenge or volume resuscitation is the first step of hemodynamic support.
<u>How the fluid challenge is usually given?</u>

- Surviving Sepsis Campaign guidelines (2012) recommend administration of 30 mL/kg crystalloid solution to be completed within the first three hours of resuscitation. Some patients may need greater amount of fluids administered at a faster rate.[1]
- Actually the volume and rate of fluid administration should be individualized. The goal is not to infuse a specific amount of fluid but to achieve normal tissue reperfusion without causing fluid overload.
- For initial fluid resuscitation, many patients require 20-30 ml of crystalloid IV fluid for per Kg body weight. Initially, 500 ml crystalloid (eg, normal saline) can be given over 30 min. The hemodynamic status should be monitored at least clinically by checking pulse, blood pressure, capillary refill time; and signs of volume overload such as pulmonary rales (due to pulmonary edema); if there is no evidence of volume overload, 1-2 liters of normal saline is generally infused over initial 1-2 hours.[2]
- About one-third of patients with hypotension and organ hypoperfusion respond to volume resuscitation with IV fluids.[2]

Which IV fluids are appropriate for sepsis associated hypotension?

1. For the initial volume resuscitation, **crystalloids are the fluids of first choice.**[1] The standard intravenous (IV) isotonic crystalloid fluids are Normal saline (NS) and Lactated Ringer's (LR) solution. Although the metabolic changes that occur with the infusion of large quantities of these two fluids (normal saline versus Lactated Ringer's solution) are somewhat different, in most cases practically the differences are not significant. **However, normal saline (0.9%NaCl) is probably the most commonly used fluid** for the initial volume resuscitation in sepsis associated hypotension.

   Isotonic crystalloid fluids expand the intravascular and interstitial fluid spaces. Usually about 30% of the infused isotonic fluid remains in the circulation. **When the crystalloid fluid requirement is high, administration of some albumin solution may be beneficial.**[1]

2. Colloids are more expensive and have no clear benefit over crystalloid, so not recommended in septic shock.
3. Hydroxyethyl starches (eg, hetastarch, pentastarch and tetrastarch) are not recommended.

Notes:

- The resuscitation measures should be started immediately and should not be delayed for ICU admission.
- In a patient with sepsis, when the blood pressure begins to fall, an ECG should also be performed immediately, especially to detect sepsis induced arrhythmia such as atrial fibrillation, which itself may cause hypotension or may aggravate sepsis-induced hypotension.

What can be done if hypotension persists after the fluid challenge?

In such cases, usually vasopressor infusion (norepinephrine initially) is added to the therapy.[1]

The target of resuscitation in sepsis-induced tissue hypoperfusion during the first 6 hours of resuscitation includes all of the followings:[1,7]

1. Central Venous Pressure (CVP) 8–12 mmHg (12-15 mmHg if the patient is on mechanical ventilation)
2. Mean Arterial Pressure (MAP) ≥ 65 mm Hg;
3. Urine output > 0.5 mL/ kg/ hr
4. Superior vena cava (central venous) oxygenation saturation ($Scvo_2$) ≥70%;
5. Normalization of the lactate level when elevated lactate was a marker of tissue hypoperfusion;

*To determine the endpoint of hemodynamic resuscitation, where $Scvo_2$ is not available, lactate normalization may be an alternative target. When both are available, target $Scvo_2$ and lactate normalization both should be achieved.[1]

B. Vasopressor therapy in septic shock (with brief description of some vasopressors and inotropes)

Indication:
Generally, when initial volume resuscitation (usually about 30 ml/kg crystalloid) alone cannot achieve target blood pressure (MAP >65 mmHg; or roughly, systolic BP >90 mmHg), vasopressors are added to the therapy.[1,7] However, in life threatening hypotension, vasopressor therapy may need to start early, even when the initial fluid resuscitation is not complete.[8]

Target BP
Generally, a low normal blood pressure (MAP 65-90 mmHg[7]; systolic BP 90 – 100 mmHg) is maintained to ensure adequate vital organ perfusion minimizing the side effects of vasopressors. CVP and central venous oxygen saturation ($Scvo_2$) should be measured when a patient needs vasopressor agents.

Generally, it is advised to infuse vasopressors through central venous lines to avoid ischemic tissue injury from extravasation.

Norepinephrine:

- In septic shock, norepinephrine is commonly considered as the vasopressor of first choice.[1]
- It acts on both arteries and veins. It is a potent α-adrenergic agonist and causes marked vasoconstriction. It has weaker β-adrenergic effect, so causes minimal increase in heart rate;[9] it is less arrhythmogenic than dopamine and epinephrine.[10] Therefore, in septic shock where vasodilation is usually the most important cause of hypotension norepinephrine is often very effective to increase mean arterial pressure with minimal adverse effects.[9]

Dose:

- Initial dose 1-2 mcg/min **(not per Kg/min)** as an IV infusion; titrate the dose to maintain systolic BP> 90 mmHg. The usual maintenance dose is 2-4 mcg/min; maximum dose is 30mcg/min; for refractory shock 10-30 mcg/min may be needed.[11]
- In the United States, 20 mcg/ min is the commonly accepted maximum dosage.[12]
- Be watchful about some side effects such peripheral ischemia, tachycardia etc. when administering higher dose of norepinephrine. An alternative agent should be sought if adverse effects occur before reaching the desired therapeutic goals.

<u>What can be done if hypotension persists (systolic BP < 90 mmHg; MAP <65 mmHg) despite fluid resuscitation and norepinephrine therapy?</u>

Various suggestions exist for these patients; you can consider the following steps:
Add low-dose hydrocortisone (200mg/day)[13,14] to the therapy, plus consider additional any one of the three steps:

- Addition of dobutamine to norepinephrine if cardiac output is low or not measured; this combination is a popular option; [8] or
- Addition of epinephrine to norepinephrine;[1] or
- Replacement of norepinephrine with epinephrine and use epinephrine as the only vasopressor and inotrope.[1, 8]

<u>The rationale behind this approach:</u>

- In vasopressor-unresponsive septic shock, early addition of low dose hydrocortisone to the vasopressor is likely to reduce both short-term and long-term mortality significantly.[13, 14]
- Dobutamine is a potent inotropic agent and increases cardiac output by increasing myocardial contractility. In severe sepsis, low cardiac output due to sepsis induced cardiomyopathy is common. In septic shock, when hypotension remains unresolved even after adequate volume resuscitation and vasopressor support with norepinephrine, low cardiac output is likely.

  Norepinephrine is not a potent inotrope; therefore, in this situation, if cardiac output is low or cannot be measured, additional inotropic support by adding dobutamine to norepinephrine is logical.

  Alternative to this combination may be: (a) addition of epinephrine (which has both strong inotropic and vasopressor effects) to norepinephrine, or (b) using epinephrine as a single agent, replacing norepinephrine. [1, 8] However, the concept of these alternative two options is relatively new and probably not widely practiced.

<u>Epinephrine:</u>

- Epinephrine is a potent α- and β-adrenergic agonist.[9] Epinephrine increases mean arterial pressure by α_1-adrenergic receptor mediated vasoconstriction and cardiac output by its β_1-adrenergic effect.
- Epinephrine is used as the first-line catecholamine in cardiopulmonary resuscitation (CPR) and anaphylactic shock.[9] However, in septic shock epinephrine is usually considered as a second-line agent and the first alternative to norepinephrine. It can be added to or substituted for norepinephrine when an additional second line drug is required to achieve and maintain target blood pressure.[1]
- Although some studies suggest epinephrine has deleterious effects on splanchnic circulation, the overall outcome is not worse.[1] However, epinephrine may increase aerobic lactate production by stimulating of β_2-adrenergic receptors in skeletal muscles, so lactate clearance cannot be used as a guide for resuscitation in epinephrine treated patients.[1]

<u>Dobutamine</u>

Dobutamine is a synthetic catecholamine with mainly β-adrenergic and only limited α- adrenergic activity.[9] Although it is a derivative of dopamine, it does not cause release of endogenous norepinephrine like dopamine, and acts directly on adrenergic receptors.[15] Dobutamine is a potent and relatively selective inotropic agent with minimal chronotropic and peripheral vascular effects.[15] It increases cardiac output by increasing mainly myocardial contractility (β_1 effect).

Unlike dopamine, which is a potent chronotrope at all doses, dobutamine causes much less increase in heart rate. **Dobutamine is less arrhythmogenic than other catecholamines used in the treatment of hypotensive states (eg, dopamine, norepinephrine and epinephrine).**[16] Dobutamine reduces systemic and pulmonary vascular resistance by its β_2 effect[9] which may be minimized partially by its limited α- adrenergic activity; and as a single vasoactive agent, its overall impact is often mild vasodilation, especially at low doses (<5μg/Kg/min).[17]

Dobutamine is the preferred vasoactive drug to treat cardiogenic shock with low cardiac output and increased afterload. In septic shock, when added to norepinephrine, dobutamine can optimize cardiac output minimizing sepsis associated myocardial depression while norepinephrine minimizes sepsis induced vasodilation by its vasopressor effect.[8] Additionally, dobutamine can increase oxygen delivery and consumption in the tissues.[18]

<u>When can I add dobutamine to norepinephrine in septic shock?</u>
Dobutamine can be added to norepinephrine in septic shock with:

1. Myocardial dysfunction (suggested by high cardiac filling pressure and low cardiac output),[1, 9] **or**
2. Ongoing evidence of tissue hypoperfusion (eg, $Scvo_2 < 70\%$ and or persistently elevated serum lactate) despite adequate volume resuscitation and achieving target mean arterial pressure.[1, 18]

<u>Dose of dobutamine</u>: 2.5-20 μgm/kg/min[17]

<u>Dopamine</u>

Dopamine acts on dopaminergic and adrenergic receptors.[17] In addition to its direct β_1-adrenergic effects on heart, dopamine stimulates endogenous norepinephrine release within the myocardium. However, dopamine has little or no β_2-adrenergic effects.

Low-dose dopamine through dopaminergic receptors present in the coronary, renal, mesenteric, and cerebral vascular beds, promotes vasodilation and increases blood flow to this tissues.[17] However, low-dose dopamine should not be used to improve renal circulation in septic shock.[1] Also, dopamine should not be used routinely in septic shock, as its use is associated with increased mortality.[1]

<u>When can dopamine be used in septic shock then?</u>
As an alternative vasopressor agent to norepinephrine, dopamine can be used only in highly selective cases such as patients with absolute or relative bradycardia and low risk of tachyarrhythmias[1]

<u>Norepinephrine versus dopamine in septic shock</u> (Information from references 1, 8, 11, 17)

Norepinephrine	*Dopamine*
1. Although norepinephrine has both α and β adrenergic effects, it preferentially acts on α receptors and increases mean arterial pressure over cardiac output.	1. Activity is dose dependent: a) At low dose (2-5 mcg/Kg/min) stimulates dopaminergic and β adrenergic receptors producing increased GFR, heart rate and myocardial contractility. b) At moderate dose (5-10 mcg/Kg/min) preferentially stimulates β adrenergic receptors resulting in increased heart rate and myocardial contractility. c) At high dose (>10 mcg/Kg/min) predominantly stimulates α adrenergic receptors resulting in peripheral vasoconstriction. [Maximum dose may be 50 mcg/Kg/min; however, in most cases a dose up to 20 mcg/kg/min is administered]
2. Norepinephrine increases mean arterial pressure (MAP) primarily by its vasoconstrictive effects, with little increase in stroke volume and heart rate.	2. Heart rate and stroke volume increase are generally more prominent compared to norepinephrine.
3. Less arrhythmogenic	3.More arrhythmogenic
4. Not suitable for improving systolic dysfunction.	4. More effective in systolic dysfunction
5. More potent to reverse hypotension	5. Less potent compared to norepinephrine to reverse hypotension
6. No significant impact on endocrine function or immunity.	6. Can affect endocrine function via the hypothalamic pituitary axis and has immunosuppressive effects.

Phenylephrine

Phenylephrine is a potent and almost pure α-adrenergic agonist with virtually no β-adrenergic effects.[1, 17] It may reduce stroke volume but is least likely to produce tachycardia.[1]

It is primarily used to correct sudden severe hypotension in neurogenic shock (eg, spinal cord injury or spinal anesthesia);[18] simultaneous ingestion of nitrate and sildenafil; or vagally mediated hypotension during some percutaneous diagnostic or therapeutic procedures.[17]

Phenylephrine can be used in the treatment of septic shock only in some special circumstances:[1]

1. When norepinephrine is associated with dangerous arrhythmias, or
2. Persistently low blood pressure despite high cardiac output, or
3. When combined inotrope/vasopressor agents and low dose vasopressin have failed to restore target mean arterial pressure.

Vasopressin[1]

- Relative vasopressin deficiency occurs in septic shock. However, conflicting results have been found with the use of vasopressin in septic shock. A Randomized Controlled Trial comparing norepinephrine alone to norepinephrine plus low dose vasopressin (0.03 units/minute) showed no difference in outcome in the intent-to-treat patients. However, vasopressin 0.03 units/minute can be added to norepinephrine either to raise mean arterial pressure to target or to reduce norepinephrine dose.
- Low dose vasopressin should not be used as a single initial vasopressor agent. Higher doses of vasopressin (>0.03-0.04 units/minute) are more likely to cause cardiac, digital, and splanchnic ischemia, so should be considered only in situations where alternative vasopressors have failed to achieve the target MAP.

C. Steroid therapy in septic shock

Severe illness and stress strongly stimulate the hypothalamic-pituitary-adrenal (HPA) axis and ultimately cause increased secretion of cortisol from the adrenal cortex. This increased cortisol release is an essential defensive mechanism of the host. Cortisol has a vital supportive role in maintaining vascular tone, capillary permeability and the distribution of total body water among various body fluid compartments.[19] But in many critically ill patients, dysfunction develops in the HPA axis resulting in insufficient cortisol release.[20] The reported prevalence of adrenal insufficiency in critically ill patients is very variable (0–77%), with up to 60% among patients with septic shock.[20]

The mechanism of this HPA axis dysfunction is complex and not clearly known.[20] Factors involved in it include inflammatory cytokines; effects of drugs; and direct damage of the gland by hemorrhage, infarction, injury, or tumor.[21] The American College of Critical Care Medicine (ACCCM) has introduced the term "critical illness-related corticosteroid insufficiency" (CIRCI) to describe the HPA axis dysfunction in critical illnesses. In many cases, CIRCI is reversible.[20]

<u>How to diagnose corticosteroid insufficiency in critical illness?</u>
It is often difficult to ascertain adrenal insufficiency in a critically ill patient;[21] absolute cortisol levels may not be low although they are low for the degree of stress of the acute illness. In this state of relative cortisol deficiency, random cortisol level and the results of the ACTH stimulation test both may be misleading.[1] **Surviving sepsis campaign does not recommend ACTH stimulation test to identify the sub-group of patients with adrenal insufficiency in septic shock.[1]**

<u>When can corticosteroid be added to the treatment of septic shock?</u>

- Intravenous hydrocortisone can be added to the treatment of septic shock when adequate fluid resuscitation and vasopressor therapy fail to achieve target blood pressure (such as systolic BP <90 mmHg after observing about one hour with IV fluid plus norepinephrine therapy).[1,14,20]
- Surviving sepsis campaign does not recommend the use of corticosteroids in sepsis without shock.[1]
- The American College of Critical Care Medicine (ACCCM) does not recommend dexamethasone to treat critical illness–associated corticosteroid insufficiency in septic shock or ARDS.[20]

<u>How can hydrocortisone be given?</u>

- Surviving sepsis campaign recommends continuous infusion of low-dose hydrocortisone (200mg/day).[1] However, hydrocortisone 50mg IV 6 hourly can also be given.[2,20]
- Bolus doses of hydrocortisone may cause more side effects especially hyperglycemia. High dose corticosteroid should not be used in septic shock, since it is generally considered harmful.

The optimal duration of corticosteroid treatment in septic shock and ARDS is unclear.[20] Hydrocortisone should be tapered when vasopressor support is no longer necessary,[1] which may take 5-7 days.

The ACCCM (American College of Critical Care Medicine) recommendation about dose and duration of hydrocortisone therapy in septic shock and early ARDS:[20]

- Hydrocortisone 200 mg/day IV in 4 divided doses; or 100-mg initial bolus followed by continuous infusion at 10 mg/hr (240 mg/d).
- *Duration:* In septic shock 7 days or longer before tapering; in early ARDS 14 days or longer before tapering;

What can be done if $Scvo_2$ remains < 70% or lactate remains high even after achieving target CVP and MAP?

- This clinical state generally indicates inadequate tissue oxygenation;
- Transfuse packed red cells (if hematocrit <30%) to raise hematocrit >30%; but if still $Scvo_2$ remains <70% or lactate remains high, add dobutamine with gradual incremental dose (to maximum 20 µgm/Kg/min)

Please see the next page for a flow chart for hemodynamic resuscitation in severe sepsis and septic shock.

Steps of hemodynamic resuscitation in severe sepsis and septic shock (simplified form)

Suspected sepsis patient with otherwise unexplained hypotension or lactate level ≥ 4 mmol/L

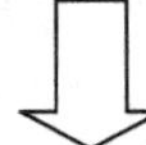

<u>Start initial volume resuscitation</u>
Infuse 30 ml/Kg crystalloid (eg, Normal saline) within the first 3 hours of resuscitation;

Hypotension persists

- Measure CVP and $Scvo_2$
- Continue crystalloid infusion until CVP >8mmHg;
- Start vasopressor support for hypotension, initially with norepinephrine;

Still hypotensive
(Despite norepinephrine support for about one hour)

Add low-dose hydrocortisone (200mg/day) plus consider additional any one of the three steps:

- Addition of dobutamine with norepinephrine if cardiac output is low or not measured; **or**
- Addition of epinephrine with norepinephrine; **or**
- Replacement of norepinephrine with epinephrine and use epinephrine as the only vasopressor and inotrope;

*<u>Achieve the target</u> CVP 8-12 mmHg and MAP >65 mmHg (systolic BP >90mmHg) within the first 6 hours of resuscitation (which includes the first three hours of initial volume resuscitation);

Other supportive measures include:

- <u>Oxygen therapy:</u> As in other acute illnesses, all patients with severe sepsis or septic shock should receive high concentration oxygen to achieve oxygen saturation between 94% and 98%, except those at risk of hypercapnic respiratory failure (eg, patients with COPD, morbid obesity, chest wall deformities, or neuromuscular disorders) where the target saturation is 88-92%.[22,23]
- <u>Ventilatory support</u> when appropriate;
- <u>Red blood cell transfusion</u> usually given for hemoglobin <7 gm/dL;[1,2] target hemoglobin: 7- 9 gm/dL.[1]

- Maintain blood glucose concentration below 180 mg/dl with insulin if needed;[1] however, tighter control with maintaining a level between 100 and 120 mg/dL could be harmful and does not improve survival.[2] Capillary blood glucose may not be accurate in this setting, so arterial or venous plasma glucose should be measured.
- Stress ulcer prevention: For stress ulcer prevention in severe sepsis or septic shock, proton pump inhibitor should be used.
- Deep-vein thrombosis (DVT) prevention:
  - DVT prophylaxis is generally considered in all patients with severe sepsis and septic shock. *Low Molecular Weight Heparin (LMWH) at prophylactic dose is probably most commonly used* unless there are any contraindications to anticoagulant use, such as active bleeding, thrombocytopenia, coagulopathy, or recent intracranial hemorrhage.
  - If possible intermittent pneumatic compression devices should be used with pharmacoprophylaxis.
  - Intermittent compression devices or compression stocking should be used if anticoagulation is contraindicated.
- Platelet transfusion: In severe sepsis, indications for platelet transfusion:[1]
  a) Counts are $\leq$ 10,000/mm^3 (10×10^9/L) even in the absence of any bleeding;
  b) Counts $\leq$ 20,000/mm^3 (20×10^9/L) when there is a significant risk of bleeding;
  c) Counts are low but still $\geq$ 50,000/mm^3 (50×10^9/L) in the presence of active bleeding or before surgery, invasive procedures etc.
- Nutritional supplementation
- Treatment of complications if any such as Acute Renal Failure, arrhythmia, ARDS, DIC, Multiorgan failure etc.

What can be done when blood pressure of an admitted patient with suspected sepsis on antibiotic(s) is falling progressively but the patient is still not overtly hypotensive?

- Look for possible causes.
- If apparently there is no cause other than sepsis, following steps can be considered:
  - Start normal saline infusion, initially 500ml over half an hour;
  - Have an ECG (particularly look for arrhythmia such as atrial fibrillation);
  - Check blood lactate
  - Review antibiotic dose and regimen
  - Monitor hemodynamic status— particularly check pulse; BP; chest for rales after starting IV fluid (sign of volume overload);

Some patients with sepsis develop hypotension due to hypovolemia during the course of their treatment and only adequate volume replacement may correct that problem.

Please see the next page for a summary of the treatment of severe sepsis and septic shock.

Summary of the treatment of severe sepsis and septic shock

- Initiate treatment as soon as possible when severe sepsis or septic shock is suspected;
- Give oxygen to maintain saturation 94-98% (for COPD patients 88-92%)
- Initiate empiric antibiotic therapy (after taking blood for culture) as soon as possible, at least within one hour of suspicion of severe sepsis or septic shock;
- Initiate hemodynamic resuscitation (see the flow chart below) immediately if the patient is hypotensive or lactate level is high;
- Take measures to control the source of infection after successful initial resuscitation;

Flow chart for hemodynamic resuscitation

Suspected sepsis patient with otherwise unexplained hypotension or lactate level $\geq$ 4 mmol/L;

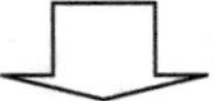

Initial volume resuscitation (to be completed within the first 3 hours of resuscitation)

- Infuse 30 ml/Kg crystalloid (eg, Normal saline);
- Check lactate

Hypotension persists or lactate remains high, > 4mmol/L; (practically, this state is considered as septic shock; these patients should be cared in ICU)

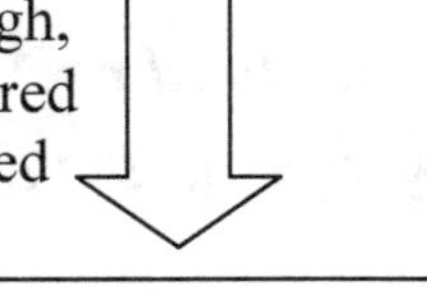

Complete the steps below within the first 6 hours of resuscitation (this 6 hours includes the first three hours of volume resuscitation)

- Measure: CVP and $Scvo_2$;
- Continue crystalloid infusion until CVP >8mmHg;
- Start vasopressor support for hypotension and continue until MAP >65 mmHg; **(For vasopressor selection see the chart below)**
- Recheck lactate (if previous lactate was high)
- If CVP and MAP targets achieved but $Scvo_2$ remains < 70% or lactate remains high, transfuse packed red cells (if hematocrit <30%) to raise hematocrit >30%; but if still $Scvo_2$ remains <70% or lactate remains high, add dobutamine with gradual incremental dose (to maximum 20 µgm/Kg/min)
- Achieve all the following targets within the first 6 hours of resuscitation: MAP >65 mmHg; CVP 8-12 mmHg; $Scvo_2$ >70%; urine output > 0.5 ml/Kg/hr; and normal lactate;

Provide other supportive treatments: ventilatory support, metabolic support, nutritional support etc. as appropriate;

Vasopressor selection:

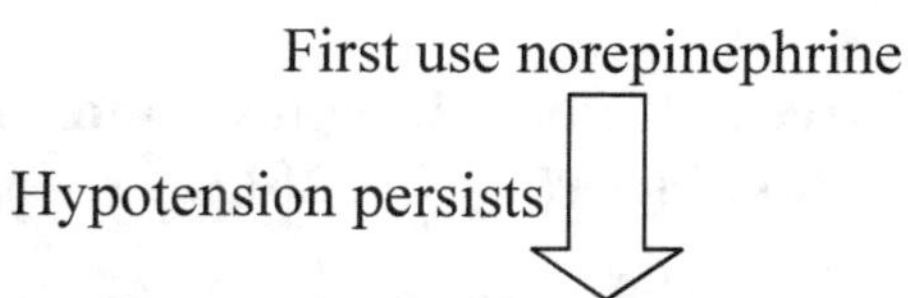

Add low-dose hydrocortisone (200mg/day) plus consider additional any one of the three steps:

- Addition of dobutamine with norepinephrine if cardiac output is low or not measured; **or**
- Addition of epinephrine with norepinephrine; **or**
- Replacement of norepinephrine with epinephrine (and use epinephrine as the only vasopressor and inotrope);

References:

1. R. Phillip Dellinger et al. Surviving Sepsis Campaign: International Guidelines for Management of Severe Sepsis and Septic Shock: 2012. **Crit Care Med 2013**. 41(2): 580-637

2. Relevant chapters of **Harrison's Principles of Internal Medicine**; 18 th edition; Dan L Longo et al (Editors). New York, McGraw-Hill 2012

3. **Antimicrobial stewardship in University of Pennsylvania Health System.** Severe sepsis/ septic shock: empiric treatment guidelines. At: http://www.uphs.upenn.edu/antibiotics/Sepsis.html

4. Andre Kalil. Septic Shock. **Emedicine**. At: http://emedicine.medscape.com/article/168402-overview#showall

5. Jessica C. Njoku. 'Double Anaerobic Coverage: What is the role in clinical practice?' Published by **Nebraska Medical Center; 2010**. Available at: http://www.nebraskamed.com/app_files/pdf/careers/education-programs/asp/doubleanaerobiccoverage.pdf

6. '3-hour bundle' on the website of **surviving sepsis campaig**n. At: http://www.survivingsepsis.org/SiteCollectionDocuments/Bundle-Three-Hour-SSC.pdf

7. Emanuel Rivers et al. Early Goal-Directed Therapy in the Treatment of Severe Sepsis and Septic Shock. **N Engl J Med 2001**; 345:1368-77

8. Relevant chapters of **Kumar &Clark's Clinical Medicine,** 8th edition; Parveen Kumar and Michael Clark (Editors). Edinburgh, Elsevier, **2012**.

9. Stefan Herget-Rosenthal et al. Approach to Hemodynamic Shock and Vasopressors. **Clin J Am Soc Nephrol 2008;** 3: 546-553

10. Relevant chapter of the book **'Pharmacology and Physiology for Anesthesia'; first edition;** Hugh Hemmings and Talmage Egan. **Elsevier 2012.**

11. Relevant chapters of **Current Medical Diagnosis and Treatment**; Maxine A. Papadakis et al (Editors). New York, McGraw-Hill, **2013**

12. Gregory S. Martin. Norepinephrine Infusion in Severe Circulatory Shock. **Medscape Critical Care 2003**; at: http://www.medscape.com/viewarticle/462579

13. Charles L. Sprung et al. Hydrocortisone Therapy for Patients with Septic Shock. **N Engl J Med 2008**; 358:111-24.

14. Djillali Annane et al. Effect of Treatment with Low Doses of Hydrocortisone and Fludrocortisone on Mortality in Patients with Septic Shock. **JAMA. 2002**; 288(7):862-871

15. John D. Stoner III et al. Comparison of dobutamine and dopamine in treatment of severe heart failure. **British Heart Journal, 1977**; 39: 536-539

16. Henry S. Loeb et al. Superiority of Dobutamine over Dopamine for Augmentation of Cardiac Output in Patients with Chronic Low Output Cardiac Failure. **Circulation, 1977**; 55(2):375-8.

17. Christopher B. Overgaard et al. Contemporary reviews in cardiovascular medicine. Inotropes and Vasopressors: Review of Physiology and Clinical Use in Cardiovascular Disease. **Circulation 2008;** 118:1047-1056

18. Michael C. Bond. Vaso-Active Agents in the Emergency Department. **On the website of University of Maryland department of Emergency Medicine.** At: https://umem.org/files/uploads/0701181837_VasopressorHandOut.doc

19. Steven W.J. Lamberts et al. Corticosteroid Therapy in Severe Illness. **N Engl J Med 1997**; 337:1285-1292.

20. Paul E. Marik et al. Recommendations for the diagnosis and management of corticosteroid insufficiency in critically ill adult patients: Consensus statements from an international task force by the American College of Critical Care Medicine. **Crit Care Med 2008;** 36 (6): 1937-1949

21. Mark S. Cooper et al. Corticosteroid Insufficiency in Acutely Ill Patients. **N Engl J Med 2003**; 348:727-34.

22. B R O'Driscoll et al. BTS guideline for emergency oxygen use in adult patients. **Thorax 2008**; 63(Suppl VI):vi1–vi68. doi:10.1136/thx.2008.102947

23. **'Sepsis Management:** National Clinical Guideline No. 6 (November 2014)' by the **National Clinical effectiveness Committee of Ireland**. At: http://hse.ie/eng/about/Who/clinical/natclinprog/sepsis/sepsis6.pdf

Section 2: Electrolyte and Acid-base disorders

Chapter 11

Hyponatremia

Hyponatremia

(Normal serum Na level: 135-145 mmol/L)
Hyponatremia, which is defined as a serum Na <135 mmol/L, is the most common electrolyte disorder in hospitalized patients[1] affecting up to 22% of them;[2] however, only 1-4% of patients with hyponatremia have serum sodium level < 130 mmol/L.[3]

Classification of hyponatremia:

A. Depending on volume status:[2]

1. Hypovolemic hyponatremia
2. Euvolemic hyponatremia
3. Hypervolemic hyponatremia

B. Depending on biochemical severity:[3,4]

1. Mild hyponatremia: Serum Sodium concentration: 130 - 135 mmol/L
2. Moderate hyponatremia: 125 - 129 mmol/L
3. Profound (Severe) hyponatremia: <125 mmol/L

*Some authors have categorized hyponatremia as moderate when serum Na concentration is between 120-129 and severe when <120 mmol/L.[5,6] Actually, the classification of hyponatremia based on serum Na level is more variable in published research, and the serum Na level used to define profound (severe) hyponatraemia ranged from 110 to 125 mmol/L.[4]

C. Depending on duration[4]

1. Acute (documented duration of hyponatremia <48 hours)
2. Chronic (documented duration of hyponatremia >48 hours)

Although the vast majority patients with hyponatremia have chronic form of the disorder, the duration of hyponatremia is often difficult to determine. When the duration of the hyponatremia cannot be ascertained, for therapeutic purpose it is safer to consider it as chronic.[6]

*Pseudo-hyponatremia (also called isotonic hyponatremia[1]):

In this rare condition plasma sodium concentration is spuriously low in the absence of real hyponatremia.[7] This occurs in severe hyperlipidemia (with increased chylomicrons, triglycerides or rarely cholesterol levels) or hyperproteinemia.[7,8] Aqueous portion of the plasma is reduced due to the presence of macromolecules of fat or protein;[8] sodium ions are confined to the aqueous portion of the plasma but its concentration is expressed in terms of total plasma volume.[7]

However, **measured** plasma osmolality (not calculated one) is not affected by the presence of fat or protein molecules. So in pseudo-hyponatremia, **measured** plasma osmolality is normal. Therefore, hyponatremia with normal **measured** plasma osmolality is suggestive of pseudo-hyponatremia.[2] However, newer Na assay techniques using ion-specific electrodes do not produce pseudo-hyponatremia.[1]Treatment of pseudo-hyponatremia is not necessary.[7]

*Transient hyponatremia (also called **hypertonic hyponatremia[1]**):

It may occur in hyperglycemia or with mannitol infusion. In these hyperosmolar states, osmotic shift of water occurs from the intracellular compartment into extracellular space.[1,8] This shifting of water increases plasma volume resulting in reduced plasma sodium concentration; thus a true hyponatremia develops.[1] In hyperglycemia, plasma sodium concentration falls by about 1.6-2.4 mmol/L for every 100 mg/dL increase in plasma glucose.[2] these transient hyponatremia are resolved after correction of hyperglycemia or discontinuation of mannitol.[1,2]

***Hypotonic hyponatremia**

It is the most commonly encountered form of hyponatremia in clinical practice. It is characterized by hyponatraemia with a low **measured** plasma osmolality (<275 mOsm/kg). Hyponatremia is considered hypotonic when non-hypotonic causes of hyponatremia described above (pseudohyponatremia and transient hyponatremia) and artefactual results are excluded.

***Artefactual result** may occur if the blood drawn from a limb where infusion of fluid with low sodium concentration is going on.[7]

Causes of hyponatremia

Causes of hypovolemic hyponatremia (↓total body water; ↓↓total body sodium):[1,2,7,8]

Extrarenal loss of Na (urinary Na concentration < 20 mmol/ L)	Renal loss of Na (urinary Na concentration >20 mmol/L)
Gastrointestinal loss- eg, vomiting, diarrhea and tube drainage; Pancreatitis Skin Na loss- sweating, burns etc.	Diuretic therapy (especially thiazides) ACE inhibitors Adrenocortical (mineralocorticoid) insufficiency Salt-losing nephropathies - Tubulo-interstitial renal disease, recovery phase of acute tubular necrosis, post-obstructive uropathy, reflux nephropathy, medullary cystic kidney etc. Osmotic diuresis (due to glycosuria, ketonuria or bicarbonaturia) Cerebral salt-wasting syndrome

Causes of euvolemic hyponatremia (water retention alone while total body sodium remains almost unchanged; no edema);[1-3,7,8]

- Syndrome of inappropriate ADH secretion (SIADH)
- Primary polydipsia
- ACTH deficiency (secondary adrenal failure)
- Beer potomania
- Endurance exercise

- Reset osmostat
- Hypothyroidism
- Excessive electrolyte free water infusion

* Potentially life-threatening symptomatic cerebral edema is characteristically develops in euvolemic hyponatremia including that due to psychogenic polydipsia.[6]

*Low serum potassium and magnesium may potentiate ADH release resulting in hyponatremia; this mechanism may also contribute to the diuretic-associated hyponatremia.[7]

Causes hypervolemic hyponatremia (occurs in edematous states; ↑↑total body water; ↑ total body sodium)[1,2,7]

- Congestive cardiac failure
- Cirrhosis
- Nephrotic syndrome
- Advanced acute or chronic renal failure (Oliguric; U_{Na}>20 mmol/L)

*In the first three causes of hypervolemic hyponatremia, urine sodium concentration is <20 mmol/L like hypovolemic hyponatremia due to extrarenal causes. In congestive cardiac failure and cirrhosis, increased plasma rennin activity (increased aldosterone secretion) and increased ADH secretion occur because of low effective circulatory volume. However, water retention (ADH activity) is disproportionately greater than Na reabsorption (aldosterone activity) in the renal tubules resulting in hyponatremia.

Clinical features of hyponatremia[1,2]

- Symptoms of hyponatremia are due to mainly cerebral edema.
- Development of symptoms depends on acuity and severity of the hyponatremia.
- In chronic cases, severe hyponatremia (even serum Na <110 mmol/L) can occur without producing significant symptoms because of adaptation of the cerebral neurons. But in acute cases, when hyponatremia develops over hours or days, moderate hyponatremia can be severely symptomatic.
- Mild hyponatremia (130-135 mmol/L) usually does not produce symptoms.

Symptoms of hyponatremia include headache, nausea, vomiting, abdominal pain, lethargy, dizziness, muscle cramp, muscular weakness, gait disorder, tendency to fall, irritability, and confusion; in more severe cases drowsiness, disorientation, stupor, seizure, coma etc. may develop.

Physical examination is particularly focused to determine volume status of the patient.

Investigations

- Plasma and urine electrolyte and osmolality
- Blood urea nitrogen and serum creatinine
- Blood glucose
- Plasma rennin activity (PRA) (if doubt about volume status)
- Investigations to find the underlying cause

Notes:

1. In most cases, only plasma and urine electrolyte and osmolality along with volume status determined clinically are usually required to classify hyponatremia.[8]
2. In some cases, where the hyponatremia has single obvious cause such acute diarrhea or vomiting in an otherwise healthy person, treatment can be given only on serum electrolyte results.
3. Urine sodium concentration <20-30 mmol/L in the absence of clinical hypervolemia (such as edema in congestive heart failure) is suggestive of hypovolemic hyponatremia.[2]
4. Confusion between hypovolemic hyponatremia and SIADH: Although typically urine sodium concentration is low (<20-30 mmol/L) in hypovolemic hyponatremia and high (>20-30 mmol/L) in SIADH, there may be considerable overlap in urine sodium concentration between hypovolemia and SIADH especially in the elderly. When doubt exist between the two conditions, a trial of normal saline infusion can be given; usually normal saline corrects hypovolemic hyponatremia but in SIADH serum sodium concentration shows some fluctuation only.[2]

Determination of volume status

Typical features of volume depletion (↓Extracellular fluid volume)

Clinical:

Dryness of mouth, increased thirst, oliguria, decreased skin turgor, sunken eyes, tachycardia, postural hypotension (in more severe cases hypotension in supine position) etc;

*Clinical assessment of volume status is not reliable in many cases as its sensitivity and specificity are low in patients with hyponatremia.[4]

Laboratory:

Raised hematocrit

Raised blood urea nitrogen (BUN)

(Although the interpretation may be complex in some cases, urine osmolality and urine sodium concentration may be helpful in determining volume status in the absence of kidney diseases or recent use of diuretics).

Treatment of hyponatremia (for quick review see the treatment summary)

Following factors need to consider before making a decision regarding treatment:

1. Volume status of the patient (Hypovolemic/ euvolemic/ hypervolemic)
2. Acute or chronic hyponatremia (Chronic- if the duration of hyponatremia is >48 hours)
3. Asymptomatic or symptomatic; if symptomatic, severity of the symptoms
4. Biochemical severity (mild/ moderate/ severe)
5. Underlying cause

Some facts and critical considerations regarding treatment of hyponatremia:

- Treatment of hyponatremia is not to infuse NaCl solution in all cases. Some patients may not need NaCl replacement at all.

- Generally, urgent correction of hyponatremia is considered when hyponatremia is associated with severe or moderately severe symptoms of hyponatremia, and in other cases, cause-specific treatment is given.
- The rate of correction of hyponatremia is very important. Although rare, overly rapid correction of hyponatremia can precipitate a potentially life-threatening condition, osmotic demyelination syndrome (ODS). (described later)
- Actually, vast majority of patients do not need urgent correction and in many centers, urgent correction with hypertonic saline is rarely used; when hypertonic saline is used it should always be given by an experienced team.
- The underlying cause should be treated in all cases, and concomitant hypomagnesemia and hypokalemia if present should be corrected cautiously.

Here treatment of hyponatremia has been described in two main sections: common considerations and cause-specific measures described with the details of specific causes.

Common considerations of the treatment of hyponatremia

A. Free water restriction (for all):

- For all patients with hyponatremia irrespective of volume status, **free** water intake and hypotonic fluid intake should be restricted.
- Patients with diarrhea and or vomiting can drink oral rehydration salt which contains NaCl instead of drinking free water.
- The degree of free water restriction varies from patient to patient and the permitted amount may be only 600 ml to 1 or 1.5 L per day.[1,8]

B. Therapeutic measures depending on volume status

1. Hypovolemic hyponatremia

Adequate volume resuscitation is required. For example:

a) Mild hyponatremia due to gastrointestinal fluid loss: oral rehydration salt along with treatment of the underlying cause may be adequate.
b) Moderate to severe hyponatremia due to gastrointestinal fluid loss:
    - Volume resuscitation with normal saline (0.9% NaCl) or lactated Ringer's solution will also correct hyponatremia.
    - Accompanying potassium depletion if any should also be corrected. Correction of hypokalemia enhances the correction of hyponatremia.
    - Concomitant acid-base abnormalities usually do not need correction.[2,7]

Considerations for special situations:

a) Patients with hemodynamic instability: Volume resuscitation should be given priority as the need for rapid volume resuscitation usually overrides the risk of an overly rapid correction of hyponatremia.[4]
b) Patients with equivocal volume status: When there is a suspicion of hypovolemic hyponatremia (eg, patients with a history of extracellular fluid loss) but clinically the volume status is equivocal, a fluid challenge with 0.5 to 1 liter[9] (in some cases 1-2 liters[6]) of isotonic saline (0.9 % NaCl) may be diagnostic and therapeutic.

2. Euvolemic hyponatremia

- Free water restriction
- Oral salt (NaCl) supplementation (eg, salt tablet)
- Correction of potassium and magnesium deficiency
- Loop diuretics may promote aquaresis[6]
- Vaptans can be considered in some cases[6]

3. Hypervolemic hyponatremia

- Free-water restriction
- Salt (NaCl) restriction[6,10]
- Loop diuretics[1, 6,10]
- Vaptans can be considered in some cases[3]
- Hemodialysis can also be considered in severe cases with renal impairment[1, 10]

Some key recommendations on therapeutic approaches from two comprehensive articles on hyponatremia:

'Clinical practice guideline on diagnosis and treatment of hyponatraemia'[4]- is one of the most comprehensive sources of information on management of hyponatremia currently available. This guideline was prepared mostly by European experts and has been mentioned as 'European guideline' in this chapter for an easy reference. Another article- 'The Challenge of hyponatremia'- by Adrogué and Madias[6] also contains very important treatment suggestions.

Some key treatment recommendations from the two articles:

a) *All patients of hypotonic hyponatremia with severe or moderately severe symptoms of hyponatremia need urgent treatment;* it is applicable for both acute and chronic hyponatremia irrespective of biochemical severity.[4] Urgent treatment should also be considered in hyponatremia associated with neurologic or neurosurgical condition of the brain, as these patients can tolerate hyponatremia poorly.[6]

b) *All other patients of hyponatremia should receive cause-specific treatment.*[4]

Please see the next page for a decision-algorithm defining therapeutic approaches for hyponatremia.

A decision-algorithm defining therapeutic approaches for hyponatremia[4,6]

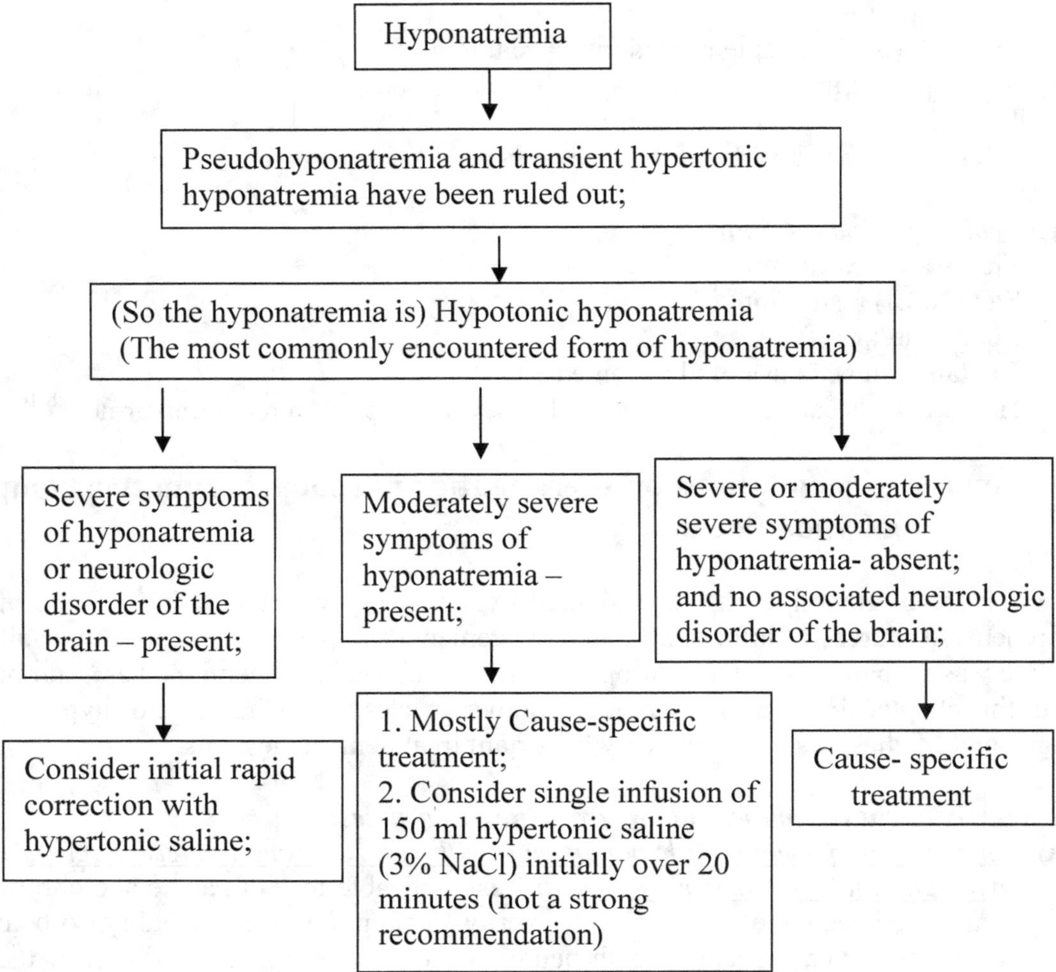

<u>Gradation of symptoms:</u>

<u>Severe symptoms include</u> vomiting, seizures, coma, cardiorespiratory distress and marked drowsiness.[4]

<u>Moderately severe symptoms include</u> headache, nausea, and confusion.[4]

*The above algorithm is applicable for all forms of hypotonic hyponatremia including both acute and chronic type irrespective of biochemical severity.

Rationale behind the approaches suggested in the above algorithm:[4,6]

Hyponatremia with severe or moderately severe symptoms of hyponatremia are dangerous conditions. Hyponatraemia with severe symptoms indicates the presence of cerebral edema, and death may occur quickly if remains untreated. On the other hand, although in hyponatremia with moderately severe symptoms, immediate threat to life is not as much as for hyponatraemia with severe symptoms, any further fall in plasma sodium level can cause rapid deterioration of the clinical state.

But rapid correction of chronic hyponatraemia may predispose osmotic demyelination syndrome, a potentially life-threatening neurologic disorder. *However, when the hyponatremia is associated with severe or moderately severe symptoms of hyponatremia, the risk of cerebral edema outweighs the risk of osmotic demyelination syndrome.*

Actually, hypertonic saline infusion may be life saving for patients with severe symptoms of hyponatremia. However, there must have sufficient reason to consider that the symptoms are due to hyponatremia, not caused by concomitant other conditions.

On the contrary, for patients without moderately severe or severe symptoms of hyponatremia, there is time for diagnostic workup and to initiate cause-specific treâtment, so rapid correction of hyponatremia is not needed.

However, *the vast majority of patients with hyponatremia do not need urgent treatment.*[6] Moreover, when and how hypertonic saline should be used is actually still unclear.[4] As a result, *in many centers, hypertonic saline is rarely used;* however, when used it should always be given by an experienced team.

* *Biochemically mild hyponatremia (Serum Na: 130 -135 mmol/L) usually does not produce moderately severe or severe symptoms;* if such symptoms are present in biochemically mild hyponatremia, other causes of the symptoms should be sought carefully, and rapid correction of hyponatremia is generally not considered in these cases.[4]

What can be done in acute hyponatraemia without severe or moderately severe symptoms?

Usually cause-specific treatment is considered.[4]

However, if the acute fall in serum sodium concentration is >10mmol/L, European guideline development group suggests a single I.V. infusion of 150ml 3% hypertonic saline or equivalent over 20min to prevent further fall in serum Na level irrespective of the underlying cause. But this is not a strong recommendation and it is very important to be ascertained that the hyponatremia is really acute.[4]

Only clinical impression is often unreliable to be sure about the duration of the hyponatremia, so time of previous serum Na assay should be available in most cases to consider the hyponatremia as acute. Then accuracy of the serum Na measurement should be checked. When a sudden fall in serum Na level is observed between two measurements, it needs to be sure that the same technique has been used for the both measurements and sometimes, serum Na may need to be rechecked using the same technique of the previous measurement.

What can be done in chronic hyponatraemia without severe or moderately severe symptoms?

1. Treatment should be cause-specific.[4]
2. In mild hyponatremia no treatment just aiming to increase serum sodium concentration is usually considered.[4]

How can hypertonic saline be infused during the initial rapid correction of hyponatremia when indicated?

For severe symptoms:

a) Suggestions of the European guideline development group:[4]

- Treatment should be initiated in a high dependency unit by an experienced team. European guideline development group suggest repeated infusion (twice in most cases) of 150 ml 3% NaCl over 20 minutes until serum sodium concentration rises by 5mmol/L or the symptoms improve, whichever occurs first.
- Serum sodium should be checked every 20 minutes during the hypertonic saline infusion. A 5 mmol/L rise in serum sodium level can be sufficient to improve symptoms in these cases.
- If the symptoms improve with a maximum 5mmol/L rise in serum sodium concentration in the first hour → stop hypertonic saline infusion → keep an IV channel open with normal saline with feasible smallest infusion rate until cause-specific treatment is started.
- After the initial rapid correction, serum sodium should be checked at least after 6 and 12hours, and daily afterwards until the serum sodium concentration has stabilized.
- In small-sized individuals, instead of infusion of fixed boluses of 150 ml hypertonic saline, weight-based boluses (each bolus of 2 ml/Kg) can be considered to minimize the risk of overcorrection.

(b) Another way of hypertonic saline infusion in hyponatremia with severe symptoms:

Adrogué and Madias[6] have suggested that instead of bolus infusion, hypertonic saline (3% NaCl) can be given as a continuous infusion to increase the serum sodium concentration by 4–6 mmol/L over 4–6 hours with close monitoring of the serum sodium concentration.

* Full recovery of the brain may take some time after optimal rise in serum Na concentration; therefore, it should not be expected that severe symptoms of hyponatremia will be resolved completely immediately.[4]

*Use of furosemide with hypertonic saline: When volume support is not needed, intravenous furosemide 20 mg can be added to the treatment with 3% NaCl infusion to limit volume expansion resulting from hypertonic saline infusion.[6] Additionally, furosemide causes disproportionately greater water diuresis than natriuresis; furosemide-induced diuresis is roughly equivalent to a one-half strength of isotonic saline, so it contributes to the correction of hyponatremia too.[11]

For moderately severe symptoms:

a) Suggestions of the European guideline development group:[4]

- European guideline development group recommends cause-specific treatment for this category of patients. However, the group suggests a single I.V. infusion of 150ml hypertonic (3% NaCl) saline or equivalent over 20min immediately.
- This approach may prevent further drop in serum Na concentration. However, guideline development group's motivation was less strong regarding the infusion of hypertonic saline in these patients than for hyponatremia with severe symptoms.
- Further correction (after infusion of hypertonic saline) should be done with a target of total 5mmol/L per 24-hour increase in serum sodium concentration. In these cases, priority is to prevent further fall in serum sodium concentration rather than a rapid increase in serum Na level.
- In these cases, serum sodium should be checked after 1, 6 and 12 hour during initial management.

(b) Adrogué and Madias[6] did not suggest hypertonic saline infusion in hyponatremia with moderately severe symptoms.

Rate of correction of hyponatremia:

European guideline development group's recommendation:[4] Avoid an increase in serum sodium concentration of >10mmol/L during the first 24hour and >8mmol/L during every 24hour thereafter in all types of hyponatremia. Check the serum sodium concentration repeatedly until it has stabilized with a stable treatment.

However, Adrogué and Madias[6] suggested total correction should not exceed 6–8mmol/L in any 24-hour period which is applicable for all types of acute and chronic hyponatremia, regardless of clinical presentation and method of treatment. They argued osmotic demyelination syndrome (ODS) can occasionally develop after an increase in serum sodium of only 9–10 mmol/L in 24 hours and no clinical advantage can be expected exceeding the threshold of 6–8mmol/L in a 24-hour period in any acute or chronic hyponatremia.

To avoid overcorrection, serum Na level can be corrected until it reaches130 mmol/L.[4]

Is there any problem if acute hyponatremia is corrected rapidly?
Although theoretically rapid correction of acute hyponatremia is not considered as a risk factor for osmotic demyelination syndrome, practically a cautious approach is generally followed and the above mentioned correction limit is usually followed in all acute cases also. Moreover, in many cases duration of hyponatremia (i.e. acute or chronic) cannot be ascertained, so they should be corrected as chronic.

Treatment of inadvertent overcorrection of hyponatremia:[2,6]

To prevent or reverse osmotic demyelination syndrome following an inadvertent overcorrection, hyponatremia can be reinduced or serum Na concentration can be stabilized safely. Infusion of 5% dextrose in aqua and/ or administration of vasopressin agonist desmopressin (DDAVP) (1–5 μg 6- to 8-hourly) can be considered for this purpose.

How can I estimate the total amount of sodium containing IV fluid needed for a particular patient with hyponatremia?

(See below 'Some useful formulas for the treatment of hyponatremia' and the examples)

During calculating fluid requirement for a patient ongoing loss (if any) should also be taken into account.

Some useful formulas for the treatment of hyponatremia

Formula for the calculation of plasma osmolality/osmolarity

Clinically the term osmolality and osmolarity can be used interchangeably.

Calculated plasma osmolarity = 2 [Na] + Glucose + Urea (all in mmol/L).

or

Calculated plasma osmolarity = 2 [Na] + 2 [K] + Glucose + Urea (all in mmol/L).

In the US, to calculate plasma osmolarity the following equation is usually used:

Plasma osmolality = 2[Na+] + [Glucose]/18 + [BUN]/2.8; when [Glucose] and [BUN] are measured in mg/dL.

Approximate total body water (as a fraction of body weight):[1,11]

Subject category	TBW (as percentage of body weight)
Non-elderly adult male	60%
Non-elderly adult female	50%
Male above 60 years	50%
Female above 60 years	40%

Of the total body water, normally 40% is extracellular and 60% is intracellular fluid.

Formulas for the correction of hyponatremia

(1) Formula for the estimation of sodium deficit (or sodium requirement)[1,11]
Sodium deficit (or sodium requirement) = Total body water (TBW) × (desired serum Na level – actual serum Na sodium level)

During initial rapid correction of hyponatremia, the desired serum Na level is generally between 125 and 130 mmol/L.[1,11]

*Loss or gain of about 3 ml of water/Kg of body weight will change the serum sodium concentration roughly 1 mmol/L.[12]

Sodium concentration of various intravenous fluids:[1,11]
3% Hypertonic saline (3% Sodium chloride): 514 mmol per liter
Normal saline (0.9% Sodium chloride in water): 154 mmol per liter
Ringer's lactate solution: 130 mmol per liter
0.45% Sodium chloride in water: 77 mmol per liter
5% Dextrose in aqua: 0 mmol per liter

An example of saline requirement to correct hyponatremia:
A 50- year old female presents with hyponatremia; her body weight is 60 kg and serum Na is120 mmol/L.

If the desired serum Na concentration is 127mmol/L, the estimated Na deficit or requirement= 30 × (127-120) = 30 ×7 = 210 mmol of Na.
(Here total body water = 50% of the body weight considering age and sex of the patient)

One liter of normal saline (0.9% NaCl) contains 154 mmol of Na; therefore, if only normal saline is used, infusion of about 1.3 liters of the saline is likely to be needed to achieve the desired serum Na level.

(2) Formulas for the estimation of correction of hyponatremia with a particular infusate:
Adrogue'-Madias formulas[11] are widely used in this regard.

The predicted change in serum sodium level following infusion of 1 liter of a sodium containing fluid:
(a) Change in serum Na concentration in mmol/L= (Infusate Na concentration– serum Na concentration) ÷ (Total body water + 1)

An example: Effect of infusion of one liter normal saline in a 50-year old man with 60 Kg bodyweight and serum sodium concentration 120mmol/L:
Increase in Serum Na= (154-120) ÷ (36 + 1) = 34 ÷37= 0. 91mmol/L

(b) If the IV fluid contains potassium, it should also be taken into account; in that case the formula will be:
Change in serum Na concentration in mmol/L= [(infusate Na concentration + infusate K concentration) - serum Na concentration] ÷ (total body water + 1)

Rationale: Most of the infused potassium will move intracelluarly with shifting Na into the extracellular fluid, contributing to increase in serum sodium concentration.

However, none of the formulas used to estimate the correction of hyponatremia is accurate and there is a risk of overcorrection of hyponatremia if they are strictly followed. For this reason, clinicians should not depend solely on them; instead, serum sodium should be checked repeatedly which is the best way to evaluate response to therapy.

Use of vasopressin receptor antagonists (Vaptans) in hyponatremia:

Indications:

- Vaptans can be used in mild to moderate euvolemic and hypervolemic hyponatremia when conventional measures fail.[6] They are effective in correcting serum sodium concentration in SIADH and hypervolemic hyponatremia due to heart failure or cirrhosis.[2,7]
- In SIADH, oral vaptan (Tolvaptan) can be considered in significant and persistent hyponatremia (such as malignancy associated) when the hyponatremia is not responding to water restriction, oral salt (NaCl) supplementation and furosemide.[2]

*Actually, data regarding vaptan use are insufficient; their indications and safety are also unclear.[4] Although Food and Drug Administration (FDA) of the USA has approved limited use of some vaptans, the European guideline development group[4] did not recommend their use.

Safety issues regarding vaptan use:

- Although vaptans do not affect sodium and potassium excretion,[7] their aquaretic effect is variable.[6] The most pronounced safety related issue is overcorrection of the hyponatremia which occurs in about 10% of cases.[2] Because this risk is highest in patients with biochemically severe (profound) hyponatraemia, the European guideline development group suggested not to use vaptans in severe hyponatremia.[4] Also, vaptans should not be used in hypovolemic hyponatremia and are not useful in immediate correction of hyponatremia during emergency.
- Fluid restriction should be liberalized (>2 Liters/day) for vaptan treated patients to minimize the risk of overcorrection, and the treatment should be started in hospital with frequent checking of serum sodium concentration.[2]

Summary of the treatment of hyponatremia

Determine the urgency:

1. If severe symptoms of hyponatremia or neurologic disorder of the brain is present: Consider initial rapid correction with hypertonic saline.
2. In patients with moderately severe symptoms of hyponatremia, initially limited amount of hypertonic saline may be infused.
3. In all other cases, the treatment should be cause-specific.

These rules are applicable for all forms of hypotonic hyponatremia including both acute and chronic type irrespective of biochemical severity.

Gradation of symptoms:

Severe symptoms include: vomiting, seizures, coma, cardiorespiratory distress and marked drowsiness.

Moderately severe symptoms include: headache, nausea, and confusion.

Therapeutic measures depending on volume status

Free water restriction is applicable for all. Patients with gastrointestinal fluid loss can take oral rehydration solution. Additional measures for different categories:

1. Hypovolemic hyponatremia

Adequate volume resuscitation is required.

Normal saline (0.9% NaCl) or any other appropriate IV fluid depending on the nature of the lost fluid may be needed.

Patients with equivocal volume status: A fluid challenge with normal saline (0.9 % NaCl) 0.5 to 1 liter over 15-30 minutes (in some cases 1-2 liters) may be diagnostic and therapeutic.

2. Euvolemic hyponatremia
Oral salt (NaCl) supplementation (eg, salt tablet)
Loop diuretics may promote aquaresis;
Vaptans can be considered in some cases

3. Hypervolemic hyponatremia
Salt (NaCl) restriction
Loop diuretics
Vaptans may be considered in some cases
Hemodialysis may be needed in severe cases with renal impairment

Other measures are largely cause-specific and have been described under specific causes. Concomitant hypomagnesemia and hypokalemia if present should be corrected cautiously.

Formula for the correction of hyponatremia
Formula for the estimation of sodium deficit (or sodium requirement):
Sodium deficit (or sodium requirement) = Total body water (TBW) × (desired serum Na level – actual serum Na sodium level)
The desired serum Na level during initial rapid correction of hyponatremia: 125 - 130 mmol/L

Sodium concentration of various intravenous fluids
3% Hypertonic saline (3% Sodium chloride): 514 mmol per liter
Normal saline (0.9% Sodium chloride in water): 154 mmol per liter
Ringer's lactate solution: 130 mmol per liter

Rate of correction: Avoid an increase in serum sodium concentration of >10mmol/L during the first 24hour and >8mmol/L during every 24hour thereafter. However, it may be better not to correct >6–8mmol/L in any 24-hour period which is applicable for all types of acute and chronic hyponatremia, regardless of clinical presentation and method of treatment.

Osmotic demyelination syndrome (ODS) or central pontine myelinolysis (CPM)

Osmotic demyelination syndrome is rare[11] but serious neurological disorder in which an acute or subacute demyelination occurs typically in the central pons; however, it often extends into other areas of the brain. A rapid rise of osmolality of extracellular fluid, particularly due to overly rapid correction of hyponatremia is the main cause.[6,7] Aggressive correction of hyponatremia by any method including water restriction alone can predispose ODS.[11]

Risk factors for the development of osmotic demyelination syndrome[4,6]

1. Chronic hyponatremia with serum Na <110 mmol/L
2. Liver disease

3. Hypokalemia
4. Malnutrition
5. Alcohol abuse
6. Orthotopic liver transplantation
7. Use of thiazide diuretic or antidepressants

*Alcoholism alone can cause ODS in patients without any electrolyte disturbances,[13] and although extremely rare ODS may develop in hyperosmolar hyperglycemic state (HHS) when serum sodium is normal.[14]

Pathophysiology

Pathophysiology of this condition is not clearly understood.[13] Some theories have been given below:
Adaptive changes in the brain in hyponatremia:[11]
Hyponatremia → decreased osmolality of extracellular fluid → in acute cases, shifting of extracellular fluid into the intracellular compartment causing cell swelling (cerebral edema) → thereafter gradual adaptation with movement of osmotically active particles (osmolytes) from intracellular compartment into the extracellular fluid →reduction of cerebral edema and establishment of osmotic equilibrium between intra-and extracellular compartment (it usually takes about 48 hours).

When hyponatremia develops gradually, usually cerebral edema does not develop, because with the fall of osmotic pressure of the extracellular fluid, intracellular osmolytes get enough time to move out to establish an osmotic equilibrium between the intra-and extracellular compartments.

Consequence of overly rapid correction: Overly rapid correction of **chronic hyponatremia** (where an osmotic equilibrium has already been established between intra-and extracellular compartment) →sudden increase in osmolality of extracellular fluid →shifting of intracellular fluid into the extracellular compartment → brain shrinkage → triggering of demyelination.[11]

Another theory: Overly rapid correction of chronic hyponatremia →sudden increase in osmolality of extracellular fluid →shifting of intracellular fluid into the extracellular compartment →shrinkage of glial cells → disruption of blood brain barrier→ entrance of harmful inflammatory mediators into the brain → damage of oligodendrocytes and myelin sheath.[14]

Clinical features:[6,11,15]

Symptoms and signs usually begin to appear 1-7 days after the correction of hyponatremia and may progress over 1-2 weeks. The symptoms and signs include dysarthria, dysphagia, paraparesis or quadriparesis, behavioral disturbances, lethargy, Parkinsonism, locked-in syndrome, seizure, delirium and coma.

The most characteristic features are those of pseudobulbar palsy (dysarthria and dysphagia) and spastic quadriplegia resulting from demyelination of corticobulbar and corticospinal tracts within the pons.

*Locked-in syndrome (LIS) is a neurological condition in which a patient is aware but cannot move or speak due to complete paralysis of almost all voluntary muscles in the body except extraocular muscles.

Diagnosis of ODS

The demyelinating lesions can be detected by CT scan or MRI of the brain; however MRI is the imaging of choice.[13]Hyperintense areas on T2-weighted MRI images indicate demyelination.[16] However, the initial MRI may be normal and the lesions may not be detectable on MRI for days to weeks after the onset of symptoms.[13] Earlier detection may be possible with diffusion-weighted imaging.

Treatment

A neurologist should be consulted as soon as the syndrome is suspected. The treatment is mainly supportive along with treatment of the underlying cause. Patients usually need extensive and prolonged physical therapy and rehabilitation.

Parkinsonian symptoms may respond to the dopaminergic drugs. Some physicians have tried corticosteroid and some other experimental therapies such as Plasmapheresis, Thyrotropin Releasing Hormone and Intravenous Immunoglobulin, but more studies are needed before their implementation in clinical practice.[13,14]

Relowering of serum Na following overly rapid correction can prevent ODS[2] and gentle reinduction of hyponatremia is effective in treating ODS if started immediately after the syndrome is suspected.[2,16]

Prognosis

Although ODS was considered as a devastating condition previously with almost 100% mortality rate,[13]recent data show that more than 50% of the patients recover either completely or with minimal residual disability. Prompt diagnosis and adequate supportive treatment is very important for a favorable outcome.[14]

Details of some specific causes of hyponatremia

Diuretic induced hyponatremia

- Diuretic induced hyponatremia is one of the most common causes of hyponatremia. About 11% of elderly patients on diuretics develop hyponatremia.[17] It is the most common cause of community-developed hyponatremia.[17]
- All types of diuretics can cause hyponatraemia including potassium sparing ones; however, thiazide or thiazide-like agents are the most common cause while loop diuretics are rarely involved,[4,17] as loop diuretics cause disproportionately greater water diuresis.[2] In fact, furosemide-induced diuresis is roughly equivalent to a one-half isotonic saline (0.45%) and it helps to correct hyponatremia like dermal and respiratory fluid losses.[11]

Risk factors for diuretic induced hyponatremia

- The major risk factors for diuretic induced hyponatremia include old age; female sex; lower body mass; hypokalemia; and concurrent use of other drugs that affect renal free water excretion, especially nonsteroidal anti-inflammatory agents.[18,19]
- Increased water intake during diuretic therapy to compensate for the diuretic induced fluid loss increases the risk of hyponatremia.[20]
- Diuretic induced hyponatremia is three times more commonly identified in women than men.[19,21] Elderly women appear to be at particularly greater risk.[21]
- The risk of developing hyponatraemia is minimal with non-thiazide diuretics and at low dose.[21]

Thiazide induced hyponatremia (TIH)

Thiazide induced hyponatremia may be acute or chronic. In 50%-90% cases, TIH develops within two weeks of starting the drug. However, it may develop any time, sometimes very rapidly, within a day or two, or even just after taking a single dose of the drug when other complicating factors, such as age-related reduction in renal function, are present.[18]

Pathogenesis:

The exact pathogenesis of diuretic induced hyponatremia is unclear.[17]Traditionally it is thought that diuretic-induced sodium or volume loss stimulates ADH secretion and hyponatremia results from ADH-induced water retention. But all patients with diuretic induced hyponatremia are not hypovolemic, and diuretics can cause a SIADH-like state with normal or slightly increased extracellular fluid volume.[4] In TIH, three main factors are possibly involved: stimulation of ADH secretion, decreased free-water clearance, and increased water intake.[20]

Clinical presentation:

- Most patients with TIH are asymptomatic and diagnosed incidentally on routine laboratory tests.[22] However, TIH can produce mild to severe life-threatening symptoms of hyponatremia such as convulsion and coma.
- One striking feature of TIH is that in susceptible individuals, the serum Na level may fall within hours of taking the first dose of the drug, and severe hyponatremia may develop within less than two days.[20] However, when a patient on diuretic presents with symptoms of hyponatremia, possible other causes for those symptoms should also be sought.

Management:

The following therapeutic measures can be considered for TIH:[18,20]

- Stopping the offending drug
- Restricting free water intake
- Oral salt supplementation
- Infusion of normal saline (0.9% NaCl)
- Infusion of hypertonic saline (rarely needed)

*Furosemide can be added to normal saline or hypertonic saline to avoid volume expansion due to saline infusion and to make the correction of hyponatremia faster when appropriate.

Therapeutic suggestions for specific categories of patients with TIH:

1. Hyponatremia with no or minimal symptoms (mild nausea fatigue etc):[18,20,22]
   - The majority of the patients with TIH fall in this group and their hyponatremia usually resolves spontaneously within 1-2 weeks with withdrawal of the offending drug and free water restriction.
   - Oral salt supplementation can also be helpful to increase serum Na concentration.
   - Normal saline infusion can be considered if hypovolemia is present.

2. Hypovolemic hyponatremia:
   - Consider infusion of normal saline (0.9% NaCl).
   - ADH inhibits free water excretion; in hypovolemic TIH, ADH secretion is stimulated by hypovolemia; normal saline infusion restores volume and suppresses ADH release.[20]

3. Hyponatremia with moderately severe or severe symptoms

Consider hypertonic saline infusion for initial rapid correction then continue specific measures for TIH.[4] For details please see the 'treatment of hyponatremia with severe and moderately severe symptoms' described earlier in this chapter.

4. Euvolemic or hypervolemic TIH:

In TIH, the volume status is variable. Most patients appear euvolemic,[20] while some are hypo- or hypervolemic[18,20]

In euvolemic and hypervolemic TIH, blood urea, creatinine and uric acid levels may be low.[18,20] The serum sodium concentration of these patients is usually not restored with infusion of normal saline. But hypertonic saline can increase their serum sodium level predictably and addition of furosemide to the hypertonic saline can make the correction faster, avoiding volume overload from hypertonic saline infusion.[20] Therefore, when patients with euvolemic or hypervolemic TIH need rapid correction of their hyponatremia (eg, severely symptomatic hyponatremia), hypertonic saline should be considered; combination of hypertonic saline and furosemide may also be used, particularly in edematous states.[18]

However, the decision of infusion of hypertonic saline should be taken by an experienced team; practically, in many centers, use of hypertonic saline is mainly restricted to hyponatremia with severe symptoms such as convulsion and coma.

Prevention of TIH:[18,20]

- Thiazides should be prescribed at low dose, particularly in elderly women and in individual with low body mass.
- Serum sodium and potassium levels should be monitored closely; for high risk patients, such as elderly women or individual with low body mass, serum Na should be checked daily for several days initially. In other cases, serum electrolytes should be checked within two weeks of starting the diuretic.
- Patients should be warned not to drink excessive fluid to compensate for the increased urine output due to diuretic. They should drink as usually or when thirsty.
- Appropriate potassium supplementation, and combining K-sparing diuretics with thiazide probably can also reduce the risk of hyponatremia.

Syndrome of Inappropriate Antidiuresis (SIAD) or Syndrome of Inappropriate Antidiuretic Hormone secretion (SIADH)

Normally hypovolemia and hyperosmolar state of plasma stimulate ADH secretion. ADH secretion is inappropriate when occurs without these physiologic stimuli. SIADH is the most common cause of euvolemic hyponatremia.

Causes of SIADH[1,2,7,8]

- Malignancy- eg, lung, colon, pancreas, thymus, lymphoma;
- Pulmonary diseases- eg, pneumonia, tuberculosis, neoplasm, obstructive lung disease;
- CNS disorders- eg, CNS infection, stroke, psychosis, brain tumor, head injury;
- Metabolic causes- eg, alcohol withdrawal and porphyria;
- Drugs-
    - Anticonvulsants-eg, carbamazepine
    - Psychotropics- eg, phenothiazines, butyrophenone (eg, haloperidol)
    - Antidepressants- eg, SSRI, TCA
    - Antidiabetics- eg, chlorpropamide, tolbutamide
    - Cytotoxics- eg, vincristine, cyclophosphamide
    - Opiates- eg, morphine
- Others- postoperative, pain, stress, nausea, hypokalemia, AIDS;
- Idiopathic

Diagnostic criteria[7,8]

1. Euvolemic state
2. Hyponatremia (Plasma Na typically <130 mmol/L)
3. Low plasma osmolality (typically <270 mOsm/Kg); (Normal: 275- 295 mOsm/Kg).
4. Urine osmolality is not appropriately low, >150 mosm/Kg (typically higher than plasma osmolality)
5. Urine sodium level not appropriately low (>30 mmol/L)
6. Plasma urea, creatinine and uric acid levels are low-normal
7. Clinical context is appropriate and there is no renal, thyroid or adrenal dysfunction or other causes of hyponatremia.

*Urine osmolality and specific gravity:

- Normal urine osmolality is usually higher than plasma osmolality. Urine osmolality is a more reliable indicator of concentration of urine than urine specific gravity.
- *Normal urine osmolality:* Random urine: 300- 900 mOsm/Kg; 24 Hour urine: 500-800 mOsm/kg.
- *Normal urine specific gravity:* 1.000 to 1.030 (Varies from Lab to Lab)

Treatment of SIADH

Underlying cause should be treated if possible.
Biochemical abnormalities of SIADH can be corrected with the following measures:

A. ***When urgent correction of the hyponatremia is not needed*:**

- **Free water restriction:** 500 ml -- 1000 ml per day; however it is difficult to tolerate; if tolerated, can correct the biochemical abnormalities in many cases.[7]
- **Oral salt (NaCl) supplementation[2,4]**
- **Oral furosemide**: 20 mg once or twice a day; higher dose may be needed in renal failure. Oral salt supplementation and oral furosemide can correct hyponatremia in many cases where strict fluid restriction was not tolerated or only fluid restriction was not adequate.[2]
- **The combination of normal saline infusion and a loop diuretic** can also raise the serum sodium level in SIADH.[18]
- **Demeclocycline** (300-600mg twice daily) can be considered in rare occasions, when persistent marked hyponatremia does not respond to water restriction, salt tablets and furosemide. Demeclocycline blunts collecting ducts responsiveness to ADH. But the drug is nephrotoxic and frequently causes photosensitive rash; it should be avoided in cirrhosis of liver.[2,7,8]
- **Oral urea** promotes water excretion by increasing solute load of the glomerular filtrate. Oral urea (30-45g/day) may be an alternative to demeclocycline but it is unpalatable.[8]
- **Use of Vasopressin receptor antagonists (Vaptans):** They are effective in correcting serum sodium concentration in SIADH. However, data regarding their use are insufficient, and their indications and safety are unclear.[4] In SIADH, oral vaptan (Tolvaptan) can be considered in significant and persistent hyponatremia (such as malignancy associated) when the hyponatremia is not responding to water restriction, oral salt supplementation and furosemide.[2] The treatment should be started in hospital with frequent checking of serum sodium concentration.[2]

B. ***When urgent correction of hyponatremia is needed:[4]***

- In patients with moderately severe or severe symptoms of hyponatremia, urgent correction of hyponatremia with 3% hypertonic saline (3% NaCl) should be considered initially. Hypertonic saline should be given by an experienced team. (*For details please see the 'treatment of hyponatremia with severe or moderately severe symptoms' described earlier in this chapter)*

*Mild lethargy, unsteadiness and falls in elderly patients are not considered as severe symptoms, so slow correction of hyponatremia (without using hypertonic saline) can be considered in such cases.

*Normal saline (0.9% NaCl) infusion (without loop diuretics) is not useful to correct hyponatremia in SIADH.[6] With normal saline infusion, infused sodium is excreted normally, as sodium excretion is normal in SIADH while some of the water may be retained, worsening the hyponatremia.[11] However, during the time of normal saline infusion, slight increase in serum sodium concentration may occur transiently, as sodium concentration of the infused fluid is higher than that of serum.

Other disorders commonly create confusion with SIADH:

- Hyponatremia in elderly frail patients: Hyponatremia is common in sick elderly frail patients due to salt and water deficit which may result from poor intake or other causes. This hyponatremia may be difficult to distinguish clinically from SIADH. In these circumstances, slow infusion of 1-2 liters of normal saline (0.9% NaCl) can be considered as a therapeutic trial. Sodium deficiency will respond with this therapy while SIADH will not.[7]

- ACTH deficiency: Its biochemical picture has many similarities with SIADH. Therefore, hypothalamic-pituitary-adrenal axis may need to be tested in some cases, particularly in patients with neurosurgical conditions; ACTH deficiency may be relatively common in neurosurgical patients.[7]

- Thiazide induced hyponatremia (TIH) (in patients with the risk factors for both SIADH and TIH): Urine sodium concentration is high in both the conditions and they may also have some other overlapping features. The two conditions can be differentiated by keeping thiazide off for 1-2 weeks then repeating urine sodium estimation. If urine sodium is still high then it is suggestive of SIADH.[2]

- Cerebral salt wasting (described later)

Primary polydipsia

It is a form of psychogenic polydipsia where patients drink excessive amount of free water (generally >10 liters/day[1]) in the absence of any abnormalities in ADH or thirst control; or any defined psychiatric diseases.

Polydipsia may be a feature of many specific psychiatric illnesses such as schizophrenia, anxiety disorders and depressive disorders. Psychogenic polydipsia may be worse when it is associated with a specific psychiatric disease. However, many psychotropic drugs may cause hyponatremia (SIADH) and patients with psychiatric illnesses may have multifactorial electrolyte disorders.

Psychogenic polydipsia is a broader term which includes both primary polydipsia and polydipsia due to specific psychiatric illnesses.

Clinical presentation of primary polydipsia

- Patients with this condition have an uncontrollable urge to drink and to pass a large volume of dilute urine.
- The patients may have symptoms of hyponatremia and drinking a huge amount of water may cause water intoxication which is characterized by symptoms of confusion, lethargy, psychosis, and seizures; and may progress eventually to death.

Investigations

- *Serum and urine electrolyte and osmolality:*
  - Serum sodium generally low-normal, or low (<135 mmol/L); plasma osmolality tends to be low (<280 mosm/Kg);
  - Urine osmolality- low, may be <100 mosmol/Kg; urine Na <20mmol/L;
- *Blood sugar:* normal
- *24-hour urine volume*- increased

- *Urinalysis*-normal
- *Blood urea, serum creatinine*- normal
- *Blood ADH level*- low or undetectable
- *Chest radiograph* (to exclude lung cancer): normal
- *Water deprivation test:* This test can be used to differentiate between diabetes insipidus (DI) and psychogenic polydipsia.
    - In psychogenic polydipsia, plasma osmolality is low at the beginning of the test. After water deprivation, ADH release is started; both plasma and urine sodium concentration and osmolality gradually come back towards normal. However, usually urine cannot be concentrated maximally, as concentrating abilities of the kidneys are somewhat impaired because of washout of solutes from renal medulla during excessive diuresis.
    - In diabetes insipidus, with water deprivation, plasma Na and osmolality increase further, but urine Na concentration and urine osmolality cannot increase.

Differential Diagnosis

- *Diabetes insipidus:*
    - The most important differential diagnosis of primary polydipsia is diabetes insipidus (DI). Polydipsia and polyuria are characteristics of both the conditions.
    - The main differentiating point- unlike primary polydipsia, DI generally causes high-normal or high serum Na (hypernatremia) and high-normal or high plasma osmolality. When the diagnosis remains uncertain, water deprivation test can be used to differentiate between the two entities.

- *SIADH:* In both SIADH and primary polydipsia, serum Na and plasma osmolality are low but urine characteristics of the two conditions are reverse of each other. In SIADH, urine Na is not low, typically >30 mmol/L and urine osmolality is also not low, usually >150 mosmol/Kg. Additionally, plasma ADH is high in SIADH.

- *Diuretic induced hyponatremia:* Withdrawal of the diuretic for 1-2 weeks may resolve hyponatremia.

Note

Causes of polyuria and polydipsia include:[1,7]

- Diabetes mellitus
- Diabetes insipidus
- Hypercalcemia
- Hypokalemia
- Drugs such as lithium
- Psychogenic polydipsia

Treatment of primary polydipsia

- Water restriction
- Behavioral therapy

- For hyponatremia with moderately severe or severe symptoms - judicious use of hypertonic saline (3% NaCl); *(For details please see the 'treatment of hyponatremia with severe and moderately severe symptoms' described earlier in this chapter)*
- Pharmacotherapy: clozapine, olanzapine and risperidone have been tried in some patients but evidence is insufficient and probably they are not approved treatment.

Exercise-associated hyponatremia

Potentially life- threatening hyponatremia can develop after endurance exercise such as marathon running. The major risk factor for this complication appears to be excessive fluid intake during preparation (pre-exercise overhydration) and or during the activity.[23] Exercise- associated hyponatremia is more common among women.[23]

Pathogenesis

- The pathogenesis of exercise induced hyponatremia is not clearly understood.[24] However, the hyponatremia is commonly dilutional, resulting primarily from consumption of disproportionately greater amount of free water and other hypotonic fluids (eg, sports drink) than the total loss fluid from the body.
- Other factors which contribute to the development of hyponatremia include Na loss in sweating, increased ADH secretion and reduced renal excretion of free water because of decreased GFR due to reduced renal blood flow.[24] During sustained strenuous exercise, splanchnic vasoconstriction delays absorption of consumed fluid and the fluid may be absorbed rapidly after the exercise when splanchnic vasoconstriction is over, lowering serum sodium concentration.[1]

Treatment of exercise induced hyponatremia

Treatment depends on volume status of the patient and severity (both clinical and biochemical) of the condition.

Mild (Serum Na: 130-135 mmol/L) asymptomatic hyponatremia:[24]
Most cases fall in this category; usually only fluid restriction and observation until spontaneous diuresis is started is required.

Patients with clear evidences of hypovolemic hyponatremia:[24]
Consider infusion of normal saline for volume resuscitation. However, normal saline infusion should be done cautiously, because delayed absorption of previously consumed fluid may cause volume overload in these patients.

Patients with symptomatic hyponatremia or serum Na <120 mmol/L:
Consider infusion of hypertonic saline.[24] Although there is no consensus on how much hypertonic saline can be infused in these patients, 100 ml (3% NaCl) over 10 minutes can be given in the field when severe symptoms of hyponatremia are present. This amount of hypertonic saline infusion is likely to raise the serum sodium level 2 to 3 mmol/L in a short period.[23,24] Hypertonic saline can also be given in severe symptomatic patients even in the presence of volume overload such as pulmonary edema. In such cases, loop diuretics can be used to overcome volume overload.[24] Exercise associated hyponatremia is often clearly acute (<48 hours duration), so rapid

correction is generally not considered unsafe.[24] However, serum electrolytes should be monitored closely.

Concomitant hypokalemia should be corrected cautiously.[24]

Endurance athletes should drink according to thirst instead of following a fixed schedule of drinking. Consumption of no more than 400 - 800 mL/h is generally recommended during the event.[23]

Beer potomania (Poton means drink, mania means akin)

Beer potomania is an unusual cause of hyponatremia, develops in heavy beer drinkers whose dietary solute intake is low.[25] The solutes in plasma are glucose, protein, urea etc. Beer is poor in electrolytes and solutes. Patients with beer potomania often have protein malnutrition. Although in normal circumstances, kidneys can excrete vast amount of ingested fluid, in beer potomania this is impaired because of low solute content of plasma.

Pathophysiology

Beer is a hypoosmolar drink, containing mostly water with a very little amount of sodium (about 2 mmol/L) and minimal solutes. Consumption of massive amount of beer with poor food intake causes fall in plasma osmolality. As a result, ADH secretion drops but diuresis is grossly affected, because reduced excretion of urinary solutes limits free water excretion [26] (↓solute concentration of plasma → ↓ renal tubular solute load →↓ free water clearance).[27] Therefore, water is retained in plasma resulting in hyponatremia.

Diagnosis

Clinical features of beer potomania are those of hyponatremia. However, presentation with severe symptomatic hyponatremia is common in beer potomania.[28]

There is no specific diagnostic test. Common biochemical features include severe hyponatremia, hypokalemia, low serum osmolality, low urine sodium[25] and low urine osmolality (may be <100 mosmol/kg).

Treatment

There is no consensus on replacement of sodium in beer potomania[27] and the management may be challenging. Various types of IV fluids such as normal saline, 5% dextrose in aqua and 3% hypertonic saline may be needed initially.

Therapeutic suggestions for specific categories of patients:

(1) <u>For patients with mild or no symptoms (irrespective of biochemical severity of the hyponatremia)</u>:

Initially only fluid restriction should be considered; serum Na should be monitored closely; in biochemically severe cases (serum Na <125 mmol/L), serum Na should be checked 2 hourly until it is fairly stable.[25,28]

(2) <u>For hyponatremia with moderately severe or severe symptoms</u>
For initial rapid correction, European guideline development group's recommendation[4] can be followed. *(Please see the 'treatment of hyponatremia with severe and moderately severe symptoms' described earlier in this chapter.)*

However, these malnourished alcoholics are at greater risk of developing osmotic demyelination syndrome (ODS)[2,27] with an approximate rate of 18%.[28] The development of ODS in these patients does not depend on hypertonic saline infusion; instead, it can develop with infusion of normal saline or even with fluid restriction alone.[27] Therefore, correction of hyponatremia in these patients should be done with extreme caution. Brisk diuresis is started with improvement of plasma osmolality. Infusion of normal saline alone can cause overcorrection of hyponatremia quickly in these patients, exceeding the daily correction limit.

<u>To keep the limit of correction within the desired level:</u>[28]
If the serum sodium concentration rises at a rate that can exceed the desired goal:

a) 5% dextrose in aqua should be started to match urine output and
b) Desmopressin may be considered if 5% dextrose in aqua is unable to achieve the goal;

Although oral feeding is important in these malnourished individuals, consider withholding it for the first 24 hours of presentation to avoid rapid correction.[28] If caloric intake is required, 5% dextrose in aqua infusion can be used.[28]

Caring team should also be aware of that these patients may develop alcohol withdrawal syndrome.

Causes of low urine osmolality (<100 mosmol/kg)
It is uncommon and seen in the following conditions:

1. Psychogenic polydipsia[4]
2. Beer potomania[4]
3. Very low dietary solute intake (eg, extreme vegetarian diet)[2]

Cerebral salt wasting (CSW)

It is a rare form of hypovolemic hyponatremia, develops in patients with intracranial disorders such as infections, tumors, cerebrovascular accidents (particularly subarachnoid hemorrhage) and CNS surgery.[1,4] The pathophysiology of this disorder is unclear;[1] brain natriuretic peptide (BNP) mediated renal sodium loss may have an important role.[4]

Clinical features of CSW include refractory hypovolemia and hypotension requiring continuous infusion of saline.[1] Hyponatremia typically starts within the first ten days of the predisposing event.

The diagnosis may be difficult, as both SIADH and secondary adrenal insufficiency are more common in this clinical setting.[4] However, <u>SIADH and secondary adrenal insufficiency causes euvolemic hyponatremia while hyponatremia in CSW is hypovolemic</u>. In both SIADH and CSW, urine osmolality and urine sodium concentration are high. The main differentiating feature between these two conditions may be the presence of clear evidence of volume depletion (eg, hypotension, decreased skin turgor, raised hematocrit and raised blood urea) which is suggestive of CSW.[4] For this reason, in confusing cases, the response to a trial of isotonic saline infusion can be used to distinguish between CSW and SIADH. With normal saline infusion, hypotension and hyponatremia of CSW will improve while hyponatremia of SIADH will remain unresponsive or may worse. However, in some cases SIADH and CSW may coexist.

The treatment of CSW is volume resuscitation with isotonic saline.[4] Oral salt supplement (salt tablets) can be given when patients are able to take orally. Mineralocorticoid such as fludrocortisone, can also be considered. Resolution usually occurs within 3-4 weeks if the predisposing condition is corrected.

Brief description of some other causes of hyponatremia

Hyponatremia in heart failure and liver failure (cirrhosis)

In both the conditions effective circulatory blood volume is reduced. In heart failure, it is due to low cardiac output and in liver failure it is due to systemic vasodilation and arteriovenous shunting of blood. Reduced effective circulatory blood volume stimulates ADH release; generally, water retention caused by increased ADH secretion plays a major role in developing hyponatremia.[4] Hyponatremia may be associated with increased mortality in both heart failure and liver failure.

Treatment of hyponatremia in heart failure and liver failure (cirrhosis)

Suggestions from European guideline development group:[4]

- *For asymptomatic mild to moderate hyponatremia:* No measures targeting only elevation of serum sodium concentration have outcome benefits. So no treatment was recommended by the group for this category of patients.
- *For asymptomatic severe hyponatremia (<125 mmol/L):* The group believed it may be reasonable to avoid further fall in serum sodium concentration in this category of patients, but it refrained from making any recommendation other than fluid restriction. The group did not recommend vasopressin receptor antagonists, demeclocycline or lithium for this patient-group. For vasopressin receptor antagonist, data were insufficient and some available ones showed unfavorable patient outcome, while side-effects of demeclocycline and lithium are high in this category of patients.

Ensuring appropriate treatment for heart failure or liver failure is very important, and probably in most cases, it is reasonable to continue the appropriate treatment despite the presence of hyponatremia.

Primary adrenal insufficiency

In this condition hyponatremia occurs mainly due to aldosterone deficiency.
Primary adrenal insufficiency → aldosterone deficiency→ renal loss of sodium and water → overall impact hypovolemic hyponatraemia. Sometimes, hyponatraemia is the first and only sign of primary adrenal insufficiency.

Secondary adrenal insufficiency

Secretion of adrenocorticotrophic hormone (ACTH) is reduced or absent→ mainly cortisol deficiency → normal cortisol induced inhibition of vasopressin (ADH) secretion impaired → increased ADH secretion → water retention → euvolemic hyponatremia

Nephrotic syndrome

The exact mechanism of hyponatremia in nephrotic syndrome is not clearly known.[1]
One possible mechanism of hyponatremia in nephrotic syndrome (underfill theory): Proteinuria → hypoalbuminemia → decreased plasma oncotic pressure → translocation of fluid out of the intravascular space → reduced blood volume → increased vasopressin release → water retention. However, this water retention is usually balanced by intense retention of sodium by the kidney, which is a primary abnormality in nephrotic syndrome. But these patients usually need considerable dose of diuretics for their edema which causes natriuresis. The combined effect of increased vasopressin release and diuretic use may cause up to moderate hyponatraemia in nephrotic syndrome.

Hypothyroidism

Hypothyroidism is a very rare cause of hyponatremia and clinically significant hyponatremia occurs only in severe hypothyroidism. The mechanism of hyponatremia in hypothyroidism is not clearly understood. Treatment of hypothyroidism with thyroid hormone corrects the hyponatremia.[2]

Reset osmostat

- In this rare form of euvolemic hyponatremia, serum sodium and serum osmolality are maintained at a lower set point.
- ADH secretion is stimulated at relatively lower plasma osmolality than usual. However, renal abilities of concentrating and diluting urine remain intact.
- Reset osmostat classically occurs in severe pulmonary diseases, neurologic conditions (eg, epilepsy, paraplegia), malignancy, pregnancy and malnutrition.
- Hyponatremia is mild to moderate (serum Na>125 mmol/L) and stable on multiple measurements.
- The diagnosis is made by exclusion of other causes of hyponatremia. During water deprivation, urine becomes concentrated while water challenge causes diluted urine.
- The hyponatremia is asymptomatic and treatment is not necessary.

References:

1. Relevant chapters of **Current Medical Diagnosis and Treatment**; Maxine A. Papadakis et al (Editors). New York, McGraw-Hill, **2013**

2. Relevant chapters of **Harrison's Principles of Internal Medicine**; 18 th edition; Dan L Longo et al (Editors). New York, McGraw-Hill 2012.

3. Eric E Simon. **Hyponatremia. Emedicine**; at: http://emedicine.medscape.com/article/242166-overview#showall

4. Goce Spasovski et al. Clinical practice guideline on diagnosis and treatment of hyponatraemia. **European Journal of Endocrinology 2014**; 170, G1–G47

5. Ramón De las Peñaset et al. SIADH-related hyponatremia in hospital day care units: clinical experience and management with Tolvaptan. **Support Care Cancer 2016**; 24:499–507

6. Horacio J. Adrogué and Nicolaos E. Madias. The Challenge of Hyponatremia. **J Am Soc Nephrol 2012**; 23: 1140–1148

7. Relevant chapters of **Kumar &Clark's Clinical Medicine,** 8th edition; Parveen Kumar and Michael Clark (Editors). Edinburgh, Elsevier, **2012**

8. Relevant chapters of **Davidson's Principles and Practice of Medicine**, 21 edition, Nicki R. Colledge et al (editors). India, Elsevier, **2010**

9. Management of hyponatremia. **General practice Notebook- a UK medical reference**; at: www.gpnotebook.co.uk/simplepage.cfm?ID=-1321926637

10. Kian Peng Goh. Management of Hyponatremia. **Am Fam Physician 2004;** 69:2387-94

11. Hyponatremia. Horacio J. Adrogué and Nicolaos E. Madias. **N Engl J Med 2000**; 342:1581-1589

12. Richard H. Sterns. Disorders of Plasma Sodium - Causes, Consequences, and Correction. **N Engl J Med 2015;** 372: 55-65

13. A. Kenneth Musana and Steven H. Yale. Central Pontine Myelinolysis: Case series and review. **Wisconsin Medical Journal 2005**; 104(6): 56-60

14. Karla Victoria Rodríguez-Velver et al. Osmotic Demyelination Syndrome as the Initial Manifestation of a Hyperosmolar Hyperglycemic State. **Case Reports in Neurological Medicine 2014**; article ID 652523, 5 pages

15. Christopher Luzzio. **Central Pontine Myelinolysis. Emedicine.** At: http://emedicine.medscape.com/article/1174329-overview#a6

16. Hideomi Yamada et al. Relowering of Serum Na for Osmotic Demyelinating Syndrome. **Case Reports in Neurological Medicine 2012**; article ID 704639, 2 pages

17. George Liamis et al. A Review of Drug-Induced Hyponatremia. **Am J Kidney Dis 2008**; 52:144-153

18. Emmanuel Eroume A Egom et al. A review of thiazide-induced hyponatraemia. **Clinical Medicine 2011**, Vol 11, No 5: 448–51

19. Eline M. Rodenburget al. Thiazide-Associated Hyponatremia. **Am J Kidney Dis. 2013**; 62(1):67-72

20. Kyu Sig Hwang et al. Thiazide-Induced Hyponatremia. **Electrolyte Blood Press 2010;** 8:51-57

21. Y Sharabi1 et al. Diuretic induced hyponatraemia in elderly hypertensive women. **Journal of Human Hypertension 2002;** 16: 631–635

22. Spiros Fourlanos et al. Managing drug-induced hyponatraemia in adults. **Australian Prescriber 2003**; Vol. 26 No. 5

23. William G. Schucany. Exercise-associated hyponatremia. **Radiology report 2007**; Proc (Bayl Univ Med Cent, Texas); 20(4):398–401

24. Mitchell H. Rosner and Justin Kirven. Exercise-Associated Hyponatremia. **Clin J Am Soc Nephrol 2007**; 2: 151–161

25. Debbie Chen et al. Beer Potomania: Don't Just Stand There, Do Nothing. On the **website of University of California, Davis Medical Center Sacramento, CA**; available at: https://www.ucdmc.ucdavis.edu/internalmedicine/education_programs/KT/Posters/2014%20ACP%20posters/BuiAlbert.pdf

26. George L Liamis et al. Mechanism of hyponatremia in alcohol patients. **Alcohol and alcoholism 2000**; 35(6): 612-16

27. Nimesh Bhattarai et al. Beer potomania: a case report. **BMJ Case Rep. 2010**; 2010: bcr10.2009.2414

28. Shalin R. Sanghvi et al. Beer Potomania: An Unusual Cause of Hyponatremia at High Risk of Complications From Rapid Correction. **American Journal of Kidney Diseases 2007;** Vol 50, No 4 (October): pp 673-680

Chapter 12
Hypernatremia

Hypernatremia

Hypernatremia is defined as a serum sodium concentration >145 mmol/L.[1,2] It is a common electrolyte disorder[2] although much less common than hyponatremia[1].

Among outpatients, it is predominantly found in individuals at the extreme of age, particularly in the elderly. In contrast, the age distribution is more general among hospitalized patients. In the elderly, it is often associated with disability or febrile illness;[2] older people are more vulnerable because of their impaired thirst mechanism, lack of access to water due to disability, or reduced intake of water due to psychiatric illness, dementia etc.

Hypernatremia invariably causes hyperosmolality of plasma,[3] and hyperosmolality is a potent stimulator of thirst.[4] Therefore, when an individual's thirst mechanism is intact and he or she has unlimited access to drinking water, usually hypernatremia cannot develop.[3,4]

Biochemical Classification of hypernatremia

There is no widely acceptable biochemical classification of hypernatremia. However, it can be categorized as follows:

1. Mild: serum Na 146-150 mmol/L
2. Moderate: 151-158 mmol/L
3. Severe: >158 mmol/L

Causes of hypernatremia[1,2,4,5]

Hypernatremia is a state of water deficit in relation to the body's Na content. Like hyponatremia, causes of hypernatremia can be divided into three major groups:

A) Hypovolemic hypernatremia

This is the most common form of hypernatremia which occurs due to hypotonic fluid loss (i.e. Na loss with disproportionately greater water loss, or pure water loss).

1. *Nonrenal causes*

- Gastrointestinal fluid loss- vomiting, nasogastric drainage, diarrhea (due to viral gastroenteritis or osmotic laxative)
- Dermal loss- excessive sweating, burns etc
- Respiratory water loss (pure water loss)- tachypnea, mechanical ventilation, fever etc
- Hypodipsia (pure water deficit)

** Diarrhea is the most frequent gastrointestinal cause of hypernatremia. Secretory diarrhea (cholera, VIPoma etc.) generally causes isotonic stool and thus hypovolemia with or without hyponatremia may develop; but diarrhea due to viral gastroenteritis or osmotic laxative (such as lactulose) usually produce hypotonic stool containing disproportionately greater amount of water than sodium and potassium, thus the greater water loss may lead to hypovolemic hypernatremia.*[1]

2. ***Renal causes*** (Urinary sodium loss with disproportionately greater water loss)

- Diuretics (particularly loop diuretics and osmotic diuretics)
- Glycosuria [especially hyperosmolar hyperglycemic state (HHS)]
- Postobstructive diuresis
- Polyuric phase of acute tubular necrosis
- Intrinsic kidney diseases

B) Euvolemic hypernatremia (pure water loss)

- Diabetes insipidus (central or nephrogenic)

C) Hypervolemic hypernatremia (occurs due to hypertonic Na gain i.e. gaining of disproportionately greater amount of sodium than water; mainly iatrogenic)

- Hypertonic saline infusion
- Hypertonic sodium bicarbonate infusion (eg, resuscitation in cardiac arrest)
- Enteral or parenteral feeding with inadequate free water
- Hypertonic saline enemas etc.

Impact of hypernatremia on brain

Hypernatremia → hyperosmolality of plasma → shifting of intracellular fluid (ICF) into extracellular compartment → intracellular dehydration → cell shrinkage (in brain it affects both neurons and vascular endothelium). In acute hypernatremia, severe cell shrinkage may cause cell death or rupture of blood vessels resulting in intracerebral or subarachnoid hemorrhage, permanent neurological damage or death.[1,2] However, the vascular complications are primarily developed in pediatric patients.[1]

Adaptive changes in brain in chronic hypernatremia:
In prolonged hypernatremia, brain cells begin to generate organic osmolytes (osmotically active molecules) in 4-6 hours of dehydration which is continued for several days→ osmolytes increase osmolality of intracellular fluid→ fluid shifts into the intracellular space → cell shrinkage minimized.[3]

In chronic hypernatremia, when the adaptive changes have established a new osmotic equilibrium between ICF and ECF, aggressive correction of the hypernatremia with hypotonic fluid can cause shifting of some the fluid into intracellular space resulting in cerebral edema which may lead to convulsion, coma or even death.[1,2]

Summary of the effects of severe acute hypo- or hypernatremia and inappropriately rapid correction of chronic hypo- or hypernatremia on the brain:

Acute severe hyponatremia → cerebral edema (Cell swelling)
Acute severe hypernatremia → brain shrinkage (Cell shrinkage)
Inappropriately rapid correction of chronic hyponatremia → Osmotic demyelination syndrome (possibly due to cell shrinkage)
Inappropriately rapid correction of chronic hypernatremia → cerebral edema (Cell swelling)

Clinical features

Symptoms of hypernatremia itself are nonspecific. Like hyponatremia, they are largely due to central nervous system dysfunction, and their development depends on acuity and severity of the hypernatremia. Elderly patients usually have few symptoms until the serum Na is >160 mmol/L.[2]

- Early features are weakness, lethargy, irritability, thirst etc.[2,3]
- In severe cases (serum Na >158 mmol/L), hyperthermia, delirium, convulsion and coma may develop.[3]
- The presence of tachycardia and orthostatic hypotension indicate hypovolemia.
- A long history of polyuria and polydipsia is suggestive of diabetes insipidus.[4]

Investigations

- For mild hypernatremia (serum Na <150 mmol/L) when the cause is obvious, no other laboratory tests may be needed for the correction of that hypernatremia only.
- In other cases, serum and urine electrolytes and osmolality measurements are usually considered along with investigations to determine the underlying cause.

Treatment

Treatment of hypernatremia involves two types of measures:

- Correction of the hypernatremia
- Treatment of the underlying cause

Here correction of the hypernatremia has been described.

Correction of the hypernatremia

Correction of the hypernatremia is done with replacement of the water deficit. The water deficit can be replaced in the following ways-

1. The best way is intake of free water orally or via feeding tube.[1,2]
2. Intravenous route should be considered when oral or feeding tube route is inadequate or not feasible.

Any of the following intravenous fluids can be used depending on the situation:[1,2,5]

- 5% dextrose in aqua
- Hypotonic saline (eg, 0.45% NaCl, 0.2% NaCl)
- Normal Saline (0.9% NaCl) in some cases during the initial correction

*In mild hypernatremia (serum Na 146-150 mmol/L), when oral intake is adequate, only oral replacement of free water may be sufficient.

IV fluid selection

- This should be based on the patient's history (eg, the type of fluid loss, history of diabetes mellitus etc) and clinical volume status.[1] Excessively rapid correction or overcorrection of hypernatremia increases the risk of catastrophic cerebral edema.
- The risk of cerebral edema rises with the volume of IV fluid used to correct the hypernatremia.[2] Therefore, an IV fluid with least percentage of Na which is appropriate for a particular type of hypernatremia should be used, so that the possible lowest amount of the infusate may be sufficient to correct serum Na concentration.

When should normal saline (0.9% NaCl) be used?
Usually normal saline is unsuitable for the correction of hypernatremia[1] and limited amount should be used only in the following conditions:

a) *In a patient with frank hypotension,* normal saline should be used for the initial volume resuscitation.[1,2,3] When the patient becomes hemodynamically stable, normal saline infusion should be stopped, and hypotonic saline (0.45% NaCl) and or 5% dextrose in aqua infusion should be started to replace the remaining water deficit.[3]
b) *In very severe hypernatremia (serum sodium >170 mmol/L),*[1,4] some physicians prefer to use normal saline initially to avoid rapid fall in serum sodium concentration.[1,4] Osmolality of normal saline (308 mosm/Kg) is lower than these patients' plasma osmolality, so it can reduce plasma osmolality.[3] However, other physicians do not support the use of normal saline in this circumstance, as adequate reduction in serum sodium concentration may not occur with normal saline infusion.[2]

Correction of specific categories of hypernatremia:

1. *Hypovolemic hypernatremia*

(a) Hypovolemic hypernatremia without frank hypotension (i.e. milder volume deficit):
For intravenous correction of this most common form of hypernatremia, 5% dextrose in aqua and or hypotonic saline (0.45% NaCl) can be used.[3] 5% dextrose in aqua is probably the most commonly used fluid in this setting; however, the fluid prescription may be more specific if the type of fluid loss is taken into account. For example:

- *Pure water loss* (eg, hypernatremia in a patient with high fever or tachypnea): The lost fluid is pure water (insensible loss); so 5% dextrose in aqua may be the most appropriate initial fluid. But, if the patient is diabetic, some extra insulin is likely to be needed; hypotonic saline (0.45% NaCl) may also be used instead of 5% dextrose in aqua.
- *Hypotonic fluid loss* (eg, hypernatremia due to diarrhea or vomiting): Hypotonic saline (0.45% NaCl) may be the most appropriate initial fluid in these cases. If the correction rate is inadequate, a hypotonic saline with relatively lower concentration of Na (0.2% NaCl) can be used.

(b) Hypovolemic hypernatremia with frank hypotension
Normal saline should be used initially until the patient is hemodynamically stable; then the remaining free water deficit can be replaced with hypotonic saline (0.45% NaCl) and or 5% dextrose in aqua.[3]

Notes:

- Decreased skin turgor, dry mucous membrane and mild orthostatic hypotension may develop in milder volume deficit.
- Concomitant hypokalemia should be corrected.

- The patient should be monitored closely with repeated blood glucose and serum electrolyte testing initially. The type of infusate or rate of infusion may need to be changed depending on the response. Insulin should be started if hyperglycemia develops.[2]

2. *Euvolemic hypernatremia:*
Diabetes insipidus generally causes euvolemic hypernatremia. The hypernatremia in diabetes insipidus may respond temporarily to water ingestion or 5% dextrose in aqua infusion.[3]

- Desmopressin (an ADH analogue with longer half-life) is the treatment of choice for central diabetes insipidus.[3,5]
- Indomethacin alone[3] or in combination with hydrochlorothiazide and or amiloride may be effective in nephrogenic diabetes isipidus.[1]
- Hydrochlorothiazide and amiloride combination is partially effective in both central and nephrogenic diabetes insipidus.[3]

3. *Hypervolemic hypernatremia:*

- In this condition excess water and Na need to be excreted from the body.
- Furosemide plus 5% dextrose in aqua can achieve the therapeutic goal.[2]
- Furosemide alone will not be adequate, as furosemide causes greater water diuresis than natriuresis aggravating the hypernatremia.[2]
- In patients with kidney disease, hemodialysis may be necessary to eliminate excess Na and water from the body in severe cases.[3]

Target serum Na level during correction of hypernatremia: 145 mmol/L[2]

The rate of correction of hypernatremia

There is no consensus on the optimal rate of correction of hypernatremia.[3] Duration of the hypernatremia is considered as a very important factor in this regard.

1. <u>Acute hypernatremia (duration no more than several hours):</u> Acute hypernatremia of up to several hours' duration can be corrected rapidly (1 mmol/L per hour) without producing increased risk for cerebral edema.[2] However, this type of hypernatremia is rare, and usually results from rapid sodium loading due to large amount of $NaHCO_3$ infusion during cardiac arrest or hypertonic saline infusion. Adequate symptomatic treatment such as anticonvulsant in seizure should also be ensured when needed.
2. <u>Hypernatremia with longer (> several hours) or unknown duration:</u> Recommended maximal rate of correction is **0.5 mmol/L per hour (maximum 10 mmol/L in 24 hours)**[2]

Although theoretically hypernatremia is considered as acute when it is of < 48 hours' duration,[1,6] for treatment purposes it may be safer to consider the condition as acute when the duration is no more than several hours.[2] However, for hypernatremia in adults, the risk of inadvertent overcorrection is much lower than that for hyponatremia, and hypernatremia in adults are frequently undertreated. Rapid correction of acute hypernatremia may prevent intracranial hemorrhage and osmotic demyelination syndrome, so it should not be avoided in adults when necessary.[7]

Typically the correction of hypernatremia takes about 48 hours; longer than 48 hours may be needed if serum Na is >160 mmol/L.[1]

How much fluid should be infused?

Fluid requirement = Free water deficit + ongoing fluid loss

Free water deficit can be roughly estimated from the following formulas:

1. Free water deficit:[1,8]
Total body water (TBW) × [(Patient's serum sodium concentration -140) ÷ 140]

Here 140 is desired serum Na concentration in mmol/L.

The two formulas below, suggested by Adrogué–Madias[2], are preferred by many.

2. Predicted change in serum Na concentration with infusion of one liter of any infusate:

Change in serum Na concentration = (Infusate Na concentration – serum Na concentration) ÷ (Total body water + 1)

3. If the infusate contains potassium, it must also be taken into account; the predicted effect of 1 liter of any infusate containing both Na and K on serum Na:

Change in serum Na concentration= [(infusate Na + infusate K) - serum Na] ÷ (total body water + 1)

*All Na concentration values are in mmol/L.

*A physician should not completely rely on any of the above formulas for estimation and correction of water deficit; instead, serum sodium should be checked repeatedly along with clinical evaluation; initially it may be 6-8 hourly or more frequently during intravenous fluid therapy. Fluid administration should be adjusted according to the assessment results.

Approximate total body water (TBW):

Subject category	*TBW (as percentage of body weight)*
Non-elderly adult male	60%
Non-elderly adult female	50%
Male above 60 years	50%
Female above 60 years	40%

Of total body water, normally 40% is extracellular and 60% is intracellular fluid.

Insensible fluid loss (Skin and lungs): the amount is very variable, may be 600-900ml/day or about 10 ml/Kg/day.
(Metabolic water production which is added to the body fluid is about 400 ml/day)

Sodium concentration of various intravenous fluids
0.9% Sodium chloride in water: 154 mmol per liter

Ringer's lactate solution: 130 mmol per liter
0.45% Sodium chloride in water: 77 mmol per liter
5% Dextrose in aqua: 0 mmol per liter

An example of calculation of fluid requirement:
A 56 years old man with body weight 70 Kg and serum sodium concentration 164 mmol/L:

Total body water: 70×0.6=42 liters

According to the formula 1 (above), estimated free water deficit= 42× [(164-140) ÷140]=42×[24÷140]
=42× 0.171= 7.2 liters (Approximately).

According to formula 2 (above), one liter 5% dextrose in aqua infusion will correct the hypernatremia of this patient by: [(0-164) ÷ (42+1)] = -164÷43= 3.8 mmol/L; therefore, if 10 mmol/L serum sodium concentration reduction is the target over the next 24 hours, 10 ÷ 3.8=2.6 liters (5% dextrose in aqua) plus the amount for ongoing loss will be needed to replace.

Summary of the treatment of hypernatremia

Correction of the hypernatremia

Correction of the hypernatremia is done with replacement of the water deficit which can be performed in the following ways-

1. The best way is intake of free water orally or via feeding tube.
2. Intravenous route should be considered when oral or feeding tube route is inadequate or not feasible.

***Any of the following intravenous fluids can be used depending on the situation*:**
a) 5% dextrose in aqua
b) Hypotonic saline (eg, 0.45% NaCl, 0.2% NaCl)
c) Normal Saline (0.9% NaCl) in some cases during the initial correction;

IV fluid selection for a particular category of hypernatremia

1. *Hypovolemic hypernatremia*
(a) Hypovolemic hypernatremia without frank hypotension (i.e. milder volume deficit):
5% dextrose in aqua and or hypotonic saline (0.45% NaCl) can be used.

- *Pure water loss* (eg, hypernatremia in a patient with high fever and or tachypnea): 5% dextrose in aqua may be the most appropriate initial fluid.
- *Hypotonic fluid loss* (eg, hypernatremia due to diarrhea or vomiting): Hypotonic saline (0.45% NaCl) may be the most appropriate initial fluid.

(b) Hypovolemic hypernatremia with frank hypotension
Initially Normal saline until the patient is hemodynamically stable; then hypotonic saline (0.45% NaCl) and or 5% dextrose in aqua;
2. *Euvolemic hypernatremia:*
5% dextrose in aqua;
3. *Hypervolemic hypernatremia:*
Furosemide plus 5% dextrose in aqua;
In patients with kidney disease, hemodialysis may be needed;

Target serum Na level during correction of hypernatremia: 145 mmol/L
Maximal rate of correction for most cases: 0.5 mmol/L per hour (maximum 10 mmol/L in 24 hours);
Fluid requirement = Free water deficit + ongoing fluid loss
Free water deficit = Total body water (TBW) × [(Patient's serum sodium concentration -140) ÷ 140]
Two other formulas preferred by many:
1. Predicted change in serum Na concentration with infusion of one liter of any infusate:
Change in serum Na concentration = (Infusate Na concentration– serum Na concentration) ÷ (Total body water + 1)
2. If the infusate also contains potassium, it must also be taken into account;
The predicted effect of 1 liter of any infusate containing both Na and K on serum Na:
Change in serum Na concentration= [(infusate Na + infusate K) - serum Na] ÷ (total body water + 1)

The patient should be monitored closely with repeated serum electrolyte and blood glucose testing initially. The type of infusate and rate of infusion may need to be changed depending on the response. Insulin should be started if hyperglycemia develops.

The underlying cause should also be treated.

References

1. Relevant chapters of **Harrison's Principles of Internal Medicine**; 18 th edition; Dan L Longo et al (Editors). New York, McGraw-Hill 2012.

2. Horacio J. Adrogué, Nicolaos E. Madias. Hypernatremia. **N Engl J Med. 2000;** 342(20):1493-99

3. Relevant chapters of **Current Medical Diagnosis and Treatment**; Maxine A. Papadakis et al (Editors). New York, McGraw-Hill, **2013**

4. Relevant chapters of **Kumar &Clark's Clinical Medicine,** 8th edition; Parveen Kumar and Michael Clark (Editors). Edinburgh, Elsevier, **2012**

5. Relevant chapters of **Davidson's Principles and Practice of Medicine**, 21 edition, Nicki R. Colledge et al (editors). India, Elsevier, **2010**

6. Ivo Lukitsch. **Hypernatremia Treatment & Management. Emedicine;** at: http://emedicine.medscape.com/article/241094-treatment

7. Richard H. Sterns. Disorders of Plasma Sodium — Causes, Consequences, and Correction. **N Engl J Med 2015;** 372:55-65.

8. Zina Semenovskaya. **Hypernatremia in Emergency Medicine Treatment & Management. Emedicine;** at: http://emedicine.medscape.com/article/766683-treatment#showall

Chapter 13

Hypokalemia

Hypokalemia

(Normal serum K: 3.5-5.0 mmol/L[1,2])

- Hypokalemia is defined as a serum potassium concentration <3.5 mmol/L.[3,4]
- Hypokalemia is found in about 20% of hospitalized patients and one-fourth of these hypokalemic patients have serum potassium levels < 3 mmol/L.[5,6] Hypokalemia is more common in women and patients with malignancy.[5]

Spurious hypokalemia or pseudohypokalemia: This can occasionally occur in patients with acute leukemia with a high WBC count (>100,000/μL) if the blood sample is allowed to stand at room temperature for several hours after collection when abnormal blood cells may take up potassium.[6,7]

Biochemical classification of hypokalemia[8]

1. Mild: 3.0- 3.4 mmol/L
2. Moderate: 2.5- 2.9 mmol/L
3. Severe: <2.5 mmol/L

Causes of Hypokalemia[1,2,4,6,9,10]

- More than 98% of total-body potassium is intracellular.[1] Hypokalemia results from increased potassium loss, inadequate intake of potassium, or shifting of potassium from the extracellular compartment into the intracellular space.[4]
- Increased potassium loss, through either the kidney or gastrointestinal tract, is the most common mechanism.[6,9]
- Reduced potassium intake rarely causes hypokalemia; however, hypokalemia may develop if potassium intake falls to <1g/day (25 mmol/day).[6] In starvation or near starvation, tissue breakdown releases potassium into the extracellular fluid, minimizing the fall in plasma potassium concentration.[6]

1. Reduced potassium intake

- Infusion of large amount of fluids without potassium;
- Dietary deficiency (eg, anorexia nervosa, "tea-and-toast" diet of the elderly etc)

2. Increased potassium loss

a) ***Nonrenal loss*** (urine potassium < 20-30 mmol/day)

- Diarrhea
- Vomiting
- Nasogastric aspiration
- Villous adenoma
- Zollinger-Ellison syndrome
- Ureterosigmoidostomy

*Urinary K loss will be higher if the nonrenal fluid loss causes hypovolemia leading to activation of the renin-angiotensin-aldosterone system.

b) ***Renal loss*** (urine potassium > 20-30 mmol/day)

- Diuretic therapy (loop diuretics and thiazides)
- Osmotic diuresis (uncontrolled diabetes, mannitol therapy)
- Renal tubular acidosis
- Carbonic anhydrase inhibitor therapy
- Post-obstructive diuresis
- Recovery from acute tubular necrosis
- Hypomagnesemia
- Liddle's syndrome

Renal K loss with increased mineralocorticoid effects

- Primary hyperaldosteronism (eg, Conn's syndrome)
- Secondary hyperaldosteronism (eg, dehydration, heart failure)
- Cushing syndrome
- Corticosteroid therapy
- Renal artery stenosis
- Bartter's syndrome
- Gitelman's syndrome
- Liquorice/ carbenoxolone

*10-40% of patients taking thiazide diuretics develop hypokalemia.[6]

3. Shifting of potassium into cells (redistributive hypokalemia)

- Alkalosis
- Drugs
    - Insulin
    - β-Adrenergic agonists (bronchodilators, tocolytics etc)
    - Theophylline, caffeine
- Acute catecholamine surge from stress (e.g., acute myocardial infarction, head injury)
- Thyrotoxic periodic paralysis
- Familial hypokalemic periodic paralysis
- Barium intoxication

* ***Nebulization of one standard dose of albuterol (salbutamol)*** can reduce serum potassium by 0.2 to 0.4 mmol/L. If a second dose is administered within 1 hour, the potassium level may drop by approximately 1 mmol/L.[11]

Mechanisms of hypokalemia in diarrhea and vomiting

The potassium concentration of gastric fluid is about 10 mmol/L whereas in intestinal fluid it is about 80 mmol/L.[2,4]

Mechanisms of hypokalemia in diarrhea:

1. Substantial amount of potassium may be lost directly with stool because of high K content of intestinal fluid;
2. Diarrhea→ hypovolemia→ secondary hyperaldosteronism→ ↑renal K loss.

Mechanisms of hypokalemia in vomiting:

It is complex.[4]

1. Direct loss of K with vomitus (much lower than direct loss in diarrhea)
2. Vomiting→ hypovolemia→ secondary hyperaldosteronism→ ↑renal K loss.
3. Vomiting → gastric HCl loss → metabolic alkalosis → shift of K from the extracellular to the intracellular space;
4. Metabolic alkalosis causes increased renal collecting tubular secretion of potassium;

Clinical features[1,2,4,6,9,10]

- Hypokalemia is often asymptomatic, especially when the condition is mild. The likelihood of symptoms is generally related to the biochemical severity and rapidity of the development of hypokalemia.
- When symptoms are present, they are nonspecific and primarily related to dysfunction of muscles and heart.
- Symptoms of mild to moderate hypokalemia include fatigue, muscular weakness and muscle cramps.
- Severe hypokalemia (serum K <2.5 mmol/L) can cause flaccid paralysis, muscle pain, diminished reflex responses, tetany, rhabdomyolysis etc.
- Constipation or paralytic ileus may develop due the effect of hypokalemia on intestinal smooth muscle.
- When serum K is <2.0 mmol/L, ascending paralysis, which may eventually involve respiratory muscles, may develop.
- Prolonged hypokalemia can cause polyuria and polydipsia by interfering with renal tubular response to ADH (nephrogenic diabetes insipidus). Chronic hypokalemia may cause interstitial nephritis.
- Hypokalemia increases the risk of digitalis toxicity by potentiating its effects, and decreasing its clearance.
- Hypokalemia increases the risk of arrhythmia in patients with heart disease. However, hypokalemia in patients without underlying heart disease, usually do not induce a serious arrhythmia.
- Hypokalemia with hypertension indicates increased mineralocorticoid effects (eg, Conn's syndrome).

Investigations

In mild or moderate asymptomatic hypokalemia when the cause is obvious, such as diuretic use and gastrointestinal fluid loss, the following investigations may be sufficient for the management of the hypokalemia:

- Plasma electrolyte, calcium, magnesium
- Some routine investigations - complete blood count, blood sugar, blood urea nitrogen and creatinine
- ECG

<u>In other cases initial investigations may include:</u>

- Serum and urine osmolality and electrolytes
- Blood urea nitrogen and creatinine
- Blood sugar

- Complete blood count
- ECG (typical ECG changes are: prominent U, flat or inverted T, ST depression)
- Serum calcium and magnesium
- Urinary pH

Additional investigations such as urinary Ca, Plasma Rennin Activity (PRA), aldosterone and thyroid function test are considered depending on suspicion about the cause.

Renal potassium excretion

In hypokalemia, estimation of renal potassium excretion is helpful to detect the route of excess potassium loss, particularly in some difficult cases. Renal potassium excretion can be assessed by several ways which include measurement of spot urine potassium, 24-hour urine potassium and Transtubular K Gradient (TTKG).[12]

Transtubular K Gradient (TTKG):

The TTKG is the ratio of potassium concentration of renal cortical collecting duct fluid to that of peritubular capillary blood (i.e. plasma K).[13]

TTKG is a simple and rapid assessment, calculated from serum and urine osmolality and K concentration.[2]
TTKG = (Urine K level ÷ Plasma K level) ÷ (Urine osmolality ÷ Plasma osmolality)

Usefulness of TTKG
TTKG is an assessment of K secretion by the cortical collecting ducts, the principal site of renal K secretion. As this renal K secretion is regulated by aldosterone (mineralocorticoid effects), ***TTKG can be considered as an indirect measurement of aldosterone (mineralocorticoid) activity on renal tubule*** in patients with hypo- and hyperkalemia.[12]

In the presence of aldosterone resistance, aldosterone level may not reflect mineralocorticoid activity. So in hyperkalemia, TTKG may be most helpful to differentiate between mineralocorticoid deficiency and mineralocorticoid resistance.[12]

Interpretation of TTKG:
Although TTKG values are related to the mineralocorticoid activity on cortical collecting duct, there are no standard cutoff values to interpret the correlation between TTKG and mineralocorticoid activity.[12] Change in TTKG values is directly proportional to the change in renal K excretion. Renal K excretion (so TTKG too) should be higher in hyperkalemia, high K intake, or with increased mineralocorticoid activity and should be lower in hypokalemia, K depletion, or with decreased mineralocorticoid activity.

1. TTKG in a normal person on normal diet is typically 8-9.
2. In hypokalemia or during K depletion[1], TTKG should be <3-4; if >4, it is suggestive of increased renal K loss (i.e. increased mineralocorticoid activity is possibly causing hypokalemia)[2]
3. In hyperkalemia or during high potassium intake, TTKG should be >10; in hyperkalemia, if <6, it indicates impaired aldosterone activity on renal tubule as the cause of hyperkalemia.[12]

Limitation: TTKG is not valid if urine osmolality is lower than the plasma osmolality, or the urine sodium is <25 mmol/L.[12]

Treatment of hypokalemia

A. Correction of the hypokalemia
B. Treatment of the underlying cause

A. Correction of the hypokalemia

Some form of K replacement is needed in most cases.[9] The dose and route of potassium replacement should be individualized. Potassium replacement policies and available potassium preparations somewhat vary among health systems. You should check with your local guidelines if any.

Some general suggestions on K replacement are given below. These suggestions are for patients with normal renal function and not applicable for redistributive type of hypokalemia or hypokalemia in diabetic ketoacidosis.

Route of potassium administration

In general, for mild to moderate hypokalemia, oral potassium supplementation may be adequate if the patient is asymptomatic or has only minor symptoms.[2,4] However, in asymptomatic moderate hypokalemia when the K loss is acute (eg, acute gastroenteritis), initially some intravenous K replacement should be considered to prevent further fall in serum K concentration.

Indications for IV potassium replacement:

- When adequate replacement is not possible orally or absorption is unpredictable.[14]
- Severe hypokalemia (Plasma K <2.5 mmol/L)[2,4]
- IV potassium replacement should also be considered even in mild or moderate hypokalemia when --
    - It is associated with significant symptoms,[4] or serious complications like paralysis or arrhythmia.[1]
    - The plasma potassium level is declining rapidly and the underlying cause cannot be corrected quickly.
    - The patient has other comorbidities where hypokalemia is potentially more hazardous (patients with heart disease, digoxin therapy, etc.), particularly if the hypokalemia is acute.

The above indications for intravenous K replacement are for the initial correction and oral replacement should be started whenever possible. IV and oral replacement can be continued simultaneously too. If the patient has acidosis, replace some potassium first before correcting the acidosis to avoid further drop in serum potassium with alkali administration.[4]

Total potassium deficit estimation

- There is no widely acceptable formula to calculate the deficit reliably.

- In the absence of abnormal K shifting into cells, plasma K level falls roughly by 0.3 mmol/L for every 100 mmol reduction in total-body potassium.[6]
- Approximately, 1mmol/L fall in plasma potassium concentration is associated with 200-400 mmol K loss from total-body stores.[1,4] However, *the response is highly variable[6] and this calculation may over or underestimate the real deficit, so plasma potassium must be measured repeatedly during K replacement.*

Types of potassium salt used for replacement

1. Potassium phosphate (oral or IV) may be more suitable when hypophosphatemia is present with hypokalemia.[1,6]
2. Potassium bicarbonate or citrate should be considered when there is accompanying metabolic acidosis.[1,6]
3. In all other cases, potassium chloride is suitable for both oral and intravenous replacement.[6]

Oral or nasogastric tube potassium replacement

- Potassium chloride is the most commonly used potassium salt for both oral and intravenous K replacement.
- The required dose of oral potassium for the treatment of hypokalemia usually varies between 40 and 100 mmol/day.[11] Often initially it is given at higher dose, and then slower correction over days or weeks is done.
- Patients are also advised to take increased fresh fruits and vegetables which are generally rich source of dietary potassium. However, potassium in foods is usually present in phosphate form and not useful to correct hypokalemia with chloride loss such as in vomiting or diuretic use; potassium chloride replacement is needed in such cases.[6,11]

Oral potassium chloride preparations

- Several forms of oral KCl are available such as effervescent tablets, slow release tablets and suspension.
- Potassium is readily absorbed regardless of the formulation used.[6]
- The suspensions are less expensive, but have a strong, unpleasant taste.[11]
- Slow-release tablets are of two types—wax matrix and microencapsulated form.[6] The slow-release tablets are generally well tolerated but may cause gastrointestinal ulceration and bleeding.[6,11] The microencapsulated preparations have no unpleasant taste and are probably associated with the lowest risk of gastrointestinal side effects.[6,11]
- *Liquid (or effervescent) form of K salt is preferably prescribed*; because of their potential side effects of gastrointestinal bleeding and ulceration, slow-release forms are considered only when liquid form or effervescent tablets are inappropriate.[15]

A simplified dose schedule for oral KCl replacement in mild to moderate hypokalemia
(Total dose of K: 40-100 mmol/day)[3,11]

Severity of hypokalemia	***Oral dose of KCl***	***Comment***
Mild (3.0-3.4 mmol/L)	20 mmol TID (60 mmol/day)	Check serum K daily and adjust dose accordingly[8]
Moderate (2.5 -2.9 mmol/L)	20 mmol QID (80 mmol/day)	Check serum K daily and adjust dose accordingly[8]

*Oral potassium should be taken with or after a meal with a full glass of water (250 ml) to minimize gastrointestinal side effects.

*Switch to intravenous K replacement if oral therapy is not tolerated.

Intravenous potassium replacement

Dose schedule for intravenous potassium replacement
Although the decision should be individualized, the following simplified dose schedule can be considered for initial intravenous K replacement via a peripheral line.

Severity of the hypokalemia	*Amount needs to be infused*	*Monitoring serum K level*
Mild (3.0-3.4 mmol/L)	30 mmol KCl initially over at least 3 hours[16]	Check serum potassium 1-2 hours after finishing the initial 30 mmol and adjust dose accordingly
Moderate (2.5-2.9 mmol/L)	40 mmol KCl initially at least over 4 hours[17]	Check serum potassium 1-2 hours after finishing the initial 40 mmol and adjust dose accordingly
Severe (<2.5 mmol/L)	40 mmol KCl BID or TID;[8] Infusion rate: up to10 mmol K/hr *In very severe cases, infusion of higher doses of K may be needed. *For difficult cases consult critical care specialists or nephrologists.	Recheck serum K after each 40mmol and adjust dose accordingly.[8] *In critical situations serum K rechecking may need to be done 1-2 hourly until the serum K has reached a safe level, eg, >3mmol/L.[18] *When serum K reaches ≥3mmol/L, consider switch to oral K replacement when feasible.

What type of intravenous potassium preparations can be used?
Premixed solution of potassium chloride should be used when available.[8,18]

In a general ward via peripheral cannula:

- If available use: pre-mixed 40mmol KCl in one liter normal saline (0.9% NaCl)
- Alternatively, minibags of pre-mixed 10 mmol KCl in 100 ml 0.29% NaCl (an isotonic solution) can be used in:[18,19]
    - Most cases of hypokalemia, particularly in acute hypokalemia or
    - Patients at risk of volume overload

How can KCl solution for IV infusion be prepared when pre-mixed solutions are not available?
The solution can be prepared in the pharmacy or ward by adding 20- 40 mmol KCl (ampoules) into one liter normal saline bag for peripheral IV infusion.
Precautions:

- During preparation of the mixture in the ward, after addition of KCl (ampoules) to the normal saline bag, the bag **must be inverted at least 10 times for proper mixing.**[18,20] Density of KCl is higher than that of normal saline. Consequently, layer may form if not properly mixed, and infusion of highly concentrated KCl from that layer may be extremely hazardous.[14,18]
- KCl should not be added to any other K containing fluid bag or any hanging IV fluid bag.[14,18]
- Glucose containing IV fluids should be avoided in hypokalemia, as glucose induced increased insulin secretion can cause transcellular shift of K from extracellular fluid into intracellular compartment aggravating hypokalemia.[1,4]

Why an IV fluid with >40 mmol KCl/L (normal saline) is not recommended for infusion via peripheral lines?
Potassium chloride at the concentration higher than 40 mmol/L in normal saline (0.9% NaCl) is significantly hypertonic and irritant to vein; phlebitis and subsequent sclerosis of the vein may develop from its use.[1,8,20]

Is there any way to infuse higher concentration of K (>40 mmol KCl/L) through a peripheral line safely?
Yes, pre-mixed 10 mmol KCl in 100 ml 0.29% NaCl is an isotonic solution, and not irritant to vein; it can be administered peripherally in general wards.[18,20] Multiple minibags of this pre-mixed fluid can be infused one after another (no more than 10 mmol K/hr) in most cases of hypokalemia when IV potassium replacement is needed.

What can be done for patients at risk of volume overload?
In some cases infusion of considerable amount of normal saline may cause volume overload, especially in patients with heart diseases. In such circumstances, multiple minibags of premixed 10 mmol KCl in 100 ml 0.29% NaCl serially or larger bags with mostly similar strength of KCl and NaCl can be infused depending on the need.

Acceptable maximum concentration of KCl and maximum rate for IV infusion:

Route	Acceptable maximum concentration of K	Acceptable maximum rate of IV K infusion
Peripheral line	40 mmol KCl per liter normal saline (0.9% NaCl)[2,9,20] Exceptions: (a) pre-mixed 10 mmol KCl in 100 ml 0.29% sodium chloride mini-bags	10 mmol/hour[2,9]

	(b) For critically ill patients, in exceptional circumstances, higher concentration of K in normal saline (eg, 30 or 40 mmol/500 ml) may be permitted through a large peripheral vein.[8,14] However, pre-mixed 10 mmol KCl in 100 ml 0.29% NaCl may be the better option.	
Central line (Central line should be used when K concentration >40 mmol/L normal saline or infusion rate >10 mmol/hr is needed)[20]	20- 25mmol K/100ml infusate (in critical care area for life-threatening complications)[1,19] *Femoral vein is the preferred site for this infusion, as infusion through internal jugular or subclavian central line may increase local K concentration abruptly affecting cardiac conduction.[1]	20 mmol K/hr (in ICU setting) with continuous ECG monitoring.[1,2] <u>Exceptions:</u> (a) Up to 40 mmol/hr in acute life-threatening complications.[4,19,21] (b) When cardiac arrest is imminent in a patient with unstable arrhythmia due to hypokalemia, initially K can be given at very high rate (2 mmol K/min for 10 min, followed by 10 mmol over 5-10 min); remember rapid bolus injection of K itself may precipitate cardiac arrest.[22]

How much total potassium can be replaced in a 24-hour period?

- If the serum potassium concentration is >2.5 mmol/L, the total K replacement in a 24-hour period should not exceed 200 mmol.[23]
- When very urgent treatment is indicated (eg, serum potassium level < 2.0 mmol/L with ECG changes and/or muscle paralysis), potassium chloride may be infused up to 400 mmol in a 24 hour period very cautiously with continuous cardiac monitoring.[23]

Notes

1. Rapid administration of K may cause hyperkalaemia, arrhythmias, heart block and cardiac arrest.[14]
2. Many physicians prefer to infuse KCl at a slower rate than the recommended maximum when possible.[14,15]
3. When KCl infusion rate is >10 mmol/hour, continuous ECG monitoring should be done.[20]
4. In redistributive hypokalemia, cautious correction of potassium level should be followed, as there is a risk of rebound hyperkalemia when the underlying cause is resolved. In severe cases also (serum K <2.5 mmol/L), urgent but cautious potassium replacement should be considered.[1] However, in mild asymptomatic redistributive hypokalemia (eg,

metabolic alkalosis induced), sometimes correction of the underlying cause may be sufficient to restore plasma potassium level without any potassium replacement.[9]

5. Hypokalemia in diabetic ketoacidosis has complex pathogenesis and should be managed according to its own guideline.
6. In patient with renal impairment, potassium must be replaced cautiously; consult nephrology team, especially if the patient has severe renal insufficiency.

Target serum K level

- Target serum potassium level is usually 4 mmol/L; but in many cases when IV replacement is used, K infusion is usually done up to 3mmol/L, then the remaining correction is done by oral route if feasible.
- Some physicians suggest K replacement when serum K is low normal (between 3.5-4.0 mmol/L), but it is controversial.

Effect of hypomagnesemia

- Hypomagnesemia can make hypokalemia refractory to treatment.[1,2]
- During treatment of hypokalemia, if adequate response is not found with potassium replacement, plasma magnesium level should be checked (if not already checked). If hypomagnesemia is revealed, magnesium should be replaced.[1,2,8]

B. Treatment of the underlying cause

The underlying cause of the hypokalemia should be treated where possible. In many cases, the underlying cause can be reversed quickly such as antibiotic therapy in infective diarrhea, withdrawal of the offending drug when the condition is drug induced. But some patients may need to continue potassium losing drugs such as patients with heart failure taking loop diuretic. In such cases, one or more of the following measures can be considered to prevent hypokalemia:

1. Addition of a potassium sparing diuretic with non –potassium sparing one;
2. Addition of angiotensin-converting enzyme inhibitor (ACEI) or angiotensin-II receptor blocker (ARB)
3. Addition of β- blocker
4. Regular oral potassium supplementation
5. Consumption of potassium rich foods

*For a patient on mild to moderate dose of non-potassium sparing diuretic, oral potassium supplement of 20 mmol/d is usually sufficient to prevent hypokalemia.[2]

Summary of the treatment of hypokalemia

Correction of the hypokalemia

Some form of K replacement is usually needed. Oral K replacement may be sufficient in asymptomatic mild to moderate hypokalemia.

Indications for IV potassium replacement:

- When adequate replacement is not possible orally or absorption is unpredictable;
- Severe hypokalemia (Plasma K <2.5 mmol/L);

- IV potassium replacement should also be considered even in mild or moderate hypokalemia when --
  - It is associated with significant symptoms, or serious complications like paralysis or arrhythmia.
  - The plasma potassium level is declining rapidly and the underlying cause cannot be corrected quickly.
  - The patient has other comorbidities where hypokalemia is potentially more hazardous (patients with heart disease, digoxin therapy, etc.), particularly if the hypokalemia is acute.

***Plasma K level falls roughly by** 0.3 mmol/L for every 100 mmol reduction in total body potassium;

Simplified dose schedule

Severity of the hypokalemia	*Dose of K*	*Monitoring serum K level*
Mild (3.0-3.4 mmol/L)	**Oral:** 20 mmol TID (60 mmol/day) **IV:** (when indicated) 30 mmol KCl initially over at least 3 hours;	Check serum K daily and adjust dose accordingly; Check serum potassium 1-2 hours after finishing the initial 30 mmol and adjust dose accordingly;
Moderate (2.5-2.9 mmol/L)	**Oral:** 20 mmol QID (80 mmol/day) **IV:** (when indicated) 40 mmol KCl initially at least over 4 hours	Check serum K daily and adjust dose accordingly; Check serum potassium 1-2 hours after finishing the initial 40 mmol and adjust dose accordingly;
Severe (<2.5 mmol/L)	**IV:** 40 mmol KCl BID or TID **Infusion rate:** up to10 mmol potassium/hr; *In very severe cases, infusion of higher doses of K may be needed. *For difficult cases consult critical care specialists or nephrologists.	Check serum K after each 40mmol and adjust dose accordingly. *In critical situations, serum K rechecking may need to be done 1-2 hourly until the serum K has reached a safe level, eg, >3mmol/L. *When serum K reaches ≥3mmol/L, consider switch to oral K when feasible.

Oral potassium should be taken with or after a meal with a full glass of water (250 ml) to minimize gastrointestinal side effects.

For IV infusion: If available use pre-mixed 40mmol KCl in one liter normal saline (0.9% NaCl). Alternatively, minibags of pre-mixed 10 mmol KCl in 100 ml 0.29% NaCl (an isotonic solution) can be used in:

- Most cases of hypokalemia, particularly in acute hypokalemia;
- Patients at risk of volume overload;

Acceptable concentration and rate for K infusion through peripheral lines: up to 40 mmol KCl per liter normal saline (0.9% NaCl) at a rate of up to 10mmol potassium/hr;

Target serum potassium level is usually 4 mmol/L; but in many cases where IV replacement is used, K infusion is usually done up to 3mmol/L, then the remaining correction is done orally if feasible;

Underlying cause should be treated where possible.

References

1. Relevant chapters of **Harrison's Principles of Internal Medicine**; 18 th edition; Dan L Longo et al (Editors). New York, McGraw-Hill **2012.**

2. Relevant chapters of **Current Medical Diagnosis and Treatment**; Maxine A. Papadakis et al (Editors). New York, McGraw-Hill, **2013**

3. A Rastergar and M Soleimani. Hypokalaemia and hyperkalaemia. **Postgrad Med J 2001**;77:759–764

4. Eleanor Lederer. Hypokalemia. **Emedicine**. At: http://emedicine.medscape.com/article/242008-overview#showall

5. B.J. Paice et al. Record linkage study of hypokalaemia in hospitalized patients. **Postgraduate Medical Journal 1986**; 62: 187-191

6. F. John Gennari. Hypokalemia. **N Engl J Med. 1998** Aug 13; 339(7):451-8.

7. Bakul I. Dalal et al. Factitious Biochemical Measurements Resulting From Hematologic Conditions. **Am J Clin Pathol 2009;**131:195-204

8. **Guideline for the Management of Hypokalaemia in Adults. Gloucestershire hospital, NHS, UK.** Approved by Drug & Therapeutics Committee June **2014**. At: http://www.gloshospitals.nhs.uk/SharePoint1/Treatment%20Guidelines/Hypokalaemia.pdf

9. Relevant chapters of **Davidson's Principles and Practice of Medicine**, 21 edition, Nicki R. Colledge et al (editors). India, Elsevier, **2010**

10. Relevant chapters of **Kumar &Clark's Clinical Medicine,** 8th edition; Parveen Kumar and Michael Clark (Editors). Edinburgh, Elsevier, **2012**

11. Jay N. Cohn et al. New Guidelines for Potassium Replacement in Clinical Practice: A Contemporary Review by the National Council on Potassium in Clinical Practice. **Arch Intern Med. 2000;** 160:2429-2436

12. Michael J. Choi et al.The Utility of the Transtubular Potassium Gradient in the Evaluation of Hyperkalemia. **J Am Soc Nephrol 2008**; 19: 424–426

13. Vidhia Umami et al. Diagnosis and Clinical Approach in Gitelman's Syndrome. **Acta Med Indones-Indones J Intern Med 2011**; 43(1): 53-58

14. **Intravenous Potassium Guideline** - edition 5. Prepared by Principal Pharmacist Clinical Governance. Approved by Medicines Management Committee – **Calderdale and Huddersfield, NHS FoundationTrust, UK** in **2011**.

15. British National Formulary; 64; September 2012

16. 'Potassium replacement' in Family Practice Note book. At: http://www.fpnotebook.com/Renal/Pharm/PtsmRplcmnt.htm

17. Mohammed Hijazi et al. Protocol-driven vs. physician-driven electrolyte replacement in adult critically ill patients. **Ann Saudi Med 2005**; 25(2):105-110

18. **Guidelines**-'Potassium Chloride: Safe use of Intravenous Potassium Chloride (Adult Patients)' by **Sydney South West Area Health Service, Australia.** Date Issued: November 2007.

19. **A clinical business rule (2011)** on 'Intravenous Potassium, Storage, Prescribing, Preparation and Administration' by **St George/Sutherland hospitals and health services, South Eastern Sydney, Australia.** At: https://stgrenal.org.au/sites/default/files/upload/Medication_Potassium_Intravenous_Wards_SGSHHS_CLIN116.pdf

20. **Policy for intravenous potassium chloride (2013). Department of Health, Government of Western Australia**. At: http://www.health.wa.gov.au/circularsnew/attachments/758.pdf

21. Guidelines on '**Adult Electrolyte Replacement Protocols'** (revised in **2008).** Prepared by the Department of Surgical Education, **Orlando Regional Medical Center** (Florida, USA) in conjunction with the Pharmacy Department. At: http://www.surgicalcriticalcare.net/Guidelines/electrolyte_replacement.pdf

22. Annette V.M. Alfonzo et al. Potassium disorders-clinical spectrum and emergency management. **Resuscitation 2006**; 70: 10-25

23. 'Potassium chloride – potassium chloride injection' on the website of **'Dailymed.' At:** https://dailymed.nlm.nih.gov/dailymed/archives/fdaDrugInfo.cfm?archiveid=28014

Chapter 14
Hyperkalemia

Hyperkalemia

There is no universally accepted definition of hyperkalemia;[1] some have defined hyperkalemia as a serum potassium >5.0 mmol/L[2,3] while others ≥5.5 mmol/L[1,4]. Here a serum K >5.0 mmol/L has been considered as hyperkalemia. Hyperkalemia develops in up to 10% of hospitalized patients; however, the serum potassium >6 mmol/L is found in about 1%.[4]

Classification of hyperkalemia

There is no universally accepted classification. It can be classified as follows-

1. Mild: Serum K 5.1 - 5.9 mmol/L[3]
2. Moderate: 6.0 - 6.4 mmol/L[1]
3. Severe: ≥ 6.5 mmol/L[1]

However, some physicians consider hyperkalemia as mild when serum K is 5.5-5.9 mmol/L[1], moderate 6-6.9 mmol/L[3,5] and severe ≥ 7.0 mmol/L[3,5].

Clinically more important thing than this biochemical classification is when to start emergency treatment for hyperkalemia which not only depends on biochemical severity of the hyperkalemia.

Pseudohyperkalemia/ spurious hyperkalemia/ factitious hyperkalemia

Pseudohyperkalemia is an artefactual increase in serum potassium concentration. It is a serious problem and particularly common in blood samples collected in primary care setting.

Causes of pseudohyperkalemia:

1. Hemolysis in the test tube can occur if the blood sample is left for a prolonged period before testing. To avoid this, the sample should be tested as early as possible, at least within five hours of collection.[6] Moreover, hemolysis can occur if the blood is squirted through the needle into the bottle (test tube) during collection or if the sample is shacked.[7] However, hyperkalemia due to intravascular hemolysis, such as in hemolytic transfusion reaction and drug induced hemolytic reaction, is true hyperkalemia.[8]
2. Prolonged tourniquet time may cause hemolysis and acidosis in the sample.
3. Repeated fist clenching during phlebotomy may cause K release from forearm muscles;[9] also hemolysis and acidosis may occur in the sample.[8]
4. Cooling of the sample causes decreased cellular uptake of K.[4]
5. Marked leukocytosis and thrombocytosis are associated with increased release of intracellular K (measure **plasma** K level instead of serum K in these situations).[2]
6. Sample from a limb receiving potassium containing IV fluid;
7. Use of wrong anticoagulant, particularly potassium EDTA (used for FBC sample), for **plasma** K measurement; (**lithium heparin** should be used as an anticoagulant for **plasma** K measurement).[6,7]
8. Uncommon genetic syndromes
   - Familial pseudohyperkalemia
   - Hereditary spherocytosis

When to suspect pseudohyperkalemia?

Pseudohyperkalemia should be suspected when serum potassium level is unexpectedly high (i. e. no known risk factors for that hyperkalemia), particularly when ECG is also not suggestive of hyperkalemia.

What should be done if pseudohyperkalemia is suspected?

1. Collect blood from a large vein with the precautionary measures that can be taken to avoid pseudohyperkalemia, and send to the lab for both **serum** and **plasma** urea; creatinine; and electrolyte (U&E) assay.[1]
2. If ECG changes of hyperkalemia are present, initiate emergency treatment of hyperkalemia after collecting the blood; do not defer emergency treatment until lab confirmation.[5,6]

It can be noted that ***lithium heparin is the recommended anticoagulant for plasma electrolyte measurement***; it is free of other ions, so does not affect plasma levels of electrolytes. However, normally serum potassium concentration is slightly higher (about 0.4 mmol/L) than plasma potassium level because of K release due to rupture of thrombocytes during clotting process.[8]

Causes of hyperkalemia[2,4,10,11]

(Hyperkalemia occurs most commonly due to impaired renal function or some drugs)
The causes can be grouped as follows:

1. Reduced renal potassium excretion

a) Impaired renal function: Acute kidney injury, chronic kidney disease;
b) Drugs: Potassium-sparing diuretics such as spironolactone and amiloride, ACE inhibitors, angiotensin II receptor blockers (ARB), NSAIDs, heparin (decreased aldosterone production), trimethoprim, cyclosporine, tacrolimus etc.
c) Primary adrenal insufficiency: e.g. Addison's disease
d) Hyporeninemic hypoaldosteronism (also known as RTA type 4)
e) Tubulointerstitial disease (may or may not have renal functional impairment): Interstitial nephritis, SLE, amyloidosis, obstructive uropathy, sickle cell anemia etc

2. Increased release of K from cells

a) Tissue/cell damage -- burns, trauma, hemolysis, rhabdomyolysis, severe infection, internal bleeding etc.
b) Acidosis
c) Hypertonicity (eg, uncontrolled diabetes, infusion of hypertonic dextrose or mannitol)
d) Insulin deficiency
e) Tumor lysis syndrome
f) Hyperkalemic periodic paralysis
g) Vigorous exercise
h) Drugs: Digitalis toxicity, β-blockers (noncardioselective), succinylcholine etc.

3. *Excessive intake of exogenous potassium*

a) Transfusion of stored blood
b) IV fluid therapy (high K containing)
c) Diet (rich in K)

*Trimethoprim's hyperkalemic effect is under-recognized.[1]

Notes

- <u>Increased intake of K and hyperkalemia:</u> In a normal person, all the consumed potassium is excreted, about 90% in the urine and 10% in the stool.[4] Kidneys have excellent abilities to increase potassium excretion depending on the dietary load. ***Excessive intake alone is a rare cause of hyperkalemia when renal function is normal*** and there is no other predisposing factor of hyperkalemia. However, excessive dietary intake can cause dangerous hyperkalemia in the presence of any other precipitating factor for hyperkalemia (eg, CKD, K-sparing diuretic use).[4]
- The drugs that cause hyperkalemia are most dangerous when used in combination or in an individual with impaired renal function.
- In CKD, K excretion in the stool is increased and many CKD patients are able to maintain a fairly normal serum potassium level.[7]

Clinical features

- Hyperkalemia interferes with neuromuscular transmission and cardiac function.
- Many patients have no symptoms and when symptoms are present, they are nonspecific.
- Muscular weakness and fatigue are the most common symptoms. [8]
- **Some patients' first manifestation of severe hyperkalemia is cardiac arrest;**[10,11] bradycardia due to heart block or other arrhythmias may develop.
- Some patients develop flaccid paralysis, ileus, paresthesia, or dyspnea due to respiratory muscle weakness; deep tendon reflexes may be diminished or absent.
- In patients with diabetes and hyperkalemia, hyporeninemic hypoaldosteronism should be suspected. They usually have low serum aldosterone; the potassium level will come back to normal within a day or two with a trial of oral fludrocortisone.[12]

*Muscle paralysis (eg, limb weakness), paresthesia and arrhythmia are alarming features and urgent intervention is needed when anyone of them is present.[1]

Investigations

Initial investigations should include the followings --

- Serum electrolytes, creatinine, urea (or blood urea nitrogen), Ca and Mg;
- FBC [looking for evidence of acute hemolysis (normocytic, normochromic anemia); thrombocytosis; and/or leukocytosis][7]
- Blood glucose (to rule out hyperglycemia)
- 12-lead ECG

Other investigations mainly depend on suspicion about the cause and severity of the condition.

*Addison's disease should be ruled out unless there is another obvious cause of the hyperkalemia.[11]

<u>ECG changes in hyperkalemia</u>

- ECG is an insensitive tool for detecting hyperkalemia; only about 50%- 60% of patients with serum potassium concentration > 6.5 mmol/L will show ECG changes [2,5] and **ECG may be normal even in the presence of life-threatening hyperkalemia;**[12]
- In hyperkalemia, the presence of ECG changes of hyperkalemia is generally suggestive of cardiac toxicity and considered as a medical emergency.[6,7]
- One reasonably large scale study shows the specificity of ECG in hyperkalemia is approximately 85%; hence, if treatment of hyperkalemia is given only based on ECG evidences, it may be mistreatment in about 15% cases.[13]
- ECG changes in hyperkalemia include:[2,4,7,14,15]
    - Tall peaked T
    - Prolonged PR interval
    - Reduced height of P and eventually disappearance of P
    - Widening of the QRS complex (>0.12 sec)
    - Bradycardia
    - ST elevation (Pseudoinfarct pattern)
    - Bundle branch block or atrioventricular block
    - Sine wave due to wide QRS complex
    - Ventricular tachycardia, ventricular fibrillation
    - Asystole

Correlation between serum K concentration and ECG changes

- In hyperkalemia, generally it is considered that the ECG changes will follow a progressive pattern with rising serum K level.[1]
- The typical ECG changes in hyperkalemia, depending on serum K concentration:[4.5]

Serum K concentration	Possible ECG changes
6-7 mmol/L	Tall peaked T wave
7-8 mmol/L	Decreased height of P/ disappearance of P; wide QRS complex;
8-9 mmol/L	Sine wave pattern of wide QRST
>9 mmol/L	Atrioventricular dissociation; ventricular tachycardia/ ventricular fibrillation

- In fact, the ECG changes do not always correlate with the biochemical severity of the hyperkalemia, especially in patients with chronic kidney disease and end stage renal disease.[4]
- At almost any level of hyperkalemia, potentially life-threatening arrhythmias can develop without warning features.[8] Cardiac conduction disturbances are more common with rapid rise in plasma potassium level.[7]
- In patients with preexisting heart disease and an abnormal baseline ECG, sometimes bradycardia is the only new ECG abnormality.[7]

*ECG changes due to hyperkalemia may improve within minutes of IV calcium administration.[6,12]

Treatment of hyperkalemia

- There is considerable variation in practice regarding the treatment of hyperkalemia.[1]
- Therapeutic decisions should be individualized. The first thing in the treatment of hyperkalemia is to determine whether the patient needs emergency treatment.[4] *(Indications for emergency treatment are given below)*
- All cases of hyperkalemia need to be confirmed by repeating laboratory tests even when ECG changes are present,[2] since pseudohyperkalemia may be more common than true hyperkalaemia.[5] Moreover, in about 15% cases, diagnosis of hyperkalemia based only on ECG may be incorrect;[13] hence presence of ECG evidences do not confirm true hyperkalemia. Therefore, blood should be sent to the lab for rechecking serum K before initiating therapy in all cases of hyperkalemia.[2,6] However, when pseudohyperkalemia is not suspected and emergency treatment is indicated according to the available most recent serum K and other features, it should be initiated immediately before the repeat test result being available.[6]
- If pseudohyperkalemia is suspected (because the hyperkalemia is unexpected) but ECG evidences of hyperkalemia are present, initiate emergency treatment of hyperkalemia just after sending blood for repeat lab test; do not defer emergency treatment for the repeat test results.[5,6]
- Take all possible measures to prevent further increase in serum potassium such as reduction of potassium intake, stopping all drugs which may raise serum K and initiation of cause-specific treatments when appropriate. *(A treatment algorithm has been given at the end of this chapter)*

Indications for emergency treatment of hyperkalemia

1. Presence of ECG evidences in any degree of hyperkalemia;
2. Serum potassium $\geq$ 6.5 mmol/L with or without ECG changes.[1,2,4,11] However, opinions vary in this regard; some physicians suggest initiation of emergency treatment when serum K is $\geq$ 6.0 mmol/L[5,12] and some when $\geq$ 7.0 mmol/L[7] if ECG changes are absent; most experts recommend to start treatment in this situation when serum K is $\geq$ 6.5 mmol/L.[1]
3. Presence of significant symptoms such as muscle paralysis or paresthesia[1,2,7]
4. Emergent treatment should also be considered when serum potassium concentration is rising rapidly.[5,6,8,12]

Emergency treatment of hyperkalemia

When emergency treatment is indicated:

a) Initiate the steps of emergency treatment given below;
b) Start continuous ECG monitoring, and
c) Contact a renal physician.

Contacting a renal physician is important because many patients may not adequately respond to the conservative emergency treatment or may develop rebound hyperkalemia following an initial response, where reduction of total body potassium by dialysis may be needed for a sustained improvement; this is especially true for patients with kidney diseases.

Step 1: Protect the heart by intravenous calcium when ECG changes are present

Give 10% Calcium gluconate 10 ml IV over 5 minutes[6,10] (some physicians prefer to infuse it over 10 minutes).

- Infusion of calcium can reduce the excitability of cardiac myocytes and thereby prevent arrhythmia.
- ECG changes improve within 1-3 minutes and persist 30-60 minutes.[1,4] If there is no improvement in ECG changes or the changes recur after initial improvement, the dose should be repeated.[4] Generally the dose of calcium gluconate (10%, 10 ml) can be repeated at 5-10 minutes interval until ECG changes normalize, maximum three doses in total (i.e. 30 ml of 10% Calcium gluconate or 6.8 mmol of elemental Ca);[1,6] 10 ml of 10% calcium gluconate contains 2.26 mmol elemental calcium.[1]
- Preferably a large vein should be used for calcium infusion.

What precaution should be taken if the patient is on digoxin therapy?

As hypercalcemia may potentiate the cardiac toxicity of digoxin, intravenous Ca should be administered at a slower rate in a patient on digoxin. You can mix 10 ml (10%) calcium gluconate with100 ml 5% dextrose in aqua and infuse over 20-30 minutes.[1,4,6] However, a recent study showed no additional risk of arrhythmias or death in patients treated with intravenous Ca in the presence of digoxin toxicity.[1]

Can I infuse calcium in hyperkalemia if there are no ECG changes?

It is a controversial issue. Some physicians suggest that IV calcium should be administered only in the presence of ECG changes of hyperkalemia regardless of serum K level.[1,5,11,12] They argue that ECG is the better predictor of cardiac toxicity than serum K concentration and calcium infusion is not free of hazards[1] (*adverse effects have been described later*).

But other physicians do not support the idea; they think ECG is an insensitive tool to evaluate the severity of hyperkalemia and ECG changes may be absent even in potentially life threatening hyperkalemia; additionally ECG interpretation may vary among interpreters;[1] therefore, they are in favor of calcium infusion in all patients requiring emergency treatment for their hyperkalemia irrespective of ECG changes.

Can I use IV calcium chloride instead of calcium gluconate?

Yes, calcium chloride can also be used instead of calcium gluconate in the emergency treatment of hyperkalemia.[1,4,7] The preference of calcium salt (Gluconate/ Chloride) largely depends on the availability, local practice and the clinical state of the patient. Both calcium gluconate and calcium chloride are available as10% solution.[1]

A comparison of different aspects of the two calcium salts:[1,7]

Points	*Calcium gluconate*	*Calcium chloride*
Elemental Ca content per 10 ml 10% solution	2.26 mmol	6.8 mmol (3 times higher than that of Ca gluconate)
Bioavailability of ionized calcium after administration	Limited, as relies on hepatic metabolism (conflicting evidence)	No limiting factors
Suitability in particular clinical states	Considered as less suitable in hemodynamic instability	More suitable than gluconate in hemodynamic instability including cardiac arrest

Tissue necrosis upon extravasation (the main adverse effects of IV Ca administration)	Considered as less toxic, so more suitable for peripheral venous route	The risk is higher than that of gluconate; ideally should be given via central access

Adverse effects of IV calcium administration include tissue necrosis on extravasation, peripheral vasodilation, hypotension, bradycardia, syncope, arrhythmias etc.[1,16]

*Calcium infusion has no effect on plasma potassium concentration, so other measures are needed to reduce the plasma potassium level.

Step 2: Rapid lowering of plasma potassium level by shifting K into cells

(a) Intravenous insulin and glucose:

- Usually 5-10 units of soluble/ regular insulin[2] are added to 50 ml of 50% glucose (25 g glucose) and infused over 15-30 minutes.[1,6]
- This preparation should always be given into a large vein as it is an irritant.[1,6]
- Serum potassium will be decreased by 0.65-1.0 mmol/L.[1,6]
- The effect starts within 15-30 minutes and reaches a peak within 30-60 minutes.[1,5]
- The effect may last up to 4-6 hours[1,2,4] following which a gradual efflux of potassium into the extracellular space begins, resulting in serum K levels as high as or occasionally even higher than that was at the outset.[6]
- This dose of insulin and glucose can be repeated if necessary.[1]
- Hypoglycemia is a common problem (incidence: 11-75%) with the insulin plus glucose infusion;[1,4] late hypoglycemia, up to 6 hours after the infusion, may develop in patients with renal failure.[1] Close monitoring of blood glucose is very important; measure blood glucose 15, 30, 60, 90, 120 minutes after initiation of insulin therapy and then hourly for at least 6 hours.[1] Some experts suggest a continuous glucose infusion (eg, 10% dextrose at 50-75 ml/ hour) following the insulin-glucose administration as a precautionary measure.[1,4]

Is it useful to infuse high-concentration glucose alone (without insulin)?
Infusion of high-concentration glucose alone (without insulin) in nondiabetic patient to stimulate endogenous insulin release is not recommended, because it does not release enough insulin required to reduce plasma potassium level; moreover, the osmotic effect of hypertonic glucose may aggravate hyperkalemia by shifting K out of cells.[1]

What should be done if the patient has preexisting hyperglycemia?
If the patient has preexisting hyperglycemia (blood glucose > 200—250 mg/dl) insulin alone should be administered (without glucose) with close monitoring of blood glucose.[1,4]

(b) Nebulized β_2-agonists [usually salbutamol (albuterol)]:

- β_2-agonists have an additive effect on serum K when used as an adjuvant therapy with insulin-glucose although they are not widely prescribed in hyperkalemia.[1,4]
- *The dose of nebulized salbutamol (albuterol):* 10-20 mg in 4 ml normal saline over 10 minutes;[2,4] this dose for hyperkalemia is much higher than that for obstructive pulmonary diseases (2.5 mg).[2]

- *Response to nebulized salbutamol (albuterol):* 10 mg nebulized salbutamol (albuterol) reduces serum potassium by 0.5-0.8 mmol/L.[1] The effect begins within 15-30 minutes,[2] reaches a peak within 60 minutes and persists for 4-6 hours.[1]
- All patients do not respond to β_2-agonists; up to 40% patients with end-stage renal disease are resistant to their action;[1] the response may be reduced in patients on digoxin or non-selective β-blockers.[1,6] For these uncertainties about the response to β_2-agonists, they should not be used as monotherapy (without insulin).[1,4]
- Side effects β_2- agonists inhalation include tremor, tachycardia, palpitation, headache, mild hyperglycemia (2-3 mmol/L increase in blood glucose) etc.
- Safety of β_2- agonists is unknown in patients with heart disease, so should be used with caution (either avoid or use at lower dose).[1,6]
- Intravenous β_2- agonists: Salbutamol (albuterol) or other β_2- agonists are equally effective when given intravenously, but the nebulized route is easier and associated with fewer adverse effects.[1] For these reasons, intravenous route is rarely used and probably not permitted in many countries.

(c) Sodium bicarbonate:

- Sodium bicarbonate should not be used routinely in the emergency treatment of hyperkalemia.[1,4] It has no proven role in lowering serum potassium level during emergency. Its use may cause hypernatremia, fluid overload (eg, pulmonary edema) and tetany in hypocalcemic patients of CKD.[5]
- It can be considered when hyperkalemia is associated with severe metabolic acidosis (when pH <7.2);[5,6] in such cases, it is actually considered for the treatment of severe metabolic acidosis, not for the hyperkalemia.[4]
- If sodium bicarbonate is used, it should not be administered as a hypertonic intravenous bolus (eg, 8.4%); instead, it should be infused as an isotonic or hypotonic fluid (isotonic: 1.26% or 1.4% sodium bicarbonate) to minimize the risk of hypernatremia.[4]
- Do not give sodium bicarbonate with IV calcium at the same time through the same IV line because of risk of precipitation.[6]

Target serum potassium (during emergency treatment) is < 6.0 mmol/L within 2 hours of initiation of treatment.[1]

Serum potassium monitoring:[1]

- Measure serum K at least 1, 2, 4 and 6 hours after initiation of treatment to evaluate the response and to detect whether there is any rebound hyperkalemia, as the effects the treatment described above lasts 4-6 hours.
- Then serum K should be rechecked at 24 hours to confirm that control has been maintained.

None of the above measures described in step1 and 2(a, b, c) can reduce total body potassium. Therefore, the measures for reduction of total body potassium are considered to maintain an acceptable plasma potassium level after emergency lowering of plasma potassium.

Lowering of total body potassium

This can be done by cation-exchange resins, diuretics or dialysis.

a) Cation-exchange resins [Sodium polystyrene sulfonate (SPS); Calcium polystyrene sulfonate (Calcium resonium/ CPS)]

- Cation-exchange resins can exchange their cations, sodium (of SPS) or calcium (of calcium resonium), for other cations including K in the gut; they are ultimately excreted with stool, thus increasing fecal excretion of K.
- The resins can be administered either orally or rectally as retention enema.[12]
- One gram SPS exchanges 1 mmol Na for 1 mmol K;[5] the efficacy of calcium resonium may be almost similar.[17] However, it is unclear whether the resins themselves or the diarrhea caused by concomitant laxative-use is actually responsible for the potassium lowering effect.[1]
- Resins' onset of action is slow; the oral form may take 4-6 hours, as the drug needs about 4 hours to reach the colon, the major site their of action;[12] however, the action of rectal form is faster and may take 1-2 hours.[5] Usually multiple doses over 1-5 days are needed to obtain their full effect.[1] Therefore, the resins are generally not useful in the emergency management of hyperkalemia.
- **Indications:**
  The resins can be considered in the following conditions:
  - In mild to moderate hyperkalemia where there are no indications for emergency correction and controlling gradually over days may be acceptable;
  - During emergency management of hyperkalemia if dialysis is delayed for more than 2-3 hours.[5]
- **Dose** (The dose is same for both SPS and Calcium resonium):[1,6,10,16]
  - Oral: 15g up to 3 to 4 times daily;
    Add resin to water (3-4 ml/ g of resin); also, the resin can be added to syrup or milk to improve palatability.
    Laxative (eg, lactulose 10 ml BID or TID) should be co-prescribed to avoid constipation.
  - Retention enema: 30g resin in 150 ml of water;
    The enema should be retained for at least 9 hours then colon should be irrigated to remove the resin.
    Rectal route is usually poorly tolerated by the patients, so consider only when oral route is not feasible.[6]
- **Side effects of the resins**
  1. Intestinal necrosis is the most serious side effect of the resins, which can occur with either route of administration, oral or rectal.[1] The resins should not be used in patients with increased risk of intestinal necrosis such post operative patients; patients with ischemic bowel disease; and patients with a history of intestinal obstruction.[4]
  2. Constipation is a common adverse effect. Use of sorbitol with the resins to decrease constipation is no longer recommended, as sorbitol is likely to increase the risk of intestinal necrosis.[1,4] Resins are contraindicated in obstructive bowel disease.[1]
  3. Calcium resonium can cause hypercalcemia and SPS may cause hypernatremia, fluid retention and hypocalcemia. Prolonged use of the either resin can cause hypomagnesaemia.

4. Resins can also cause anorexia, nausea, vomiting etc.

***Resins should be used only when clearly indicated.**

***For CKD patients, calcium resonium may be the better resin than SPS**; CKD patients are at risk of developing hypocalcemia, which is countered at least partially by the hypercalcemic effect of calcium resonium. Additionally, calcium resonium does not worsen edema and hypertension in these patients, since it does not cause Na and water retention like SPS.[17]

b) Diuretics

Furosemide 40-160 mg IV can be given if the patient has good renal function;[2] for volume depleted patient furosemide plus normal saline can be considered.[11] However, the use of diuretics in hyperkalemia is controversial[7] and patients with impaired renal function are relatively resistant to its effect. Diuretic use may be more justified when the patient has other comorbidity where diuretic is indicated such as congestive cardiac failure.[7]

c) Dialysis

Dialysis is the definitive treatment of hyperkalemia in renal failure. Dialysis is also a last resort in the treatment of hyperkalemia due to other causes when more conservative measures have failed. Hemodialysis is better than peritoneal dialysis in this regard.[4] In fact in hyperkalemia, all the medical measures described so far are used for buying time either to correct the underlying cause or to arrange dialysis for removal of potassium from the body.[8,10]

****Potassium-lowering therapies can be stopped when serum potassium level comes back to normal (i.e. <5 or 5.5 mmol/L).[6,8,16]***

Please see the next page for hyperkalemia treatment algorithm.

Treatment of hyperkalemia (Algorithm)

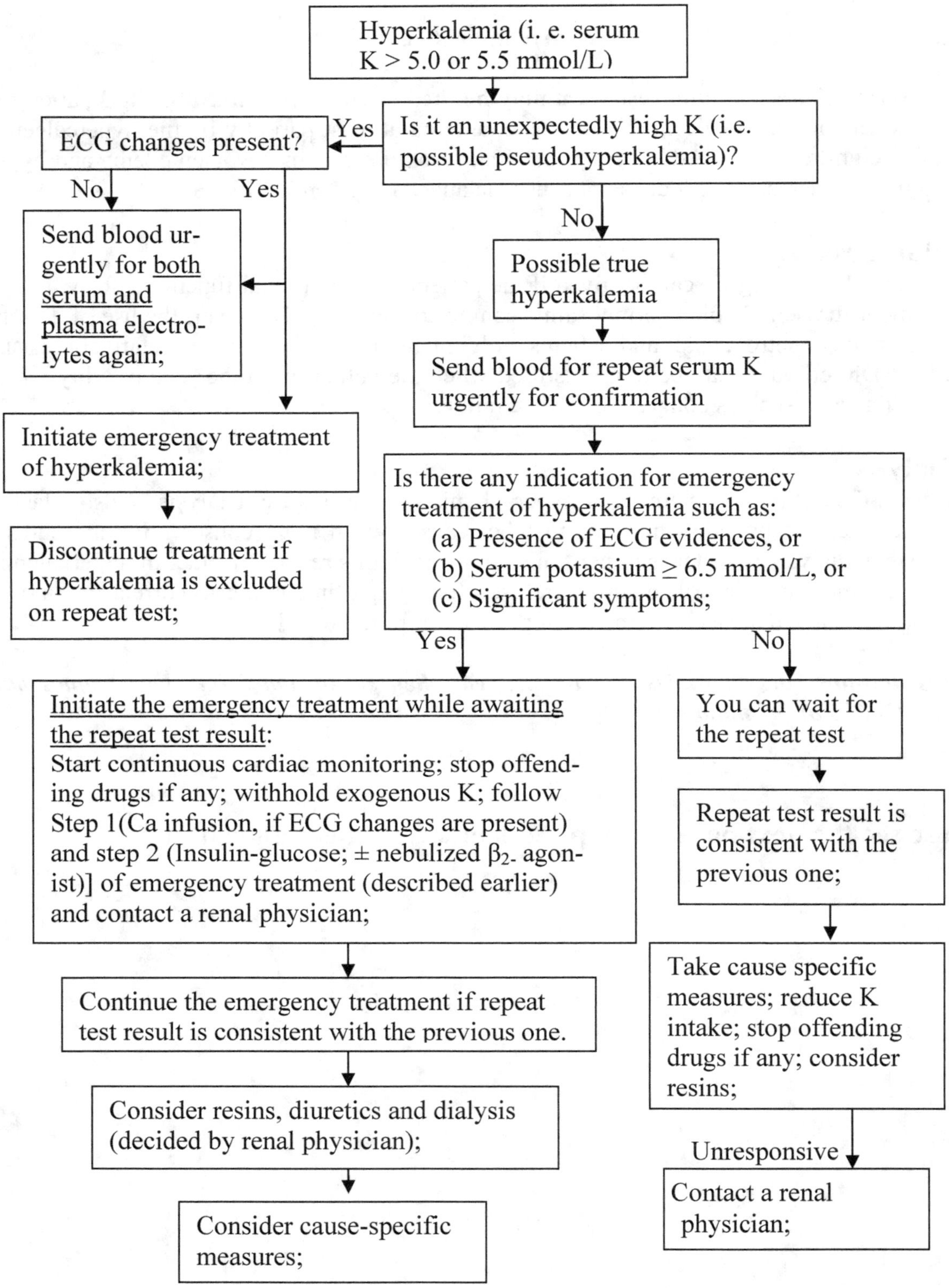

Hyperkalemia (i. e. serum K > 5.0 or 5.5 mmol/L)

↓

Is it an unexpectedly high K (i.e. possible pseudohyperkalemia)?

- Yes → ECG changes present?
  - No → Send blood urgently for <u>both serum and plasma</u> electrolytes again;
  - Yes → Send blood urgently for <u>both serum and plasma</u> electrolytes again; and → Initiate emergency treatment of hyperkalemia; → Discontinue treatment if hyperkalemia is excluded on repeat test;
- No → Possible true hyperkalemia → Send blood for repeat serum K urgently for confirmation → Is there any indication for emergency treatment of hyperkalemia such as:
  (a) Presence of ECG evidences, or
  (b) Serum potassium $\geq$ 6.5 mmol/L, or
  (c) Significant symptoms;
  - Yes → <u>Initiate the emergency treatment while awaiting the repeat test result</u>: Start continuous cardiac monitoring; stop offending drugs if any; withhold exogenous K; follow Step 1(Ca infusion, if ECG changes are present) and step 2 (Insulin-glucose; ± nebulized β_2- agonist)] of emergency treatment (described earlier) and contact a renal physician;
    → Continue the emergency treatment if repeat test result is consistent with the previous one.
    → Consider resins, diuretics and dialysis (decided by renal physician);
    → Consider cause-specific measures;
  - No → You can wait for the repeat test
    → Repeat test result is consistent with the previous one;
    → Take cause specific measures; reduce K intake; stop offending drugs if any; consider resins;
    → Unresponsive → Contact a renal physician;

* Drug induced mild or moderate hyperkalemia may resolve after stopping or reducing the dose of the offending drugs.

References

1. Clinical Practice Guidelines: Treatment of acute hyperkalaemia in adults. **UK renal association 2014;** at:http://www.renal.org/docs/default-source/guidelines-resources/joint-guidelines/treatment-of-acute-hyperkalaemia-in-adults/hyperkalaemia-guideline---march-2014.pdf?

2. Kerry C. Cho. 'Disorders of potassium concentration' in **Current Medical Diagnosis and Treatment;** Maxine A. Papadakis et al (Editors). New York, McGraw-Hill, 2013, pp 877-881.

3. Julie R. Ingelfinger. A new era for the treatment of hyperkalemia? **N Engl J Med 2015**; 372 (3): pp 275 -77; http://www.nejm.org/doi/pdf/10.1056/NEJMe1414112

4. David B. Mount. 'Fluid and electrolyte disturbances' in **Harrison's Principles of Internal Medicine,** 18 th edition; Dan L Longo et al (Editors). New York, McGraw-Hill, 2012, pp 341-359.

5. Peter Ahee et al. The management of hyperkalaemia in the emergency department. **J Accid Emerg Med 2000**; 17(3):188-191

6. Guideline for the management of acute hyperkalaemia in adults; Revised 2013; on the website of **Nottingham University Hospital (NHS trust, UK)**. The guideline is registered with the trust. At: https://www.nuh.nhs.uk/handlers/downloads.ashx?id=41671

7. 'Hyperkalaemia' on the website of **'Patient', UK;** at: www.patient.co.uk/doctor/hyperkalaemia

8. David Garth. Hyperkalemia in Emergency Medicine. **Emedicine;** at http://emedicine.medscape.com/article/766479-overview

9. Jaya R Asirvatham et al. Errors in potassium measurement: A laboratory perspective for the clinician. **N Am J Med Sci. 2013;** 5(4): 255–259.

10. MM Yaqoob. 'Disorders of potassium concentration' in **Kumar &Clark's Clinical Medicine**, 8th edition; Parveen Kumar and Michael Clark (Editors). Edinburgh, Elsevier, 2012, pp 651-656

11. M. J. Field et al. 'Disorders of potassium balance' in **Davidson's Principles and Practice of Medicine,** 21st edition; Nicki R. Colledge et al (editors). India, Elsevier, 2010, pp 438-441

12. Joyce C. Hollander-Rodriguez et al. Hyperkalemia. **Am Fam Physician 2006**; 73: (2) 283-90. At: http://www.aafp.org/afp/2006/0115/p283.pdf

13. Wrenn KD et al. The ability of physicians to predict hyperkalemia from the ECG. **Ann Emerg Med. 1991** Nov; 20(11):1229-32.

14. Brian T. Montague et al. Retrospective review of the frequency of ECG changes in hyperkalemia. **Clin J Am Soc Nephrol. 2008** Mar; 3(2): 324–330.

15. Daniel B. Petrov. An electrocardiographic sine wave in hyperkalemia. **N Engl J Med 2012**; 366 (19): 1824

16. Calcium salts. **British National Formulary 64, September 2012**

17. Kiran Nasir et al. Treatment of hyperkalemia in patients with chronic kidney disease: A comparison of calcium polystyrene sulphonate and sodium polystyrene sulphonate. **J Ayub Med Coll Abbottabad 2014**; 26(4):455-58

Chapter 15

Acid-base disorders

Acid-base disorders

The optimal pH of arterial blood is 7.4. The range of pH which is compatible with human life is 6.80 to 7.80.[1] However, normally the pH is strictly maintained between 7.35 and 7.45. This is accomplished by different chemical buffers along with respiratory and renal controlling systems.[2,3]

Arterial Blood Gas (ABG) analysis: reference range[3,4,5]

	pH	*PCO2 (mm Hg)*	*HCO3- (mmol/L)*
Reference range	7.35 - 7.45	35-45	22-28
Optimal level	7.4	40	24

Terms related to acid-base disorders:

Acidemia – arterial blood pH below the normal range (< 7.35)
Alkalemia – arterial blood pH above the normal range (>7.45)

Acidosis and alkalosis:
Acidosis is the process in which the hydrogen-ion concentration rises and alkalosis is the process in which the hydrogen-ion concentration is decreases.[1] So the terms acidosis and alkalosis indicate in which direction the pH is changing, towards acidemia or alkalemia. Although usually acidosis leads to acidemia and alkalosis leads to alkalemia, *in mixed acid-base disorders coexistence of multiple acid base disturbances may give rise to normal pH.*

An acid-base disorder is not a diagnosis, instead only a manifestation of the underlying disease process.

Primary acid-base disorder and secondary response: Primary acid-base disorder is the initial acid-base abnormality and the change that occurs as a compensatory response to the initial acid-base abnormality is the secondary response.

Types of acid-base disturbances[1,2,5]

A. Types of primary acid–base disorders: There are four recognized primary acid–base disorders- two metabolic and two respiratory disorders:

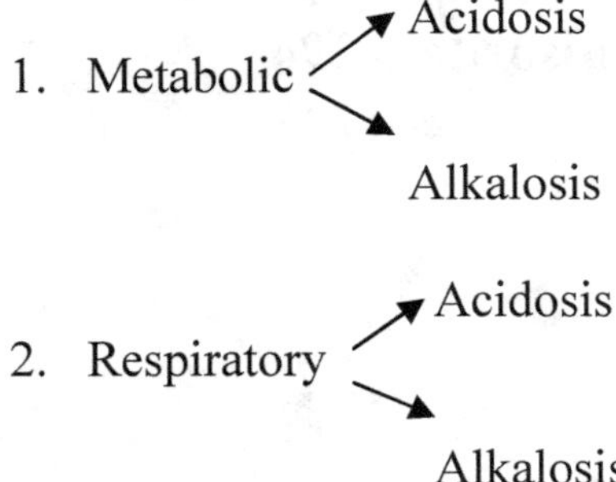

B. Simple or mixed acid-base disorder:

1. Simple acid-base disorder : presence of only one of the above mentioned four primary acid-base disorders;

2. Mixed acid-base disorders: simultaneous presence of more than one primary (not compensatory) acid-base disorders; however, two primary respiratory acid-base disorders (i.e. respiratory acidosis and respiratory alkalosis) cannot coexist; therefore, **maximum three primary acid-base disorders can coexist.**

Basic concepts of simple acid-base disorders and compensatory changes

To understand acid base disorders, it is important to understand the relationship between PCO2 and HCO3- in the Henderson Hasselbalch equation or Kassirer-Bleich equation. Of the two equations, Kassirer-Bleich equation given below is probably a bit easier to understand. However, an in-depth knowledge of acid-base physiology is generally not essential for solving clinical acid-base problems.[6]

Kassirer-Bleich equation: **[H+] = 24 × (PCO2 / [HCO3-])**

It is evident from this equation that the ratio of dissolved CO2 to HCO3- (not their actual concentrations in plasma) determines the hydrogen ion concentration (i.e. pH) of blood.[4]
A fall in [HCO3-] or a rise in PCO2→ increased PCO2 / [HCO3-] ratio → increased H+ concentration (i.e., fall in pH) or acidosis. Conversely, a rise in [HCO3-] or a fall in PCO2 leads to a drop in H+ concentration (i.e. rise in pH) or alkalosis.

In metabolic acid-base disorders primary change (i.e. the original defect) occurs in [HCO_3-] (low or high)
In respiratory acid-base disorders primary change occurs in PCO2 (low or high)

The direction of plasma HCO3- and PCO2 changes in simple acid-base disorders and their compensatory responses:

Acid-base disorder	Primary Change	Compensatory change
Metabolic Acidosis	↓ HCO3-	↓ PCO2
Metabolic Alkalosis	↑ HCO3-	↑ PCO2
Respiratory Acidosis	↑ PCO2	↑HCO3-
Respiratory Alkalosis	↓ PCO2	↓ HCO3-

How do the compensatory responses work?
The compensatory responses work as an effort to maintain the PCO2/ [HCO3-] ratio of the Kassirer-Bleich equation. When one variable (PCO2 or HCO3-) is changed by a disease process, body tries to readjust the other in an attempt to maintain the PCO2/ HCO3- ratio. For example,

when plasma HCO3- is reduced in metabolic acidosis, respiratory compensation occurs by reducing PCO2 through hyperventilation so that the PCO2/ HCO3- ratio can be maintained.

In simple acid-base disorders, although compensatory mechanisms can minimize the change in pH, they cannot restore a normal pH.[5] However, sometimes, in mixed acid-base disorders, the opposing actions of different acid-base disorders on pH may give rise to a completely normal pH.

Simple acid-base disorders: main characteristics and compensation calculation[1-5]

In metabolic acid base disorders respiratory compensation is started almost immediately. On the other hand, in respiratory acid base disorders, acute compensation by intracellular buffers is started within minutes but chronic compensation through kidneys usually begins after 6- 12 hours and takes 2-5 days to finish.[1,3,4,5]

Metabolic acidosis:[1,2,4]

Main characteristics: pH of arterial blood < 7.35 and plasma $HCO3^-$ < 22 mmol/L
Primary defect: low HCO3-
Compensatory response: respiratory (hyperventilation) → ↓PCO2
Predicted full compensation: for each 1 mmol/L HCO3- decrease, PCO2 will decrease 1.2 mmHg from 40 mmHg.

Other formulas for compensation calculation:

1. **Winter's Formula:** PCO2 = (1.5 × [HCO3-]) + 8 ± 2 mmHg
2. PCO2 = ([HCO3−] + 15) mm Hg (not a commonly practiced formula)
3. PCO2 = last 2 digits of pH (not commonly practiced)

Respiratory compensation is started immediately and completed in 12-24 hours.[1]
If patient's PCO2 is higher or lower than the predicted value, superimposed respiratory acidosis or alkalosis may be present respectively.[1]

Example: A patient with metabolic acidosis has pH 7.29, plasma $HCO3^-$ 12 mmol/L and PCO_2 26 mmHg. Is this patient's respiratory compensation is adequate?
Calculation:
Here HCO3- reduction = 24 (optimal plasma HCO^{3-}) – 12 (patient's $HCO3^-$) = 12 mmol/L
Therefore, expected PCO2 reduction = 12 × 1.2 = 14.4
So the expected PCO2 = 40 (optimal PCO2) – 14 = 26 mmHg
Patient's PCO2 is also 26 mmHg, so the respiratory compensation is adequate.
Alternative calculation
Winter's formula: Expected PCO2 = (1.5 × 12) + 8 ± 2
= 26 ± 2 (i.e. 24-28 mmHg)
So the respiratory compensation is adequate.

Metabolic alkalosis:

Main characteristics: pH >7.45 and [HCO3−] >28 mmol/L
Primary defect: High HCO3-
Compensatory response: Respiratory (hypoventilation) → ↑PCO2

Predicted full compensation: for each 1 mmol/L HCO3- increase, PCO2 will increase 0.7 mmHg from 40mmHg. This is the most commonly practiced calculation.
Another formula:
PCO2 = ([HCO3−] + 15) mm Hg

Respiratory compensation is completed within 24–36 hours.[1]

If patient's PCO2 is higher or lower than the predicted value, superimposed primary respiratory acidosis or respiratory alkalosis may be present respectively.[1]
(Compensatory PCO2 increase usually does not exceed 55 mmHg)[5]

Example: Plasma HCO3- of a patient with metabolic alkalosis is 36 mmol/L. What would be the expected PCO2?
Calculation:
HCO3- increase = 36 - 24 = 12 mmol/L
So PCO2 increase = 0.7 × 12 = 8.4 mmHg
Therefore the expected PCO2 = 40 + 8 = 48 mmHg

Respiratory acidosis:

Main characteristics: pH <7.35 and PCO2 >45 mmHg
Primary defect: Reduced alveolar ventilation → High PCO2
Compensatory response: ↑HCO3-

Predicted compensation:
Acute (by intracellular buffers such hemoglobin and intracellular proteins): ↑ HCO3- ;
HCO3- will increase 1 mmol/L for each 10 mmHg increase in PCO2 above 40 mmHg
Chronic: Renal compensation → ↑HCO3-;
HCO3- will increase 4 mmol/L for each 10 mmHg increase in PCO2 above 40 mmHg.[2]

Intracellular buffering starts within minutes of the onset of respiratory acidosis.[4]
Renal compensation is usually started 6- 12 hours after the acute increase in PCO2.[5]
The kidneys generate more HCO3- and excrete acid as NH_4Cl.
Complete compensation usually takes 2-5 days.[1]

If patient's HCO3− is higher or lower than the predicted value, superimposed metabolic alkalosis or metabolic acidosis may be present respectively.
(Serum HCO3- usually does not exceed 38 mmol/L due to compensatory responses)[2]

*Renal excretion of NH4Cl causes hypochloremia.
*If the chronic respiratory acidosis is corrected suddenly, metabolic alkalosis may develop which may persist until the kidneys excrete excess HCO3- over 2-3days.[5]

Example: PCO2 of a patient with respiratory acidosis is 70 mmHg. What would be the expected HCO3-?
Calculation:
Here PCO2 increase = 70 – 40 = 30 mmHg
If the change is acute: HCO3- rise will be $1 \times 30/10 = 3$ mmol/L
Therefore, the expected HCO3- = 24 + 3 = 27 mmol/L
But if the change is chronic: HCO3- rise will be $4 \times 30/10 = 12$ mmol/L
Therefore, the expected HCO3- = 24 + 12 = 36 mmol/L

Respiratory alkalosis:

Main characteristics: pH >7.45 and PCO2 <35 mm Hg
Primary defect: Hyperventilation → Decreased PCO2
Compensatory response: ↓HCO3-

Predicted compensation:
Acute (by intracellular buffers): ↓HCO3-
HCO3- will decrease 2 mmol/L for each 10 mmHg decrease in PCO2 below 40 mmHg[1,2,5]
Chronic: Renal compensation → ↓HCO3-
HCO3- will decrease 4-5 mmol/L for each 10 mmHg decrease in PCO2 below 40 mmHg.[1]

This renal compensation is done by reduced HCO3- reabsorption and reduced excretion of ammonium chloride (i.e. acid)[4]
Like respiratory acidosis, complete compensation usually takes 2-5 days.

If the patient's HCO3− is higher or lower than predicted value, superimposed metabolic alkalosis or metabolic acidosis may be present respectively.
(Serum HCO3- usually does not fall below 15 mmol/L due to compensatory changes and a level < 15 mmol/L indicate the possibility of the presence of a concomitant metabolic acidosis)[5]

*Metabolic acidosis may develop if chronic respiratory alkalosis is corrected rapidly as these patients have low plasma HCO3- due to renal compensation.[4]

Example:
PCO2 of a patient with respiratory alkalosis is 30 mmHg. What would be the expected HCO3-?
Calculation:
Fall in PCO2 = 40 – 30 = 10 mmHg
If the condition is acute, HCO3- fall will be 2 mmol/L.
Therefore, the expected HCO3- will be 24 – 2 = 22 mmol/L.
But if the condition is chronic HCO3- fall will be about 4 mmol/ L.
Therefore, the expected HCO3- will be 24 – 4 = about 20 mmol/L.

During compensation calculation, for a metabolic disorder, if the predicted PCO2 does not match with the patient's PCO2, a separate respiratory disorder may be present; similarly, for a respiratory disorder if the predicted HCO3- does not match with the patient's HCO3-level a separate metabolic disorder may be present.

Brief description of simple acid-base disorders

Metabolic acidosis:

Metabolic acidosis is characterized by decreased plasma HCO3- (< 22 mmol/L) and low pH (arterial blood pH < 7.35).

Some basic information on metabolic acidosis:

- **Metabolic acidosis can occur due to** accumulation of any acid other than carbonic acid in the body[3], which may result from: increased acid production or acid ingestion, loss of HCO3- from the gastrointestinal tract or kidneys, or decreased renal acid excretion.[2]
- **The impact of loss of HCO_3^- from the body** is equal to the addition of equimolar amount of H^+ (i.e., acid);[7(metabolic acidosis)] therefore, like addition of acid, loss of HCO3- also causes drop in pH or acidosis.
- **Effect of drop in pH** → stimulation of the respiratory centers → hyperventilation → ↑removal of CO2 (i.e. acid) from the body → pH goes up towards normal.
- **HCO3- is the principal buffer for noncarbonic acids** in the body; so its concentration falls in the presence of excess of these acids;[4] kidneys regenerate HCO3- to replace HCO3- used in H^+ neutralization by bicarbonate buffer system.

<u>**Anion gap (AG)**</u>

Plasma is electrically neutral (i.e. the sum of all positive ion charges = the sum of all negative ion charges). For clinical purposes, all the ions in plasma are generally not measured; there is a difference between the total concentration of commonly measured major cations and anions which is called anion gap.[1]

Calculation of anion gap:[2,5]

Anion gap= $Na^+ - (Cl^- + HCO3^-)$

<u>Normal Anion Gap:</u> 12 ± 4 mmol/L; with current auto-analyzer, it may be 6 ± 1, mainly due to high Cl- values.[5]

Some labs include serum potassium concentration to calculate anion gap. Probably the calculation including potassium is common in the UK while excluding potassium is common in the USA.

AG calculation including potassium[3,8]

Anion gap = $(Na^+ + K^+) - (Cl^- + HCO3^-)$

<u>Normal Anion Gap for these cases:</u> 14 ± 4 mmol/L

<u>Normal major unmeasured cations:</u> Ca, Mg and gamma globulins[4]

Normal major unmeasured anions: Albumin, phosphate, sulfate, lactate and anions of other organic acids.[5,8]

Albumin and anion gap:
Normally, albumin may account for the largest portion, up to 75%, of the anion gap.[1] The negative charge of 1g/L albumin is about 0.25 mmol/L, so a fall in the plasma albumin level from the normal 40 g/L to 30 g/L (i.e. 1 g/dl) will decrease anion gap by approximately 2.5 mmol/L.[1,8]

Correction of the anion gap in hypoalbuminemia: for every 1 g/dl decline in serum albumin (from normal 4gm/ dl), increase calculated anion gap by 2.5 mmol/liter.[1]

Why is anion gap important?

1. Anion gap is helpful to categorize the causes of metabolic acidosis.
2. An anion gap > 20 mmol/L is suggestive of metabolic acidosis irrespective of the pH and serum HCO3- level.[5,9]
3. Sometimes, increased anion gap (by >5mmol/L) may be the only biochemical clue to an underlying a mixed acid-base disorder when other important parameters such as pH, HCO3- and PCO2 are within reference range.[1]
4. In an alcoholic patient, a high anion gap with a normal lactate may be an important clue to the alcoholic ketoacidosis diagnosis, as nitroprusside test for ketone may be false negative in these patients.[1] *(For explanation see below)*

***The diagnosis of alcoholic ketoacidosis** may be missed in some cases, because the nitroprusside test which is widely used for the detection of ketonuria may be negative. In alcoholic ketoacidosis, β-hydroxybutyrate is the primary ketone body, but nitroprusside reacts only with acetoacetate, not with β-hydroxybutyrate; as a result, the test may be false negative. The pH of blood of these patients may also be deceptively normal or high because of concomitant metabolic alkalosis due to vomiting; or respiratory alkalosis due to liver disease, sepsis or high fever. In such cases, if serum lactate is also normal, high anion gap (which is otherwise unexplained) may be an important clue to the diagnosis of alcoholic ketoacidosis.[1]

What are the limitations of anion gap?

1. Errors in interpretation: As noted above, anion gap will be decreased in the presence of hypoalbuminemia, so it needs to be adjusted. Misinterpretation may also occur with hypo or hypernatremia and some antibiotics use (eg, Carbenicillin is an anion; polymyxin is a cation).[5]
2. Anion gap may be low or negative in hyperchloremia resulting from the presence of high levels of unmeasured cations which are seen in disorders with high Ca or Mg levels; monoclonal IgG gammopathy; lithium toxicity etc.[1] A negative anion gap can also occur due to pseudohyperchloremia in bromide or iodide intoxication.[1]

   Although bromide and iodide are negatively charged and their accumulation theoretically should increase the serum anion gap, they actually cause a low or even negative anion gap. This effect occurs because bromide and iodide interfere with chloride measurement, resulting in a spurious elevation in Cl- level.[10]

3. The reference range for anion gap is quite broad (anion gap vary by as much as 6 to 10 mmol/L in an individual laboratory) and the baseline value for an individual patient is generally unknown; as a result, actual deviation from the individual's usual may be difficult to ascertain.[10]
4. In about 50% cases, a high anion gap is due to lactic acidosis which usually results from shock or tissue hypoxia. But nearly half of the patients with serum lactate levels 3.0 - 5.0 mmol/L (normal 0.6 - 2.4 mmol/L)[3] have an anion gap within the reference range. Therefore, normal anion gap does not exclude the presence of lactic acidosis.[1]

Causes of metabolic acidosis

A. Metabolic acidosis with normal anion gap[5,8]
[This is most commonly results from diarrhea or renal tubular acidosis (type 1, 2 and 4)].

- ↑Gastrointestinal bicarbonate loss
    - Diarrhea
    - Small bowel fistula/ ileostomy
    - Ureterosigmoidostomy
- ↑Renal bicarbonate loss
    - Proximal renal tubular acidosis (type 2)
    - Tubular damage by heavy metals, paraproteins or drugs
    - Acetazolamide therapy
- ↓Renal hydrogen ion excretion
    - Distal type1 and type 4 renal tubular acidosis
- Addition of inorganic acid
    - Therapeutic infusion of or poisoning with ammonium chloride or HCl;

*In normal anion gap metabolic acidosis, when HCO_3^- is lost in urine or stool, equivalent amount of chloride is retained to maintain electrical neutrality of plasma, as a result anion gap remains normal and hyperchloremia may develop.[8]

B. Metabolic acidosis with increased anion gap
(It most commonly results from renal failure, lactic acidosis, ketoacidosis or exogenous toxin intake)

- Renal failure (acute and chronic), (mainly sulfate and phosphate accumulation due to their ↓renal excretion)[8]
- Lactic acidosis (accumulation of L-lactate or D-lactate)
- Ketoacidosis
    - Diabetic (acetoacetate acid and β-hydroxybutyrate accumulation)
    - Alcoholic (mainly β-hydroxybutyrate accumulation)
    - Starvation induced (acetoacetate and β-hydroxybutyrate accumulation)
- Drugs and toxins
    - Salicylate (accumulation of salicylate and lactate)[5]
    - Ethylene glycol (oxalate and glycolate accumulation)

- Methanol (formate accumulation)
- Propylene glycol (D-lactate, L-lactate)

Urine anion gap (UAG)

Urine anion gap can be used to differentiate between renal and extra-renal causes of normal anion gap metabolic acidosis when clinical differentiation is not possible.[9,11]

UAG = Urine Na + Urine K - Urine Cl

Interpretation of UAG values:[9,11]

1. Normal UAG = -10 to +10 mmol/L;
   It represents the concentration of unmeasured anions in urine which include sulfates, phosphates, bicarbonates and organic anions such as lactate and citrate.[9]
2. UAG in extrarenal causes of normal anion gap metabolic acidosis = <-10
3. UAG in renal causes of normal anion gap metabolic acidosis = >+10

Urine anion gap is an indirect measurement of urinary ammonium (i.e. acid) excretion.[9] Extra-renal causes of normal anion gap metabolic acidosis (in an individual with normal renal function), markedly increase NH4+ excretion by the kidneys, usually in the form of NH4Cl;[4,9] consequently, urine Cl- level increases and urine anion gap becomes negative.[4] On the other hand, in renal causes of normal anion gap metabolic acidosis (eg, RTA), the kidneys cannot generate ammonium; as a result, urinary Cl- concentration cannot increase and urine anion gap becomes largely positive (> +10).[4,9]

However, in most cases, the cause of normal anion gap metabolic acidosis (such as diarrhea) is clinically obvious and estimation of the urine anion gap does not require.[4]

Clinical features of metabolic acidosis:[2,5,8]

The symptoms and signs of metabolic acidosis are nonspecific, and clinical features of the underlying disorder predominate. The clinical manifestations of metabolic acidosis can be grouped as follows:

- Respiratory features: Compensatory hyperventilation is a striking feature and in severe cases Kussmaul respiration (regular, deep, sighing respiration) may develop.
- Cardiovascular features:
  - Peripheral arteriolar vasodilation and myocardial depression → hypotension;
  - Central venoconstriction → reduced central and pulmonary vascular compliance → pulmonary edema with minimal fluid overload.[2]
- CNS features: headache, lethargy, stupor, confusion, convulsion, coma etc.
- Other features: Anorexia, nausea, vomiting, glucose intolerance etc.

Metabolic alkalosis

Metabolic alkalosis is a common acid-base disorder.[8] It is characterized by increased plasma HCO3- (>28 mmol/L) and increased plasma pH (>7.45).[3] Compensatory hypoventilation causes increased PCO2. Associated hypokalemia and hypochloremia is common.[5]

Causes of metabolic alkalosis

(Metabolic alkalosis most commonly results from loss of gastric secretion or use of diuretics.) The causes of metabolic alkalosis can be grouped as follows:

A. <u>Hypovolemic and saline-responsive metabolic alkalosis</u> <u>(Urine Cl <25 mmol/L)</u>[1,3,5]
It is also called chloride-depletion alkalosis and is usually characterized by chloride loss as well as concurrent loss of sodium, potassium, and fluid.[12] Although these patients are usually normotensive despite some fluid loss, hypotension or orthostatic hypotension may be found.[3] *Chloride loss, even without volume deficit, accelerates bicarbonate reabsorption.*[7] Administration of fluids containing sodium chloride (usually along with potassium chloride) can correct hypovolemia, hypokalemia, metabolic alkalosis as well as chloride deficiency in these patients.[1,2,4]

<u>Causes of hypovolemic and saline-responsive metabolic alkalosis</u>
Gastrointestinal origin (loss of gastric HCl)

- Vomiting
- Nasogastric suction
- Gastrocolic fistula

Renal origin

- Use of loop or thiazide diuretic
- Posthypercapnia (Rapid correction of chronic respiratory acidosis)

*In diuretic induced metabolic alkalosis, urine chloride concentration is high during active diuretic use; gradually the concentration decreases to a level <25 mmol per liter after withdrawal of the diuretic.[1] However, diuretic induced metabolic alkalosis may not resolve with withdrawal of the diuretic alone until the maintenance factor of the alkalosis such as chloride deficiency is corrected.[8]

B. <u>Euvolemic (or hypervolemic) and saline-resistant metabolic alkalosis</u> (Urine Cl > 40 mmol/L)[1,2,3,5]
<u>Hypertensive</u> (mineralocorticoid activity↑)

- Primary hyperaldosteronism (eg, adrenal adenoma, hyperplasia and carcinoma)
- Cushing syndrome
- Corticosteroid therapy
- Liddle's syndrome

<u>Normotensive</u>

- Severe hypokalemia (Serum potassium < 2mmol/L)
- Bartter's syndrome (Very rare disease, 1 in 1 million)
- Gitelman's syndrome (Rare disease, 1 in 40,000)
- Severe hypercalcemia
- Severe hypomagnesemia

C) <u>Miscellaneous</u>

- Exogenous alkali load[4,9]
    - Administration of NaHCO3; sodium citrate, gluconate or acetate
    - Excessive use of lactate containing IV fluid such as Ringer's lactate solution
    - Massive blood transfusion (citrated blood)
    - Taking large amount of antacids
- Poorly reabsorbable anion therapy- carbenicillin, penicillin etc
- Licorice
- Carbenoxolone

* Metabolism of lactate, citrate, gluconate, acetate and ketones generates HCO3-.[2,5]

Pathogenesis of metabolic alkalosis

Normally the kidneys are very efficient at excreting excess HCO3- and an alkalotic state cannot be maintained unless there is some sort of renal impairment affecting HCO3- excretion. Therefore, ***in a sustained metabolic alkalosis usually two processes are involved***:[1,7,12]

1. Initiation/ generation factor for the alkalosis -- increased alkali load (usually endogenously produced, occasionally exogenous)
2. Maintenance factor – Some sort of impaired HCO3- excretion of by the kidneys which may occur in-[2,5,8]
    - Chloride deficiency
    - Secondary hyperaldosteronism
    - Hypokalemia
    - Extracellular fluid volume contraction (the role of this one is controversial).

Sometimes the same factor is involved in both initiation and maintenance of the metabolic alkalosis.

****Normally chloride and bicarbonate are the only anions present in abundant amounts in the extracellular fluid, so the deficiency of one lead to an increase in the other to maintain electrical neutrality of the plasma.***

The exact pathogenesis of metabolic alkalosis varies depending on the underlying cause. Brief description of some cause-specific pathogenesis is given below.

A) Metabolic alkalosis in gastric secretion loss

Initiation factor: Loss of H+ from vomiting or nasogastric aspiration causes retention of equivalent amount HCO3- in plasma → metabolic alkalosis.[2,4]

Maintenance factors:

1. *Hypovolemia* is the most common maintenance factor. It can maintain metabolic alkalosis in the following ways:
    a) Hypovolemia → ↓GFR →↑ renal tubular reabsorption of Na and HCO3- proximally to restore extracellular fluid volume → metabolic alkalosis enhanced.[2-5]

b) Hypovolemia → secondary hyperaldosteronism → aldosterone stimulates reabsorption of Na+ in exchange for K+ and H+ secretion in collecting duct → hypokalemia and alkalosis.

2. *Hypokalemia* is another maintenance factor (details given below).

B) Hypokalemia induced metabolic alkalosis:

Potassium depletion may cause modest metabolic alkalosis.[12]

1. Severe hypokalemia causes metabolic alkalosis primarily by shifting H+ into the intracellular fluid.[8,12] ↓ K^+ in ECF → K^+ moves out of cell and H^+ moves into the intracellular space in exchange.[7]
2. Hypokalemia independently increases bicarbonate reabsorption in the proximal tubule.[8,12]
3. Hypokalemia also increases $NH4^+$ production which in turn enhances net acid excretion by the kidneys.[8,12]

C) Diuretic induced metabolic alkalosis

Chloruretic agents such as thiazides and loop diuretics directly induce the urinary loss of chloride, sodium and fluid. These losses promote metabolic alkalosis by the following possible mechanisms:

1. Contraction alkalosis (in acute cases): Use of loop or thiazide diuretics → loss of extracellular fluid (with Na, K and Cl) without HCO3- loss → ↑ plasma HCO3- concentration as the same total HCO3- is dissolved in the less amount of extracellular fluid.[2,4,5] But there is a controversy whether contraction alkalosis truly exists. Recent study showed that contraction alkalosis is actually chloride depletion alkalosis, and it can be corrected by chloride administration without volume replacement.[13]
2. Chronic use of loop or thiazide diuretic →↑distal Na delivery →↑Na reabsorption with ↑tubular secretion of K^+ and H^+ → hypokalemia and alkalosis.[2,8,13]
3. ECF volume contraction → secondary hyperaldosteronism → ↑reabsorption of sodium with ↑secretion of K+ and H+ in the collecting duct → hypokalemia and alkalosis[12]
4. Diuretic associated hypokalemia augments metabolic alkalosis.[12]

D. Posthypercapnia metabolic alkalosis

- Chronic respiratory acidosis → renal compensation with ↑HCO3- reabsorption →↑ plasma HCO3- concentration. Rapid correction of chronic respiratory acidosis (which may occur with assisted ventilation) → rapid fall in PCO2 and rise in pH; but elevated plasma bicarbonate level persists until sufficient chloride is not available → metabolic alkalosis.[2]
- Hypercapnia increases renal excretion of NaCl by directly decreasing NaCl reabsorption in the proximal tubule; the NaCl and accompanying fluid loss can cause hypovolemia.[5] ***Infusion of normal saline can correct both hypovolemia and alkalosis***.

Clinical features of metabolic alkalosis

- Metabolic alkalosis has no specific clinical features and usually features of the underlying cause dominate.

- Plasma ionized calcium level falls with rise of pH due to increased binding of calcium to albumin, and neuromuscular features like that of hypocalcemia such as paresthesia, muscle cramping, tetany and seizure may develop.

Respiratory acidosis

Respiratory acidosis occurs due to CO2 retention resulting from alveolar hypoventilation. It is characterized by increased PCO2 (>45 mmHg) and decreased pH (<7.35).

The causes of respiratory acidosis include-

1. Intrinsic lung diseases (such as obstructive airway diseases)
2. Neuromuscular lesion anywhere from brain to the respiratory muscles affecting ventilation;
3. Drugs causing respiratory centre depression or respiratory muscle paralysis (e.g. sedatives and anesthetics).

* Possible opioid overdose should be considered when there is no obvious cause of hypoventilation; a diagnostic and therapeutic trial of naloxone should be considered in such cases.[5]

Clinical features of respiratory acidosis:

Clinical features of the underlying cause usually dominate. Symptoms and signs of respiratory acidosis (hypercapnia) may overlap with those of hypoxemia which often coexists.
Clinical features of -

1. *Acute respiratory acidosis include:* drowsiness, anxiety, irritability, restlessness, confusion, disorientation, psychosis, asterixis, myoclonus, coma etc.
2. *Less severe chronic respiratory acidosis include:* sleep disturbance, day time somnolence, fatigue, memory dysfunction, personality changes, incoordination, tremor etc.

Hypercapnia causes cerebral vasodilation and increases cerebral blood flow;[14] severe hypercapnia can increase intracranial pressure, cerebrospinal fluid pressure; and features of raised intracranial pressure such as headache, vomiting, papilledema etc may develop.[5] Superficial facial and conjunctival blood vessels may be dilated and more conspicuous.

Respiratory alkalosis

Respiratory alkalosis always results from sustained hyperventilation (↑alveolar ventilation). It is characterized by decreased PCO2 (<35 mmHg) and increased pH (>7.45).

Causes respiratory alkalosis:[2,5,15]

A. Hyperventilation via CNS stimulation

1. Hyperventilation syndrome or psychogenic hyperventilation (the most common cause of respiratory alkalosis)
2. Pain

3. Fever
4. Stroke
5. CNS infection- eg, meningitis and encephalitis
6. Head injury
7. Brain tumor
8. Some endogenous chemicals
    - Sepsis - various cytokines
    - Hepatic failure - some toxins
9. Drugs and hormone
    - Salicylate intoxication
    - Xanthines (aminophylline, theophylline etc)
    - Pregnancy (progesterone)
10. Heat exposure
11. Recovery from metabolic acidosis

B) **Hypoxia induced hyperventilation**

1. Lung diseases: Pneumonia, acute asthma, interstitial lung disease, pulmonary embolism etc.
2. Pulmonary edema
3. Severe anemia
4. High altitude
5. Hypotension

C) Excessive mechanical ventilation

*Respiratory alkalosis is the commonest acid-base disorder in chronic liver disease and the severity correlates with the degree of hepatic impairment.[15]
* Fairly well compensated mild respiratory alkalosis is usual in pregnancy.[15]

Clinical features of respiratory alkalosis

- Like other acid-base disorders, in respiratory alkalosis also clinical features of the underlying cause usually dominate. The features of respiratory alkalosis itself vary depending on duration and severity.
- Acute respiratory alkalosis (sudden drop of PCO2) → cerebral vasoconstriction → ↓cerebral blood flow →development of neurological symptoms including dizziness, light-headedness, confusion, seizures and syncope.
- Like metabolic alkalosis, symptoms of hypocalcemia (due to ↓ plasma ionized Ca level) such as paresthesia, circumoral numbness, muscle cramping and tetany may develop.

Investigations of acid-base disorders:

To determine the acid-base status of a patient, most commonly performed tests are-

1. Serum electrolytes
2. Arterial Blood Gas analysis

Urine electrolyte levels are needed if urine anion gap (given below) calculation is required; urine chloride is helpful to distinguish between the saline responsive and saline unresponsive causes of metabolic alkalosis.

Other investigations depend on the suspected underlying cause and severity of the condition.

During determination of the acid-base status, verification of the accuracy of HCO3- values is important. How can it be done?
During arterial blood gas analysis, pH and PCO2 are directly measured but **HCO3- is calculated** using Henderson-Hasselbalch equation. The total venous CO2 measurement is a more direct estimation of plasma HCO3- concentration.[5] The difference between the values of the calculated HCO_3^- of arterial blood gas analysis and the measured HCO_3^- (i.e. total venous CO_2) of serum electrolyte tests should not be more than 2 mmol/L. If it is >2mmol/L, there may have a laboratory error or the samples may not have been taken simultaneously.[2]

Traditionally for the detection of acid-base disorders, Arterial Blood Gas (ABG) analysis is done. Could it be useful if Venous Blood Gas (VBG) is analyzed instead?[5, 16,17,18]
Yes, it could be. Generally, the differences between the values of arterial and venous gas analysis are small, and many physicians now believe routine use of arterial blood gas analysis is not necessary for the determination of acid-base disorders; for acid-base disorders due to metabolic causes, VBG analysis may be as useful as ABG analysis. However, VBG analysis may not be adequate for patients with cardiopulmonary disorders or on mechanical ventilation, where ABG analysis results would be more reliable. This area needs more studies.

The approximate differences between the values of arterial and venous gas analysis:
1. <u>pH:</u> generally venous blood pH is 0.02-0.04 units lower than arterial blood pH.[5,17]
2. <u>PCO2:</u> usually venous blood PCO2 is 5- 8 mm of Hg higher than that of arterial blood.[5,17]

Step-by-step diagnosis of acid-base disorders

[During step-by-step analysis of a patient's data to determine the acid-base status, if you find the data are not useful for a particular step, proceed to the next step. For example, in mixed acid base disorders, sometimes pH, HCO3- and PCO2 all these are normal, so step 2 and 3 of this stepwise approach will not be useful, and you need to proceed to step 4 (anion gap calculation)]

<u>Step 1:</u> Determine clinically what type of acid-base disorder may be present.

<u>Step 2:</u> Determine the primary (original/ main) acid-base disorder

<u>Look at the pH first, then HCO3- and PCO2, and follow the flow chart below.</u>

First, you are likely to find acidemia (pH < 7.35) or alkalemia (pH>7.45).

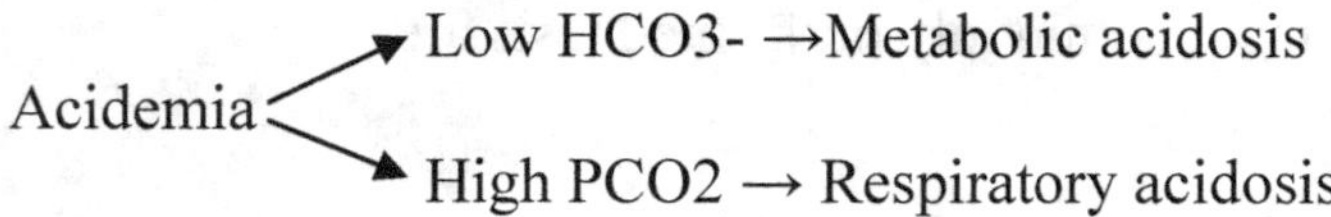

Alkalemia → High HCO3- →Metabolic alkalosis
Alkalemia → Low PCO2 → Respiratory alkalosis

According to the chart, if the patient has acidemia, you are likely to find either low HCO3- or High PCO2; if the patient has low HCO3-, arrow of the chart indicates metabolic acidosis is the primary acid base disorder; but if your patient has high PCO2, respiratory acidosis would be the primary acid base disorder. For a patient with alkalemia, the chart can be used similarly.

From abnormal HCO3- and PCO2 values how can we identify which one is the primary change?

The value which is consistent with the abnormal pH should be considered as the primary change and the other should be considered as the compensatory change. Suppose, a patient has high pH (i.e. alkalemia), high HCO3- and high PCO2; according to the above chart, the high HCO3- matches with the abnormal pH (alkalemia), so high HCO3- is the primary change, i.e. the patient has metabolic alkalosis; the high PCO2 is the result of respiratory compensation by hypoventilation.

Can the direction of HCO3- and PCO2 change help in differentiating simple from mixed acid-base disorders?

Yes, but not always. In simple acid-base disorders with appropriate compensation, always both the HCO3- and PCO2 levels are changed from the normal in the same direction (i.e. either both the values are increased or decreased). For example, in a patient with metabolic acidosis, primary change is ↓HCO3- and respiratory compensation by hyperventilation causes ↓PCO2. However, sometimes in mixed acid- base disorders, the similar trend of deviation of HCO3- and PCO2 values (i.e. in the same direction from the normal) may be found. Therefore, the change of the two parameters in the same direction indicates a simple acid-base disorder is more likely but not confirmed.

Step 3: Estimate the compensation

For respiratory acid base disorder, acute and chronic can be distinguished from the degree of compensation. (See the compensation calculation described earlier)

Step 4: Calculate the anion gap

(See the anion gap described earlier)

An anion gap > 20 mmol/L is suggestive of metabolic acidosis irrespective of the pH and serum HCO3- concentration.[5,9]

The diagnosis of simple acid-base disorders can be done with the above steps; and if the anion gap is normal, further steps are not necessary. But when the anion gap is increased further step (step 5) described below will be needed to determine whether the acid-base disorder is mixed one.

When to suspect mixed acid-base disorders

Suspect mixed acid base disorders in the following conditions:[1,4,6]

a) Absence of appropriate compensatory response (i.e. when the predicted compensatory change does not match with the patient's value).

b) Values of HCO3- and PCO2 are abnormal in the opposite direction (i.e. one value is increased while the other is decreased from normal). In a simple acid-base disorder, always both the values are abnormal in the same direction.[4] However, sometimes in mixed acid-base disorders also, the values may be changed in the same direction as in a simple acid-base disorder.

c) When pH is normal but anion gap is increased by >5mmol/L (PCO2 and HCO3- may be normal or abnormal),[1] i.e. high anion gap may be the only biochemical clue to the diagnosis of mixed acid-base disorders.

<u>**Step 5:**</u> **When anion gap is high**, calculate either **corrected bicarbonate**[5,19] (or starting bicarbonate[20] or **delta ratio**[4,15] described below.

Before calculating corrected bicarbonate or delta ratio, first we need to calculate the followings:

(a) Δ AG (Delta anion gap):[1,4] It is the increase in anion gap from normal.

Δ AG (Delta anion gap) = Anion gap – 12 (i.e. patient's anion gap – normal anion gap)

(b) ΔHCO3⁻ (Delta bicarbonate):[1,4] It is the change (decrease/ increase, often decrease) in serum bicarbonate from normal.

In most cases of mixed acid-base disorders, the patient's HCO3- is lower than the normal serum HCO3-.
Therefore, ΔHCO_3^- (Delta bicarbonate) = 24 – patient's HCO_3^- (i.e. normal serum HCO3- – patient's HCO3-)

<u>**The corrected HCO3- (or Starting HCO3-)**</u>

Corrected HCO3- (or Starting HCO3-) = Delta anion gap (i.e., increase in anion gap) + patient's HCO3-

Some other terms such as 'calculated HCO3-'[9] and 'excess anion gap'[11] have also been used by some authors instead of 'corrected HCO3-'

<u>*Interpretation* of the corrected HCO3- (or Starting HCO3-) values:</u>[9,11]

Corrected HCO3- value	*Acid-base status*
23- 30 mmol/L	Pure high anion gap metabolic acidosis
<23 mmol/L	High anion gap metabolic acidosis + non-anion gap metabolic acidosis
>30 mmol/L	High anion gap metabolic acidosis + metabolic

	alkalosis

I.e. when the corrected HCO3- is higher than normal serum HCO3-, there is concomitant metabolic alkalosis and when it is lower than normal, there is concomitant nonanion gap metabolic acidosis with high anion gap metabolic acidosis.

The Delta ratio

Delta ratio = Increase in Anion Gap / Change in serum bicarbonate[1,4,15]
i.e., Delta ratio = Delta anion gap/ delta HCO3-

Some authors have used the term 'delta gap' to instead of the term 'delta ratio'.[1]

Interpretation of delta ratio[4,15]

a) Delta ratio between 1 and 2: pure high anion gap metabolic acidosis

b) Delta ratio >2: high anion gap metabolic acidosis **Plus** either metabolic alkalosis or compensated chronic respiratory acidosis.

c) Delta ratio <1: high anion gap metabolic acidosis **Plus** nonanion gap metabolic acidosis; *Example*: diarrhea → HCO3- loss in stool → nonanion gap metabolic acidosis; concomitant fluid loss in diarrhea → shock → lactic acidosis (i.e. superimposed high anion gap metabolic acidosis)

*Be aware of the over-interpretation of delta ratio; always check for other evidences to support the diagnosis, particularly for an unexpected value.[15]

Explanation of increase in anion gap and delta ratio in high anion gap metabolic acidosis

Addition of acids with unmeasured anions (i.e. acids with anion other than HCO3- or Cl-) to the ECF → dissociation of the acid molecules into H^+ and anion → one H^+ is buffered by one HCO3- (producing CO_2 and H_2O) → decrease in bicarbonate (by one HCO3- for one H^+) → the reduction of negative charge resulting from one bicarbonate ion loss is compensated by one released anion of the added acid to maintain electrical neutrality of the plasma. The anion gap is increased due to the presence of extra anions of the added acid in plasma, as these anions are not measured.

In high anion-gap metabolic acidosis, there is a correlation between the increase in anion gap (i.e. the delta AG) and the decrease in the bicarbonate ions (i.e. delta HCO3-).[1] If all the added acids (with unmeasured anions) are buffered in the ECF by bicarbonate, the increase in the anion gap will be equal to the decrease in HCO3- level, so the delta ratio should be one.[4]

But actually, in most cases of high anion gap metabolic acidosis, all the hydrogen ions of the added acids are not buffered by bicarbonate buffer system in the ECF; instead, a considerable proportion of the H+ is buffered intracellularly and by bone. Therefore, the fall in plasma bicarbonate ions is not equal to the addition of hydrogen ions, rather a lesser degree of fall in plasma HCO_3^- occurs than asummed[1,4]

On the other hand, most of the anions of the added acid remain in the ECF, as anions cannot cross the cell membrane easily. Consequently, the increase in the anion gap (i. e. delta anion gap) often exceeds the decrease in the plasma HCO_3^- (delta bicarbonate), so the delta ratio becomes >1.[4]

The delta ratio in lactic acidosis is about1.6, but in ketoacidosis it is generally close to 1; this difference may be due to decreased renal clearance of lactate compared to keto-anions. [1] In ketoacidosis (compared to lactic acidosis), more anions (keto-anions) are lost in urine, so increase in anion gap is relatively less prominent, resulting in a delta ratio close to 1.

Currently, there is no ideal method for the evaluation of acid–base disorders. The physicochemical and base-excess methods are also used by many, but the physiologic approach described so far here is the simplest and most comprehensive approach. A brief description of base excess has been given below.

Base excess

It is defined as the amount of acid needed to add to each liter of blood to return its pH to normal at a $PaCO_2$ of 40 mmHg and normal body temperature. Base excess is the reflection of the metabolic component of acid-base balance. It is a calculated value derived from pH and $PaCO_2$ of arterial blood.[21]

Interpretation of base excess values:[11]
Reference range: -2 to +2 mmol/L

Metabolic alkalosis: if > +2 mmol/*L*
Metabolic acidosis: if <−2 mmol/L

However, the use of base excess in interpreting blood gas results is controversial.[21]

Summary of the step-by-step diagnosis of acid-base disorders

[During step-by-step analysis of a patient's data to determine the acid-base status, if you find the data is not useful for a particular step, proceed to the next step]

Step 1: Determine clinically what type of acid-base disorder may be present.

Step 2: Determine the primary (original/ main) acid-base disorder.

Look at the pH first, then HCO_3^- and PCO_2; and follow the flow chart below.

First, you are likely to find acidemia (pH < 7.35) or alkalemia (pH>7.45).

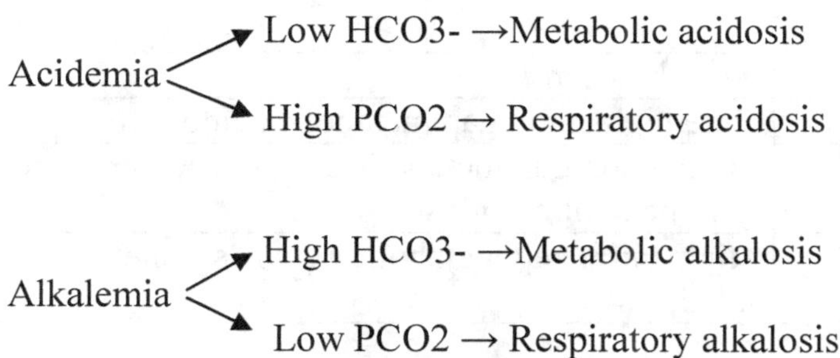

According to the chart, if a patient has acidemia, you are likely to find either low HCO3- or High PCO2; if the patient has low HCO3-, metabolic acidosis is the primary acid base disorder; but if your patient has high PCO2, respiratory acidosis would be the primary acid base disorder. For a patient with alkalemia, the chart can be used similarly.

Step 3: Estimate the compensation

Metabolic acidosis: Winter's Formula: PCO2 = (1.5 × [HCO3-]) + 8 ± 2 mmHg
Metabolic alkalosis: for each 1 mmol/L HCO3- increase, PCO2 will increase 0.7 mmHg from 40mmHg.
Respiratory acidosis: Acute: HCO3- will increase 1 mmol/L for each 10 mmHg increase in PCO2 above 40 mmHg; chronic: HCO3- will increase 4 mmol/L for each 10 mmHg increase in PCO2 above 40 mmHg;
Respiratory alkalosis: Acute: HCO3- will decrease 2 mmol/L for each 10 mmHg decrease in PCO2 below 40 mmHg; chronic: HCO3- will decrease 4-5 mmol/L for each 10 mmHg decrease in PCO2 below 40 mmHg.

Step 4: Calculate the anion gap.

Anion gap= Na^+ – (Cl- + HCO3-)
Normal Anion Gap: 12 ± 4 mmol/L
An anion gap > 20 mmol/L is suggestive of metabolic acidosis irrespective of the pH and serum HCO3- level.

The diagnosis of simple acid-base disorders may be done with the above steps and if the anion gap is normal further steps are not necessary. But when the anion gap is increased further step described below will be needed to determine whether the acid-base disorder is mixed one.

Step 5: When anion gap is high, calculate either **corrected bicarbonate** (or starting bicarbonate) or **delta ratio**.
Before calculating corrected bicarbonate or delta ratio, first we need to calculate the followings:

a) Δ AG (Delta anion gap) = Anion gap – 12 (i.e. patient's anion gap – normal anion gap);

b) ΔHCO3- (Delta bicarbonate) = 24 – patient's HCO3- (i.e. normal serum HCO3- – patient's HCO3-)

The corrected HCO3- (or Starting HCO3-)
Corrected HCO3- (or Starting HCO3-) = Delta anion gap + patient's HCO3-

Interpretation:

Corrected HCO3- value	*Acid-base status*
23- 30 mmol/L	Pure high anion gap metabolic acidosis
<23 mmol/L	High anion gap metabolic acidosis + non-anion gap metabolic acidosis
>30 mmol/L	High anion gap metabolic acidosis + metabolic alkalosis

The delta ratio
Delta ratio = Delta anion gap/ delta HCO3-
Interpretation of delta ratio:

a) Delta ratio between 1and 2: pure high anion gap metabolic acidosis;

b) Delta ratio >2: high anion gap metabolic acidosis **Plus** either metabolic alkalosis or compensated chronic respiratory acidosis.

c) Delta ratio <1: high anion gap metabolic acidosis **Plus** nonanion gap metabolic acidosis

Case discussion

Case 1 (simple acid-base disorder):

A 22-year-old man with type 1diabetes mellitus presents with increasing polyuria, polydipsia, nausea, diffuse abdominal pain and drowsiness since the previous day. He was diagnosed with type 1 diabetes mellitus three years ago and has been on insulin but has not taken insulin for three days. His is physical examination is remarkable for deep sighing respiration, orthostatic hypotension, and dry mucous membranes.

Initial laboratory values include: blood glucose 24.0 mmol/L (432 mg/dL), sodium 130 mmol/L, potassium 4.5 mmol/L, chloride 90 mmol/L, bicarbonate 10 mmol/L; serum creatinine 120 micromol/L (1.3 mg/dL); serum ketones strongly positive.

ABG: pH 7.3, PCO2 23 mmHg, HCO3- 10 mmol/L

What is the acid-base disorder?

Answer: (Step-by-step analysis)

Step 1: Clinical impression

High anion gap metabolic acidosis due to diabetic ketoacidosis ± lactic acidosis

(Lactic acidosis may develop due to tissue hypoxia resulting from hypotension)

Step 2: determine the primary acid-base disorder

Look at pH, PCO2 and HCO3- and follow the flow chart below.

First, look at pH; here pH= 7.3; i.e. acidemia is present
Now look at HCO3- and PCO2.
Here the patient's HCO3- (10 mmol/L) and PCO2 (23 mmHg) both are low; which one is consistent with acidemia?
The chart below shows that a patient with acidemia should have either low HCO3- or high PCO2; When HCO3- is low, the primary acid-base disorder is metabolic acidosis; on the other hand, if PCO2 is high the diagnosis is respiratory acidosis.

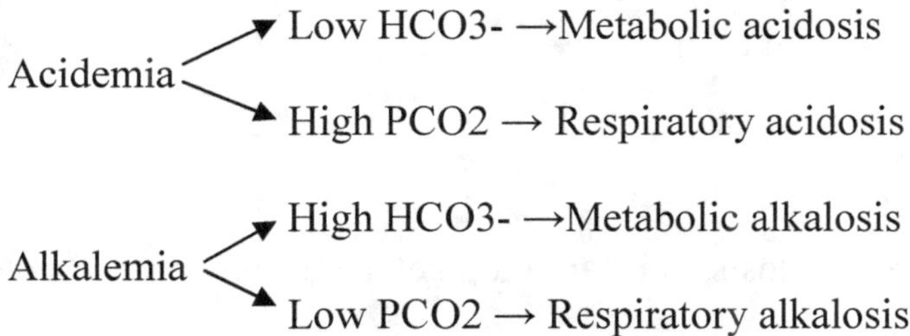

Here the low bicarbonate is consistent with acidemia; so metabolic acidosis is the primary acid-base disorder. Here the patient's low PCO2 is not consistent with pH (acidemia); therefore it may not be the primary change; instead, it is possibly due to respiratory compensation by hyperventilation.

<u>Step 3:</u> Estimate the compensation
Here the predicted PCO2 = (1.5 X [HCO3-]) + 8 ± 2 = (1.5 X 10) + 8 ± 2 = 21-25 mmHg
The patient's PCO2 is 23 mmHg; so the respiratory compensation for the metabolic acidosis is appropriate, i.e. the patient has no separate respiratory acid-base disorder.

<u>Step 4:</u> Calculate the anion gap

Anion gap = Serum Na – (Serum Cl + Serum HCO3-) = 130 – (90+10) = 30 mmol/L
It is greater than 16, so the patient has high anion gap metabolic acidosis.

<u>Step 5</u>: Since the anion gap is high, calculate either corrected bicarbonate (or starting bicarbonate) or delta ratio to determine whether there is concomitant any other acid-base disorders.
Δ AG (Delta anion gap) = Anion gap – 12 = 30-12=18

ΔHCO3ˉ (Delta bicarbonate) = 24 – patient's HCO3=24-10=14

Corrected HCO3- (or Starting HCO3-) = Delta anion gap + patient's HCO3- =18+10=28
As the corrected HCO3- is between 23-30 mmol/L, the patient has pure high anion gap metabolic acidosis.

You can calculate delta ratio instead of corrected HCO3- (or Starting HCO3-).
The delta ratio = Delta anion gap/ delta HCO3- =18/14=1.28
As the delta ratio is between 1 and 2, the patient has pure high anion gap metabolic acidosis.

Acid-base status of the patient: pure high anion gap metabolic acidosis

Case 2 (mixed acid-base disorders)

A 48 -Year-old alcoholic man presents with a five-day history of heavy drinking and vomiting; he has taken little foods over the last several days. His serum electrolyte shows Na 134 mmol/L, K 3.0 mmol/L, HCO3. 17 mmol/L and Cl 85 mmol/L; the results of ABG analysis reveal pH 7.4, PCO_2 32 mmHg and HCO3. 17 mmol/L.

What is the acid-base disorder?

Answer: (Step-by-step analysis)

Step 1: Clinical impression:

Metabolic acidosis (due to alcoholic ketoacidosis and starvation ketoacidosis)
Plus
Metabolic alkalosis (due to vomiting)

Step 2: Determination of the primary acid-base disorder:

To determine the primary acid-base disorder first we look at pH, then HCO3- and PCO2. Here the pH is normal; although HCO3- and PCO2 are abnormal, we cannot use step 2 and 3; so we cannot determine which one is the primary change only from the values of these three parameters. However, this type of values indicates the presence of mixed acid- base disorders. Now we have to skip step 2 and 3 of the step-by–step diagnostic approach, as they are not useful here, and proceed to step 4 (i.e. calculation of the anion gap).

Step 4: Anion gap calculation

Anion gap = 134- (85+17) = 134- 102 = 32
Anion gap > 20 is suggestive of metabolic acidosis irrespective of pH and HCO3- values. So this patient has high anion gap metabolic acidosis possibly due to alcoholic ketoacidosis and starvation ketoacidosis.

Now we can calculate the respiratory compensation for the metabolic acidosis.
The predicted PCO2 = (1.5 X [HCO3-]) + 8 ± 2 = (1.5 X 17) +8 ± 2 = 33.5 ± 2 = 31- 35 mmHg
The patient's PCO2 = 32 mmHg; therefore, the respiratory compensation for the metabolic acidosis is appropriate, i.e. the patient has no separate respiratory acid-base disorder.

Now Step 5: As the patient's anion gap is high, we have to calculate either 'corrected (or starting HCO3-)' or delta ratio.
Corrected (or starting HCO3-) = delta anion gap + patient's HCO3-
Delta anion gap = Anion gap – 12 = 32 - 12= 20
So Corrected (or starting HCO3-) = 20 + 17= 37 mmol/L

As the corrected HCO3- is > 30 mmol/L, so concomitant metabolic alkalosis is there (due to vomiting). It means that the patient had high HCO3- due to metabolic alkalosis from vomiting upon which metabolic acidosis was superimposed;

Alternative to corrected (or starting) HCO3- calculation is the calculation of the delta ratio.

Delta ratio = Delta anion gap/ Delta HCO3-
Delta HCO3- = 24 (optimal HCO3-) – patient's HCO3- = 24 -17 = 7
Therefore, the delta ratio= 20/ 7 = 2.8

The delta ratio is >2, which indicates the presence of concomitant metabolic alkalosis or compensated chronic respiratory acidosis; in this case, according to clinical features, the delta ratio >2 is most likely due to metabolic alkalosis from vomiting.

Diagnosis of the acid-base disorder: High anion gap metabolic acidosis plus metabolic alkalosis

Treatment of acid base disorders

- Treatment of acid base disorders depends on the underlying cause.
- In metabolic acidosis, administration of intravenous bicarbonate is not a commonly needed; it should be administered only when specifically indicated.
- In respiratory alkalosis due to hyperventilation syndrome, rebreathing in a paper bag is no longer recommended; it does not correct PCO2, instead can reduce PO2.[5] Death may occur if patients with acute myocardial infarction, pneumothorax or pulmonary embolism is misdiagnosed with hyperventilation syndrome and treated with paper bag rebreathing.[7] Reassurance may be adequate for a hyperventilating anxious patient; if not, sedation with benzodiazepines can be considered. However, hyperventilation often stops spontaneously, as respiratory muscles (with other muscles of the body) become fatigue by alkalemia.[5]

References

1. Kenrick Berend et al. Physiological Approach to Assessment of Acid–Base Disturbances. **N Engl J Med 2014;** 371:1434-45.

2. Relevant chapters of **Harrison's Principles of Internal Medicine**; 18 th edition; Dan L Longo et al (Editors). New York, McGraw-Hill 2012.

3. Relevant chapters of **Davidson's Principles and Practice of Medicine**, 21 edition, Nicki R. Colledge et al (editors). India, Elsevier, **2010**

4. 'Acid-base online tutorial' on the website of **the University of Connecticut**, **USA**. At: http://fitsweb.uchc.edu/student/selectives/TimurGraham/Welcome.html

5. Relevant chapters of **Current Medical Diagnosis and Treatment**; Maxine A. Papadakis et al (Editors). New York, McGraw-Hill, **2013**

6. Anthony M. Herd. An approach to complex acid-base problems: Keeping it simple**. Can Fam Physician 2005;** 51:226-232.

7. Relevant topic in **'Emedicine'.** At: http://emedicine.medscape.com

8. Relevant chapters of **Kumar &Clark's Clinical Medicine,** 8th edition; Parveen Kumar and Michael Clark (Editors). Edinburgh, Elsevier, **2012**

9. AK Ghosh. Diagnosing Acid-Base Disorders. **J Assoc Physicians India 2006**; 54:720-4. At: http://www.japi.org/september2006/R-720.pdf

10. Jeffrey A. Kraut et al. Serum Anion Gap: Its Uses and Limitations in Clinical Medicine **Clin J Am Soc Nephrol 2007;** 2: 162–174

11. Relevant topic in **Family Practice Notebook.** At: http://www.fpnotebook.com/legacy/Renal/Lab/UrnryAnGp.htm

12. John H. Galla. Metabolic Alkalosis. **J Am Soc Nephrol 2000**; 11: 369–375

13. Robert G. Luke and John H. Galla. It Is Chloride Depletion Alkalosis, Not Contraction Alkalosis. **J Am Soc Nephrol 2012**; 23: 204–207

14. Ito H et al. Changes in human cerebral blood flow and cerebral blood volume during hypercapnia and hypocapnia measured by positron emission tomography. **J Cereb Blood Flow Metab. 2003**; 23(6):665-70.

15. Relevant topic in 'Acid-base physiology' on the website of **Anesthesia MCQ**. At: http://www.anaesthesiamcq.com/AcidBaseBook/ABindex.php

16. Parvaiz A. Koul et al. Comparison and agreement between venous and arterial gas analysis in cardiopulmonary patients in Kashmir valley of the Indian subcontinent. **Ann Thorac Med. 2011;** 6(1): 33–37

17. Sunnie Kim. Is a VBG just as good as an ABG? **The NYU Langone Online Journal of Medicine; July 13, 2012**; at: http://www.clinicalcorrelations.org/?p=5608

18. G Malatesha et al. Comparison of arterial and venous pH, bicarbonate, PCO2 and PO2 in initial emergency department assessment. **Emerg Med J 2007**; 24:569–571.

19. 'Arterial Blood Gas Analysis Part 2: mixed disorders' on the website of **the university of California, San Francisco**, USA. At: http://missinglink.ucsf.edu/lm/abg/abg2/mixed.html

20. Student manual on 'Acid-base disorders' on the website of **Michigan State University**; at: http://echt.chm.msu.edu/BlockIII/Docs/CoreComp/B3CCTherABStudentManual.pdf

21. Abhishek K Verma et al. The interpretation of arterial blood gases. **Aust Prescr 2010**; 33:124–9

About the author

- Basic medical degree: MBBS, obtained in 1991 from Rajshahi Medical College, Bangladesh;
- Postgraduate qualification: MRCP (General Medicine) from Royal College of Physicians of Ireland;
- Passed USMLE (United States Medical Licensing Examination) Step 1 and step 2;
- Had been a postgraduate research student at Yamaguchi University Hospital (Japan) for two years;
- Current professional level: Consultant General Medicine in Bangladesh

www.ingramcontent.com/pod-product-compliance
Lightning Source LLC
Chambersburg PA
CBHW081141180526
45170CB00006B/1880

* 9 7 8 1 5 4 5 0 9 3 5 4 2 *